Acknowledgements

Grateful thanks are due to the publishers and editors of the following journals for their generosity in giving permission for reproduction of figures: Acta Biologica Hungarica, Brain Research, Experimental Brain Research, Japanese Journal of Physiology, Journal of Physiology, Perspectives in Biology and Medicine, Progress in Brain Research, Zeitschrift für Anatomie und Entwicklungsgeschichte.

Contents

Introduction

Ever since their first detailed investigations on the structure of the central nervous system, the neuroanatomists, and particularly RAMÓN Y CAJAL, have been meditating on the mode of operation of the complex patterns of neuronal arrangements that they were discovering. These patterns appeared to be so different in the various regions of the nervous system, yet there seemed to be some underlying principles of organization which could dimly be perceived. RAMÓN Y CAJAL himself did not hesitate to draw conjectural diagrams of all the major neuronal assemblages that he investigated, and he proposed many modes of neuronal interaction. But inherent in all these diagrams of neuronal pathways was the fatal defect that inhibitory synaptic action was as yet not recognized. In his diagrams all synaptic actions were assumed to be excitatory. One can now contrast his operational diagrams of the cerebellar cortex (RAMÓN Y CAJAL, 1911, Figs. 103, 104; reproduced in Fig. 25) with those of Figs. 119, 120 and 121 below.

Neuroanatomists have, I think, generally recognized that the cerebellum provides the greatest challenge in our initial efforts to discern functional meaning in neuronal patterns, because there is such a beautiful geometrical arrangement of its unique neuronal constituents. Presumably, it is for this reason that we are fortunate in possessing the most refined knowledge of microstructure that is available in the central nervous system. The pioneer investigations of RAMÓN Y CAJAL have led in recent times to fascinating developments concerning microstructure, geometrical arrangements, and numerical assessment. These developments will be described in appropriate places throughout this book.

When one considers the cerebellum in relation to the rest of the nervous system, interesting speculations in the field of comparative morphology can be developed. It appears that the unique neuronal organization of the cerebellum originally arose in relation to the vestibular and lateral line receptor organs of primitive vertebrates (JANSEN and BRODAL, 1958). With each further evolutionary development of the brain, this same cerebellar organization seemed to be a necessary adjunct, presumably because it possessed some unique mode of processing information. Hence, these newly evolved components of the brain colonized or developed areas of the cerebellum for this purpose; and most lately of all, the cerebral hemispheres have called forth the great development of the cerebellar lobes. With the evolutionary growth of the brain, the cerebellar hypertrophy has matched the hypertrophy of the cerebrum. This evolutionary story certainly gives rise to the concept that there is some highly significant and unique functional meaning in the neuronal organization of the cerebellum and in the processing of information that is accomplished thereby.

The theme of this book can be succinctly stated as being to discover the functional meaning of the patterns of neuronal connexion in the cerebellum, both in the cortex and in the various nuclei on its efferent pathways, for it will emerge that all of these structures are organized into very remarkable operational entities. Essentially the cerebellum is constructed of stereotyped and relatively simple neuronal arrangements which we can regard as "neural machinery" designed to process the input information in some unique and essential manner. This term "neural machinery" is particularly pertinent when it is recognized that the neuronal components of the cerebellar cortex are arranged in a beautiful geometrical pattern which is essentially a laminated array of a rectangular lattice (BRAITENBERG and ATWOOD, 1958).

Since the detailed structure of the cortex is virtually the same for all parts of the cerebellum in respect both of the component cells and the afferent fibers, it has been deemed sufficient for present purposes to attempt an experimental analysis of cortical responses for the region most easily investigated, namely the vermis of the anterior lobe; but so far as investigated, other regions of the cortex display similar responses. The efferent pathway from all regions of the cerebellar cortex is solely by the axons of Purkinje cells, but there are considerable differences in the manner of distribution of the Purkinje cell axons to the subcerebellar nuclei, as will appear in Chapters XIII and XIV, though all Purkinje cells are functionally homologous.

This monograph is not concerned with such important problems as the topographical organization of the cerebellum or the interaction of the diverse sensory inputs in any particular cortical region. Also it is not concerned with the classic methods of studying cerebellar function by observing the effects of localized lesions of the cerebellar cortex, and by attempting to locate the zones for the various sensory inputs using for this purpose local surface electrodes either for recording or stimulating. The great book by Dow and MORUZZI (1958) gives a most complete account of the immense literature on all these types of investigation into cerebellar function. The defect of almost all of such investigations has been that they have made little reference to the magnificent anatomical studies on the cerebellar cortex by RAMÓN y CAJAL and his successors. Too often the physiological descriptions are restricted to a kind of phenomenology of wave forms and polarities and latencies; and even where interaction experiments are attempted, there is still this same tendency to talk of depressions of potential responses without making testable postulates about the mode of production of the responses and the mode of operation of the inhibitory mechanisms.

The investigations on the structural features of neuronal organization can be considered as a dialogue between the observations of light microscopy including the Golgi and Nauta techniques on the one hand, and on the other the powerful new technique of electronmicroscopy. We would stress the necessity for the closest correlation and interpenetration of observations and ideas derived from these two complementary techniques.

The most striking feature of the electrophysiological investigations described in this book is the remarkable agreement with the structural investigations. All the histologically recognized types of neurones have been studied by unitary recording and in response to the various excitatory and inhibitory inputs by the histologically recognized synapses. The geometry of the patterns of neuronal distribution is in good accord with the analytical studies utilizing the potential fields plotted by systematic microelectrode recordings. Furthermore, intracellular recordings from the larger neurones — Purkinje cells, Deiters neurones, neurones of the intracerebellar nuclei and of the red nucleus, etc. — have given evidence that is essential for the construction of the operational diagrams not only of the cerebellar cortex but also for all the efferent pathways.

Undoubtedly the most surprising feature revealed by these investigations is the dominant role of postsynaptic inhibition. Not only is inhibition dominant in the cerebellar cortex itself with the powerful inhibitory actions of the basket, outer stellate and Golgi cells, but more remarkable is the discovery that the whole output from the cerebellar cortex is inhibitory, for all Purkinje cells are inhibitory in action. These investigations on the cerebellum have fully corroborated the so-called DALE's Principle. Postsynaptic inhibition is produced by special cells, the basket, outer stellate, Golgi and Purkinje cells, and all of the synapses made by these cells are inhibitory. For example, the Purkinje cells inhibit the cells of the intracerebellar nuclei and Deiters nucleus, but their axon collaterals are also inhibitory in their action on cells in the cerebellar cortex. Besides the conventional synaptic excitatory and inhibitory actions, these investigations reveal good examples of what we may call second order synaptic actions, disinhibition giving an effective excitation and disfacilitation an effective inhibition.

In conclusion it can be stated that this analytical study of cerebellar structure and function has been most rewarding in the insights it has given into the design and mode of operation of neural machinery. In the final chapter there will be an attempt to see how the operational units are organized so as to give the unique performance of the cerebellum as a coordinator of information in its role in providing the fine control of movement. The present monograph is very largely restricted in time to investigations over the last three years, and in place to the laboratories of the three authors, and also to other laboratories pursuing similar kinds of investigations.

Chapter I

General Survey of the Structure

A. The Cerebellar Cortex

The cerebellar cortex is a convoluted sheet of grey matter consisting of three layers: 1. the outermost molecular layer, 2. the ganglionic or Purkinje cell body layer and 3. the granular layer. This grey matter is twisted around relatively thin lamellae of white matter.

1. The Molecular Layer

The molecular layer has the thickness of about 300 μ[1] in the adult cat (310 to 400 μ in man) and is built up principally of dendritic arborizations and densely packed thin axons, running parallel with the longitudinal axis of the folium, hence called parallel fibers. The density of nerve cells in this layer is rather low. The cell bodies of only two types of neurons are localized in the molecular layer: the basket and the outer stellate cells. Both are local elements, no processes of either cell type leaving the grey matter. The dendritic ramifications of both neurons are confined to the molecular layer, so are the axons of the outer stellate cells. The axon ramifications of the basket neurons are situated both in the molecular layer and the Purkinje cell layer, penetrating for some tens of microns into the granular layer.

2. The Ganglionic or Purkinje Cell Layer

The ganglionic or Purkinje cell layer is a single sheet of beet shaped cell bodies with a vertical diameter 50—70 μ and a transversal diameter 30—35 μ that are arranged at distances of 50 μ in the longitudinal and 50—100 μ in the transversal direction of the folium. Besides Purkinje cell (P-cell) bodies this layer contains several kinds of axons either ascending or descending, and the ascending dendrites of Golgi cells. Occasionally the cell bodies of basket cells may be wedged between P-cell bodies, and the initial parts of their lower dendrites may pass between P-cell bodies before ascending into the molecular layer.

3. The Granular Layer

The granular layer is of uneven thickness, being even less than 100 μ in the depth of the furrows and 400—500 μ at the top of the folia. It is exceptionally densely packed with small nerve cells, the granule neurons. The number of granule cells is 2.4×10^6 per mm^3 in the monkey (Fox and Barnard, 1957). A considerable portion of the granular layer space is occupied by the cerebellar isles or glomeruli, the synaptic articulation arrangements being mainly between mossy fibers and

---

[1] All quantitative data given, if not specified otherwise refer to the cerebellar cortex of the adult cat.

granule cell dendrites. From cursory measurements made by planimetry from micro-photographs of Cajal-stained preparations one arrives at the estimate that the glomeruli occupy 31 % of the total space. Besides axons descending and ascending from and to the upper layers, there are the Golgi cells, several different kinds of which are usually distinguished.

For the purpose of a general survey it will be best to consider briefly first the chief cell types and secondly the terminations in the cortex of the afferent systems.

The finer details of the synaptic architecture are of crucial functional importance, and will be treated in the main chapters dealing with the respective synaptic systems.

B. Cell Types of the Cerebellar Cortex

Five different neuron types are found in the cerebellar cortex (Fig. 1.), all of which are rather specific in dendritic and axonal ramification patterns as well as in

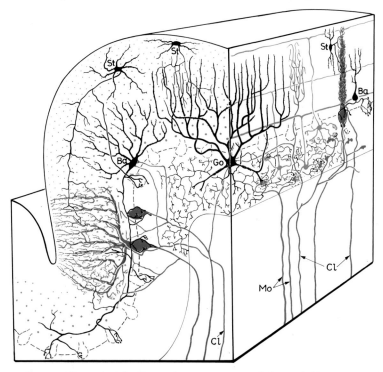

Fig. 1. Stereodiagram illustrating the five main neuron types of the cerebellar cortex and the two kinds of afferents with their main interconnexions. The afferents — both climbing (*Cl*) and mossy (*Mo*) fibers — are indicated in blue. The outlines of cerebellar glomeruli are drawn with black dotted lines. Granule neurons and parallel fibers in green, Purkinje neurons and their axons in red, the three main kinds of interneurons: stellate cells (*St*), basket cells (*Ba*), and Golgi cells (*Go*) are shown in black

their locations. The most characteristic in shape and the only true efferent elements are 1, *the Purkinje neurons;* the most numerous type, and located on the input side are 2, *the granule neurons.* The remaining three types are specific interneurons:

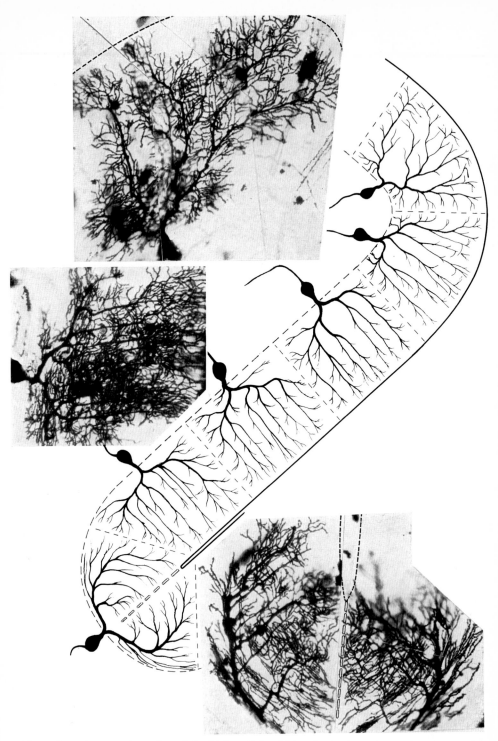

Fig. 2. Cartesian transformation of Purkinje cell dendritic arborizations due to changing curvature of the folium. Dashed lines separate fields of approximately equal areas, showing that the dendritic arborizations of Purkinje cells cover strikingly uniform areas of the molecular layer transectional surface. — "Neutral" line separating the dendritic trees in the depth of the fold-valleys is indicated by empty dashes. — Photomicrographs are giving typical examples of Purkinje cell dendritic arborizations of cells situated at the summit (above), at the side (left), and in the fold-valley (below). Human adult, Golgi-Cox procedure. Cerebellar surface indicated by dotted line

3, *the basket;* 4, *the outer stellate;* and 5, *the Golgi neurons.* With the exception of the Golgi neurons all other cell types are strictly uniform with only very slight variations in dendritic or axonal arborization patterns and in localization. The Golgi cells can be subdivided into at least three subgroups with characteristically different properties. Only one of these, however, is considered as "typical" and incorporated into the diagram (Fig. 1).

1. Purkinje Neurons

The Purkinje cells are one of the most characteristic examples of a highly differentiated neuron both with respect to the specific beauty of their dendritic arborizations as well as with respect to the many different kinds of synaptic relations they have. They are arranged in a single sheet with beet-like, bottle-shaped or pear-like cell bodies, lined up in the ganglionic layer. They are more densely arranged at the convexities of the folia than in the depth of the furrows. The axon takes its origin at the deep side of the body, rather abruptly without an axon hillock, and runs radially towards the medullary lamina. The dendritic tree arises from the bottle neck with a large primary dendrite, which varies in its branching according to the position of the cell. In the depth of the furrows it branches immediately at a broad angle (close to 180°, Fig. 2). At the convex parts of the folium it ascends for some tens of microns before branching at a more acute angle into the principal dendritic branches. The most remarkable feature of the dendritic arborization is that it is strictly confined to the transversal plane of the folium. In Golgi sections cut in the longitudinal plane of the folium, therefore, the Purkinje cell presents itself in the shape as seen in Fig. 3 A. Strangely, particularly in the cat, on often sees Purkinje cells with double dendritic sheets that appear in the longitudinal section as double spiked forks (Fig. 3 B). However, this

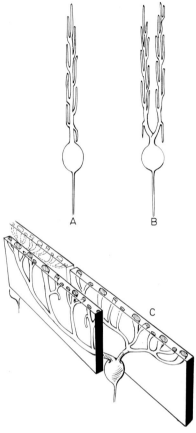

Fig. 3 A—C. Diagram to show the dendritic tree of the Purkinje cell as presenting itself in longitudinal sections of the folium. (A) typical transverse section of the dendritic sheet. (B) very common view in the thick (60—80 μ) Golgi sections, and (C) its three dimensional explanation. The sheets of arborization of the two main branches may not be in the same transversal plane, but be shifted slightly in longitudinal direction

is due simply to a slight shift in longitudinal direction between the planes of the dendritic sheets of the two primary branches as diagrammatically shown in Fig. 3 C. This is thus no exception to the principal design of the molecular layer of flat dendritic sheets arranged in parallel within the transversal plane of the folium, but it

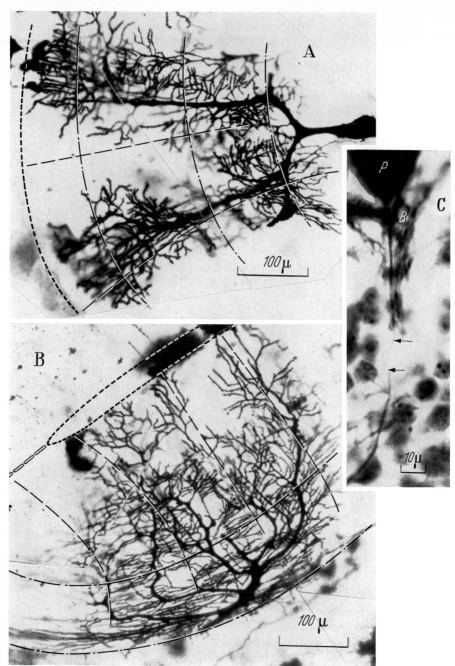

Fig. 4 A—C. The Purkinje cell. (A) from the summit of the folium and (B) neighboring fold-valley. Adult human, Golgi-Cox procedure. The cerebellar surface is indicated by dotted lines. Lines of tangential stress of the tissue matrix — due to folding — are indicated by "dash-dot" lines, radial stresses by "dashed" lines. Dendritic branches are predominantly arranged according to these lines. Arrangement of dendritic branches in direction perpendicular to "neutral line" in the depth of fold-valley can be seen in lower photomicrograph of Fig. 2. — (C) Origin of the axon at lower pole of Purkinje (P) cell body partly hidden in the basket (B). Initial part of axonal process thins down (between arrows) before assuming its final caliber and becoming myelinated. Dejnek method, cat

gives some opportunity for more intimate interdigitation of the dendritic sheets of neighbouring Purkinje cells. The primary and secondary dendritic branches are with rare exception ascending and have a smooth surface. The tertiary branches are termed *spiny branchlets* by Fox and BARNARD (1957) and are characterized by their short rather thick spines densely and regularly distributed all over the surface (Fig. 27 A, B, C).

The differences in shapes of the dendritic trees are apparently Cartesian transformations corresponding to the geometric determinations at the convexities and concavities of the cortex. According to the investigations of FRIEDE (1955) all differences in axonal and dendritic arborizations are secondary to the changes in the dendritic trees of the Purkinje cells. The diagram in Fig. 2 explains the changes in form and arborization pattern by assuming that the dendritic tree ought to cover an equal surface area of the transverse plane of the folium and that the borders between dendritic arborizations ought to be approximately perpendicular to the surface, that is radial to the curvatures. As seen from the diagram the distances between Purkinje cell bodies become smaller at the folium tops and larger in the depth of the sulci[2]. The photomicrographs attached to various regions of the diagram are giving characteristic examples of dendritic arborization patterns in Purkinje cells of various positions. The predominant directions of the tertiary (spiny) branches are nicely indicating the "lines of stresses" that are brought about in the cortex by the folding [Figs. 2 and 4 (indicated by "dashed" and "dash-dot" lines)].

HERNDON (1963) has described the fine structure of the Purkinje cell as seen under the electron microscope. There is a rather dense ergastoplasm and a prominent Golgi membrane system. Very often, so-called "lamellar bodies" occur in the cytoplasm composed of rather coarse membranes closely pressed together which may continue into the dendrites (Figs. 5 and 6) though they may be artefacts because it is quite difficult to get good plasma fixation of the Purkinje cells. The principal dendrite has a similar plasma structure with a very strong tubular system gradually becoming apparent and dominating the picture completely in the smooth primary and secondary dendritic branches (Fig. 6). This tubular system disappears abruptly in the spiny branchlets. It is replaced by a system of rather wide dendritic vacuoles, which are connected occasionally with irregular tubular channels that continue into the spines and terminate in a small vacuole in the head of the spine. The structure of spiny branchlets will be considered in more detail in Chapter III in connection with the parallel fiber synapses. The surface of the cell body and of the larger dendrites is thoroughly separated from the environment by a layer of Bergmann glia processes. Synaptic axon terminals are admitted to the cell body only at its base (the basket synapses, Chapter VI), and on the main dendrites there are: the climbing fiber synapses (Chapter II); the stellate axon synapses (Chapter VI) and the ascending basket axon collateral synapses (Chapter VI).

The axon of the Purkinje cell originates from its lower pole and gradually becomes thinner over the first 30 microns or so. Then quite abruptly its diameter

---

[2] This side of cerebellar cortex structure — especially with respect to general geometrical aspects of the problem — has been considered and lucidly discussed by BRAITENBERG and ATWOOD (1958).

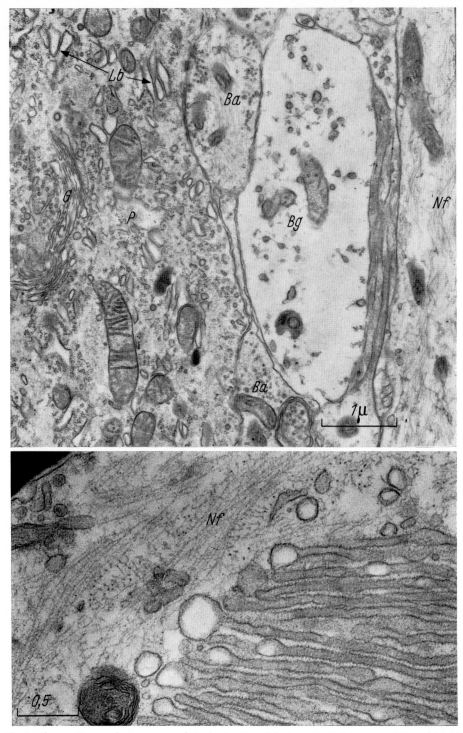

Fig. 5. Above: Plasma ultrastructure of Purkinje (*P*) cell body with Golgi system (*G*) and lamellar bodies (*Lb*). Longitudinal section of region just below the equator with branches of basket axons (*Ba*) beginning to attach themselves to cell body. Cell surface otherwise covered by Berg-

increases (Fig. 4 C) to the normal thickness and it becomes myelinated. The Purkinje axons have abundant recurrent collaterals, that according to CAJAL (1911) participate in two tangential plexuses, the infraganglionic below the Purkinje cell bodies and the supraganglionic immediately above them. The collaterals are myelinated and probably most of the myelinated axons immediately above and below the Purkinje cell bodies can be considered as Purkinje axon collaterals. These collaterals have been generally (CAJAL, 1911) supposed to terminate on the principal dendrites of the Purkinje cells. This important question will be considered in detail in Chapter IX. Under the electron microscope this initial portion of the axon looks more like an elongated part of the cell body because it contains not only neurofilaments but also an endoplasmic reticulum and numerous ribosomes that usually are absent in axons. It has therefore been proposed (HÁMORI and SZENTÁGOTHAI, 1965) that this initial segment be called the "pre-axon", and that the axon begins at the myelinated thicker part, which has true axonal structure. A peculiar system of tubules described by KOHNO (1964) in the initial segments of frog Purkinje axons can be observed also in the cat (Fig. 10). According to most recent observations by GRAY (1966, personal communication) these systems, however, are not specific for the Purkinje axon. Recently HÁMORI and SZENTÁGOTHAI (1967) have shown that the strange membrane systems first described by ANDRES (1965) in myelinated fibers of the cerebellar cortex are specific for Purkinje axons (Fig. 5). They occur not only in the main axon but also in its collaterals and even in their terminals. This enigmatic membrane system may be used therefore as a criterion for identification of Purkinje axons and their endings. Unfortunately, only a fraction of Purkinje axons have this system; hence only its presence can be used as evidence of identification and not its absence. Since it has been found in the rat (ANDRES) and in the cat as well as in human material (HÁMORI, unpublished), the membrane system can be considered as a general structural property of Purkinje axons.

2. Granule Neurons

The granular layer of the cerebellar cortex is densely packed with small neurons having spheroid nuclei of 5—8 μ diameter. The nucleus is surrounded by a thin poorly differentiated cytoplasm with a thickness of only 0.5—1 μ according to the measurement made on EM pictures. It contains small mitochondria, a small Golgi system, few and thin endoplasmic reticulum sacs, or tubuli and is rather densely packed with ribosomes. The number of granule cells per mm³ of granular layer has been found to be 2.4 million by Fox and BARNARD (1957). The average granule cell has 3—5 dentrites, 1—7 in the extreme (Fig. 7), which may branch once or rarely twice before breaking up into their characteristic claw-shaped terminal ramifications. The synaptic relations of granule cells will be discussed in detail in Chap-

Fig. 5.

mann glia (Bg) processes. Filamentous axon (Nf) at extreme right is probably a climbing fiber (see Chapter II and Fig. 23) differing from the equally filamentous basket axons by not having the strange transverse membrane systems shown in Fig. 10. — Below: peculiar membrane system characteristic of Purkinje axons. Myelin sheath can be seen in upper right corner. Nf = neurofilaments. From chronically isolated cerebellar cortex of adult cat, in which the only persisting myelinated axons are Purkinje axons

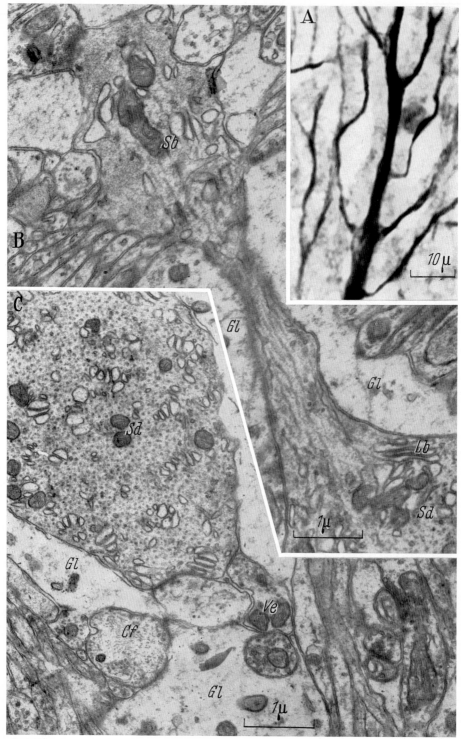

Fig. 6 A—C. Secondary dendrites and origin of tertiary branches of Purkinje dendrites. (A) Light photomicrograph of secondary dendrite giving rise to much thinner tertiary branches: the "spiny

ter VII. The dendrites are of 10—30 μ length, 0.7 μ in diameter, and, in addition to a few ribosomes, characteristically there is a rather strong tubular system. The thin axon takes its origin from either the cell body or more often from one of the dendrites. It ascends to the molecular layer where it bifurcates in T-shape manner to give rise to the so called parallel fibers, that run strictly parallel with the axis of the folium. The axons of those granule cells located in the outer zone of the granular layer ascend to the surface of the molecular layer and contribute to the superficial strata of the parallel fibers (Fox, SIEGESMUND and DUTTA, 1964). These axons according to CAJAL (1911) are much finer (0.2 μ diameter according to Fox and BARNARD, 1957) than the parallel fibers of deeper strata (1 μ diameter) that originate from granule cells located progressively deeper in the granular layer.

The initial parts of the parallel fibers, immediately after the bifurcation, are smooth; at larger distances they have short hooked side branches (Fox and BAR-NARD, 1957; Fox, SIEGESMUND and DUTTA, 1964). The length of the parallel fibers has been grossly overestimated by the classical descriptions, for example CAJAL (1911) thought that they reached to both ends of the folium. From the geometrical viewpoint this is highly improbable, for one would have to assume that there were more parallel fibers and granule cells in folia of larger length, and fewer in short folia. Since the sizes of both the molecular layer and the granular layer are completely independent of the folium length, and since the densities of parallel fibers and of granule cells do not show appreciable differences, one has to assume a priori that the parallel fibers must be of fairly uniform and rather short length in comparison with the length of the folia (c. f. also reasoning and calculation of BRAITEN-BERG and ATWOOD, 1958). Fox and BARNARD (1957) have traced parallel fibers in both directions from the point of bifurcation for 1—1.5 mm, which would justify the conclusion that the average length of parallel fibers might be 2 mm and the maximum length about 3 mm. Similar conclusions are reached on the basis of an experimental approach. In the molecular layer of chronically isolated slabs of a folium about 3 mm diameter there is no appreciable reduction of the density of parallel fibers in the middle part of the slab if compared with that in the neighbouring normal folium. If the total length of the parallel fibers would exceed 3 mm one would expect a considerable reduction.

Fox and BARNARD (1957) calculate in the monkey the number of parallel fibers that cross the dendritic tree of any Purkinje cell as being 208,000 to 278,000. Our own calculation in the cat based on fiber counts in EM micrographs led to the number of 209,000. From the uniform thickness of the molecular layer (FRIEDE,

Fig. 6 A—C.

branchlets" of the Golgi picture. The spines are not visible in this Bielschowsky stain of adult cat cerebellar cortex. (B) shows the origin of spiny branchlet (Sb) from secondary dendrite (Sd) having both the characteristic longitudinal tubuli and lamellar bodies (Lb) of the large (smooth) dendrites. Most of the dendrite surface is covered by glial processes (Gl). — (C) Transverse section of secondary dendrite (Sd) with strong longitudinal tubuli and lamellar bodies. The glial processes surround the main dendrite almost completely, only few axonal profiles: filamentous climbing fibers (Cf) (Chapter II, Figs. 23, 24) and "vesicular" (Ve) terminals of stellate and ascending basket axon branches being admitted to establish synaptic contacts. Electron micrographs from adult cat

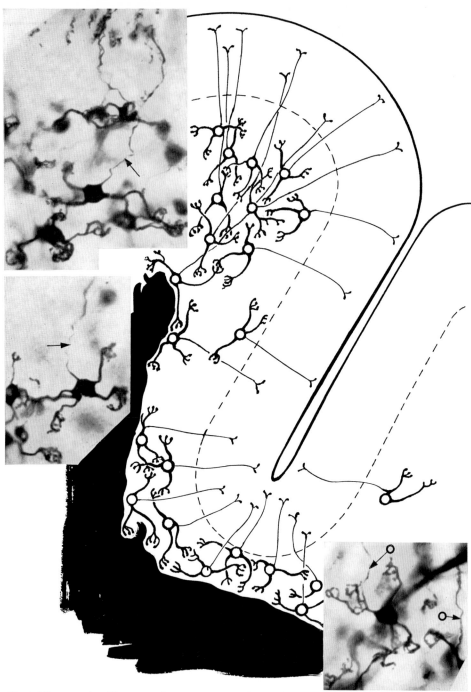

Fig. 7. Diagram that illustrates the arrangement of granule cells and their axons ascending into the molecular layer. Since the axons are diverging at the summit of the folium and converging in the depth of the interfolial grooves, the amount of granular layer tissue required to fill in the molecular layer with equal densities of parallel fibers — assuming equal sizes and densities of neurons and their processes in all regions — must be obviously much larger at the summit than in the valleys. Inset micrographs show granule neurons and their ascending axons that may originate either from the cell body (arrows) or from one of the dendrites (ringed arrows). Perfusion Kopsch procedure, adult cat

1955) and the roughly equal size of the dendritic trees of Purkinje cells one may gather that there can be little variation of these numbers in different parts of the cerebellar cortex. If this is so, one has again to assume from simple geometrical reasoning (Fig. 7) that the number of granule cells would be largest at the convexities of folia and smallest at the concavities between folia in order to supply the very different amount of molecular layer space with an equal density of parallel fibers both on the concavities and the convexities. This is indeed so, the thickness of the granular layer being 400—500 µ at the top, 200 µ at the flat sides of the folia and 100 µ in the depth of the furrows (FRIEDE, 1955).

3. Basket Neurons

The basket neurons are stellate nerve cells of lower medium size, about 20 µ diam. (Fig. 8) situated predominantly in the lower third or lower half of the molecular layer, and are slightly more numerous, by about 15—20 %, than the Purkinje cells. The dendritic tree arborizes predominantly in the lower two thirds of the molecular layer. The initial part of some of their lower dendrites descend into the ganglionic layer and then generally ascend again to terminate in the molecular layer. There is no specific pattern of arborization excepting that the dendritic tree lies in the transverse plane of the folium, exactly as with Purkinje cells. The dendrites have characteristic spines, which are much sparser, more irregularly distributed, longer and thinner than those of the Purkinje dendrites (Fig. 27 E), and are very often hooked. Under the EM the cell body of the basket cell shows an unusually irregular, almost rugged surface (Fig. 9), making it impossible to trace the surface membrane clearly for longer distances, because the plane of sectioning becomes often tangential to the deep depressions or elevations of the surface. The nucleus is also unusually irregular in surface configuration. These irregularities of surface both of the cell body and of the nucleus may be real, but, alternatively may be artefacts due to some special distortion of these cells during fixation. At any rate in EM pictures they can be used conveniently as criteria to distinguish basket cells from stellate cells. The plasma structure is rather dense on account of the numerous ribosomes and large mitochondria. This density of structure continues into the dendrites, which can be distinguished from larger Purkinje cell dendrites because they lack the characteristic tubular apparatus of the latter. The smaller basket dendrites can be recognized from their density (Fig. 9), which is in contrast to the light structure of the spiny branchlets of Purkinje cells. The smaller basket dendrites seem to have synaptic contacts with parallel fibers exclusively by means of their spines (Figs. 9 and 30) (HÁMORI and SZENTÁGOTHAI, 1964). The cell body surface is densely covered with synapses (Figs. 9 and 36).

The axon of the basket cells originates from the cell body with a rather thin initial segment (Fig. 8 B). After thickening to its normal caliber of 3 µ in the deeper strata of the molecular layer, the basket axon runs strictly in the transverse plane of the folium and parallel to the cortical surface. The axon usually does not begin to give side branches in the immediate neighborhood of the cell body, the first descending branch being given to the second Purkinje cell body. From here on, one descending branch is given to practically every Purkinje cell situated within the same transverse plane to an average distance of about 10 Purkinje cells or about 1 mm. These descending branchlets are also distributed to the P-cells that are situated in several adjacent transverse planes, as will be described in Chapter VI (Fig. 54). At about the level of the "bottle neck" of the Purkinje cell the descending collaterals of the axons divide in a brush-like manner, and the so-called Purkinje

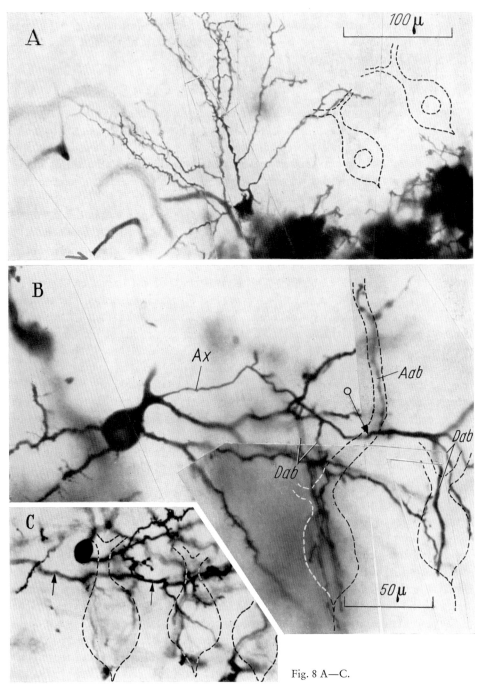

Fig. 8 A—C.

cell baskets are formed by the terminal arborizations of several basket axon collaterals converging upon the body of that Purkinje cell. As seen under the EM, the axons participating in the Purkinje baskets do not in general have synaptic contacts with the upper part of the P-cell body. True synaptic contacts are established only with the base of the P-cell and particularly the initial part of the P-axon (Figs. 10, 55, 56), or as it has recently been termed, the "pre-axon" (HÁMORI and SZENTÁ-GOTHAI, 1965). The basket does not terminate around the base of the P-cell, but continues downwards for about 20—30 µ and surrounds the pre-axon in a beard-like fashion. The basket axons are very rich in neurofilaments, but synaptic vesicles are concentrated mainly at the immediate region of synaptic attachment (Figs. 55, 56). The basket axons can be differentiated from climbing fibers, which are also rich in neurofilaments (see Chapter II), on the basis of their strange transverse membrane systems (Figs. 10, 55).

The basket axon has also numerous ascending collaterals (Fig. 8) both during its course and especially at its terminal arborization. The possible synaptic connexions of these ascending collaterals will be discussed in Chapter VI.

4. Outer Stellate Neurons

The stellate neurons (Fig. 11) in the outer half or probably more exactly the outer two thirds of the molecular layer differ from the basket neurons mainly with respect to the course and ramification of their axons. Their cell body is smaller and their dendritic ramifications span considerably smaller distances. The dendrites are otherwise similar, though perhaps with somewhat denser secondary and tertiary ramifications. They have spines essentially similar in size, distribution and form to those of the basket cell dendrites (Fig. 27 D). As with the Purkinje and basket cells, the dendritic tree is confined to the transversal plane of the folium. Under the EM the outer stellate cells differ in a spectacular manner from the basket cells, having a spheroidal cell body with smooth contours, a light plasma structure, and a spherical nucleus usually with a single deep tongue-shaped invagination of the nuclear membrane. Their mitochondria are characteristically empty, having but few cristae. On the surface of the cell body there are few synapses, but probably these do not belong to the parallel fibers that can be seen running for long distances along the cell surface without synaptic differentiations (Fig. 12).

Fig. 8 A—C. Golgi picture of a basket neuron: (A) low magnification showing dendritic arborization of the basket cell with an abundance of irregular spines. Ganglionic layer is indicated by the outlines of two Purkinje cells, below them are granule cells stained *en masse;* (B) Medium power view of another basket cell showing origin of axon with characteristic thin caliber *(Ax),* which in some distance suddenly (ringed arrow) increases to its normal caliber. Descending axon branches *(Dab)* participate in the pericellular baskets. For better understanding the outlines of Purkinje cell bodies and their main dendrites are indicated by dotted lines: ascending axon branch *(Aab)* is seen to terminate in close relation to a principal Purkinje dendrite. (C) Same basket cell axon (arrows) at the distance of 600—800 µ gives further descending branches to Purkinje cell baskets. In comparison to the density seen in Bielschowsky or Cajal silver stains (Fig. 55 A) and in spite of the much thicker sections the baskets are poor in the Golgi stain, when only one or two basket axons are stained. This indicates a considerable degree of convergence (Chapter VI) from many basket neurons to the same basket

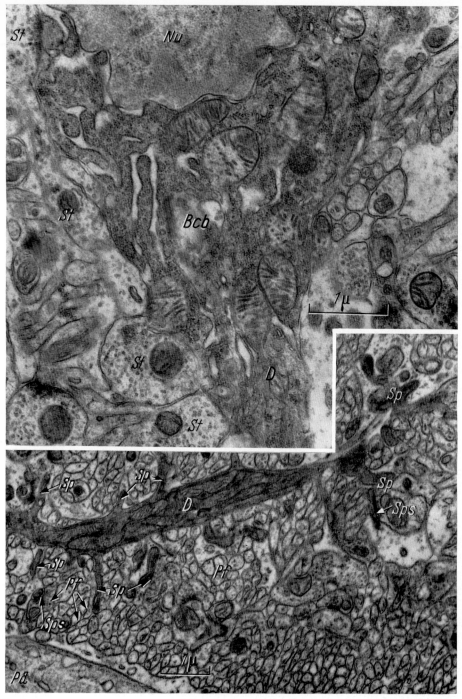

Fig. 9. Electronmicroscope structure of basket cell body (above) and of smaller spiny dendrite (below). The basket cell body (*Bcb*) has a very dense plasma structure, large mitochondria, relatively wide endoplasmic cisterns, an irregular cell body surface, covered with numerous synaptic terminals (*St*) and an irregular surfaced nucleus (*Nu*). Dendrite (*D*) of similar dense structure takes origin at lower pole of the cell. — Small basket cell dendrite (*D*) in lower photograph has equally dark plasma structure and irregular long and thin often hooked and arborizing (at upper right) spines (*Sp*) that establish synapses (*Sps*) with parallel fibers (*Pf*), here cut transversally. Primary dendrite of Purkinje cell (*Pd*) is seen at lower left separated completely from parallel axons by light glial plasma layer. Upper figure from the cat and lower from human cerebellar cortex

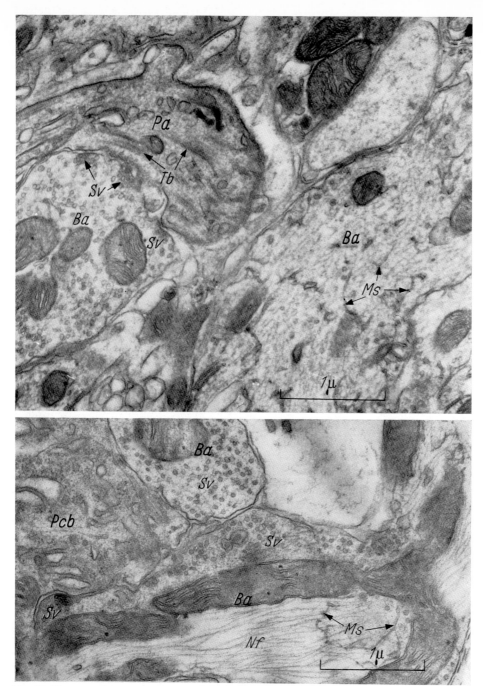

Fig. 10. Electron microscope structure of the basket axon. The basket axon as well as its terminal branches (*Ba*) are always devoid of myelin, contain numerous neurofilaments (*Nf*) and a strange irregular membrane system (*Ms*), usually arranged transversally. This membrane system can be used for differentiation of the equally filamentous climbing fibers, as they have no such membrane system (compare with Figs. 5 and 23). In upper photograph an initial part of Purkinje axon (preaxon, *Pa*) can be seen having characteristic synaptic contacts with terminal bulges of a basket axon, containing accumulations of synaptic vesicles (*Sv*). The strange tubular structures described by KOHNO (1964) in the initial segments of frog Purkinje axon can be recognized also in the cat (*Tb*). — In lower photograph a region of a Purkinje cell body (*Pcb*) very close to the axonal pole is shown, having synaptic contact with basket axon branch (*Ba*) passing by, which is descending towards the depth of the basket. Surface in both pictures is towards the left; cat

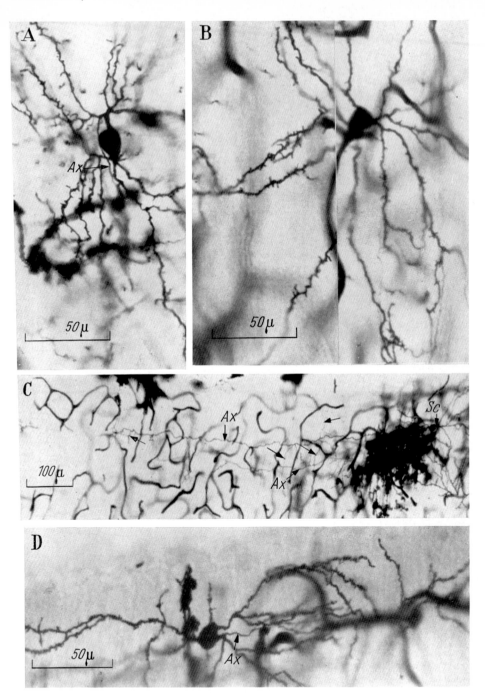

Fig. 11 A—D. The stellate neuron in the Golgi picture (A) and (B) type "a" stellate neurons with initial part of descending axon (*Ax*) seen in (A). Dendrites show rather large spines irregularly distributed. — (C) Two horizontal axons (*Ax*) of type "b" stellate neurons, one of the cells (*Sc*) can be recognized at extreme right emerging from the precipitate. Terminal side branches (arrows) of horizontal axon are vertically oriented. — (D) Type "b" stellate neuron from immediately below the surface with horizontal axon (*Ax*) originating from main dendrite

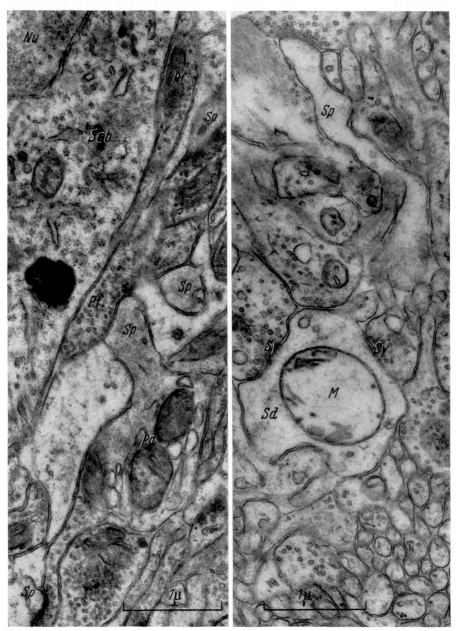

Fig. 12. Electron microscopic details from stellate neurons. — At left cell body (*Scb*) has smooth contours, relatively light plasma and mitochondria having few cristae. The nucleus (*Nu*) is spheric with generally a single tongue-shaped invagination. Synaptic contacts on cell body are rare. Parallel fibers (*Pf*) although in immediate apposition do not show synaptic differentiations, which they have in abundance with spines (*Sp*) of tertiary Purkinje dendrites (*Pd*). — For detailed description of spines and their contacts see Chapter III. — Right: characteristic light dendrite of stellate neuron (*Sd*) with large "empty" mitochondrium (*M*), having numerous axo-dendritic synapses (*Sy*) presumably with thickened parts of parallel fibers. Long spine (*Sp*) that presumably originates from this dendrite has synapse at top of the figure. Purkinje dendrites (see for example left side of this figure and Figs. 28, 29) do not have spines of such lengths (Chapter III)

21

The dendrites of the outer stellate cells can be identified under the EM with fair probability on the basis of their large mitochondria with unusually few cristae (Fig. 26), their long hooked spines (Fig. 12) and a considerable number of direct (non-spine) axo-dendritic synapses (Figs. 12, 26).

On the basis of the ramification pattern of their axons, two main outer stellate cells can be distinguished, there being two varieties of type a: a_1) the smallest cells are characteristic Golgi II type neurons with a very delicate axon having a dense arborization in the close neighbourhood of the cell and with a predominantly vertical course of their terminal branches: a_2) Somewhat larger neurons, located generally deeper than the former ones, with descending and/or ascending axon ramifications. The descending branches can be traced occasionally to the bottle neck of P-neurons, but not deeper into the baskets. The b-type cells have horizontal axons (Fig. 11 C) that can be traced for distances up to 900 μ strictly in the transversal plane of the folium. The b-type cells located closer to the surface are generally smaller, their axons being more delicate and shorter than the axons of those lying somewhat deeper. The terminal branches of these horizontal axons are short and ascend or descend vertically. In general the terminal branches of all outer stellate axons run preferentially in the vertical direction, which might be interpreted as an adaption to the vertical course of the secondary and tertiary P-cell dendrites. The possible synaptic relations of the outer stellate axons will be discussed in Chapter VI.

In the middle of the molecular layer, or somewhat deeper, there is a kind of stellate cell that was initially mentioned by CAJAL (1911, Fig. 23 C). It appears to be a transition between outer stellate and basket neurons. This type of cell has a delicate, rather short axon of horizontal course, which otherwise arborizes in a manner essentially similar to that of type "b" of the true stellate neurons, but with the difference that it has some descending branches which participate in the pericellular baskets of the P-cells. Taking into consideration the large number of very thin horizontal axons encountered in good neurofibrillar preparations with descending branches entering the baskets, one may assume that this transitional cell type is not rare and that most of the stellate cells situated in or immediately below the middle zone of the molecular layer belong to this type. Very occasionally nerve cell bodies are met with in the middle stratum of the molecular layer which cannot be classified either as of basket or of outer stellate character. It may well be that the form of the cell body gradually changes in shape and character when not localized either in the inner third or the outer half of the molecular layer.

5. Golgi Neurons

The Golgi neurons, or large stellate neurons, are situated with their cell bodies in the granular layer. The greater part of their dendritic tree, however, is usually embedded in the molecular layer. They can be recognized most easily in reduced silver stained preparations (CAJAL or BIELSCHOWSKY). The number of typical Golgi cells is slightly above 10 % of the Purkinje cells[3] with the atypical Golgi

---

[3] Ratios determined on midsagittal section of the anterior vermis in adult cat (modified Cajal stain), having 2287 P-cells, 232 typical G-cells and 36 atypical ones.

cells making an additional 1—2%. The cell body of the typical Golgi cell is fairly large — in most cases somewhat smaller than the Purkinje cell, but some may be considerably larger. It is characteristically located beneath the row of Purkinje cells in the upper stratum of the granular layer.

Unlike other cell types in the molecular layer, the dendritic tree is not confined to the transverse plane of the folium, but it expands equally in all directions. It

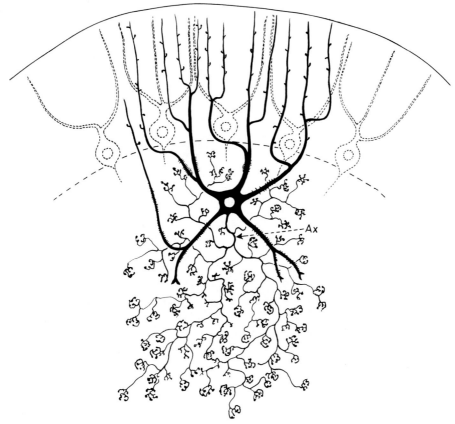

Fig. 13. Golgi neuron having typical localization; slightly diagrammatic drawing, into which characteristic features are condensed from many individual cells observed in Golgi pictures. Note "stiff" arborization of ascending dendrites and their relatively sparse spines. The Golgi cell looks similar irrespective of whether it is cut in the longitudinal or the transverse plane of the folium. The axon (*Ax*) branches regularly — but not always — in the space of the granule layer corresponding to the space occupied in the molecular layer by the ascending dendrites. "Spiny" appearance of dendrites in the granule layer — especially of the descending dendrites — is adapted from the EM picture

has a considerably wider span than the average Purkinje dendritic tree — about three times as wide. Most of the dendrites, even those that originate in the descending direction, turn towards the surface. After one or two branchings these dendrites ascend through the ganglionic layer and have further rather sparse branchings through the entire depth of the molecular layer. Immediately after branching off from a larger dendrite, the secondary and tertiary dendrites run for a short distance in horizontal directions and then turn at right angles into their dominant vertical course. This gives the dendritic tree a peculiar stiff appearance (Fig. 13). The smaller

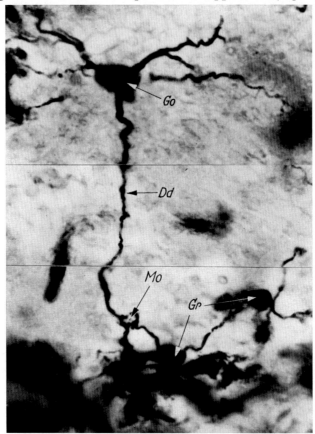

Fig. 14. Golgi cell of typical localization (*Go*) with initial parts of the ascending dendrites in focus. Descending dendrite (*Dd*) participates with typical claw-shaped dendrite of granule cell (*Gr*) in a glomerulus. Site of mossy fiber (*Mo*) is left unstained (for details of the glomeruli see Chapter VII). Adult cat, rapid Golgi stain (HÁMORI-SZENTÁGOTHAI, 1966 b)

Fig. 15 A—D. The Golgi cell in Golgi and neurofibrillar silver stains. — (A) Nearly complete staining of Golgi cells (G) in a young kitten, showing their fairly regular distribution and their typical localization in a row slightly below the Purkinje cell body layer. Some Purkinje cell bodies are indicated in dotted outlines: in the adult the Golgi cells are shifted somewhat to the depth. The Golgi axon neuropil of the granule layer is completely stained. At the surface the outer granule layer (*Og*) still persists. — As seen in (B) this layer is invaded by the upper parts of the dendrites (zone above the horizontal dashed line): Whereas the lower parts of the Golgi cell dendrites engage in contacts with the already developed lower parallel fibers by growing out primitive spines, these are lacking completely in the outer molecular layer, where there are still no parallel fibers at this early age. Arrows indicate glomeruli with Golgi axon terminal ramifications. — (C) Typical Golgi cell (G) in a Dejnek neurofibrillar stain of the adult cat cerebellar cortex. Bottom of Purkinje cell (*P*) and basket (*B*) can be seen at top of photograph. Glomeruli (*Gl*) are strongly stained with this procedure. While typical Golgi cells are not connected with the baskets, "fusiform cell" (*F*) in part (D) of this figure is approached and surrounded by numerous terminal branches (blank arrows) from the baskets (*Ba*) of two Purkinje cells (*P*), the axons of which are indicated by ringed arrows

dendrites in the molecular layer have sparse blunt and stiff spines that are irregularly distributed. There are, however, always dendrites that arborize in the granular layer and do not even reach the ganglionic layer. This is particularly so with

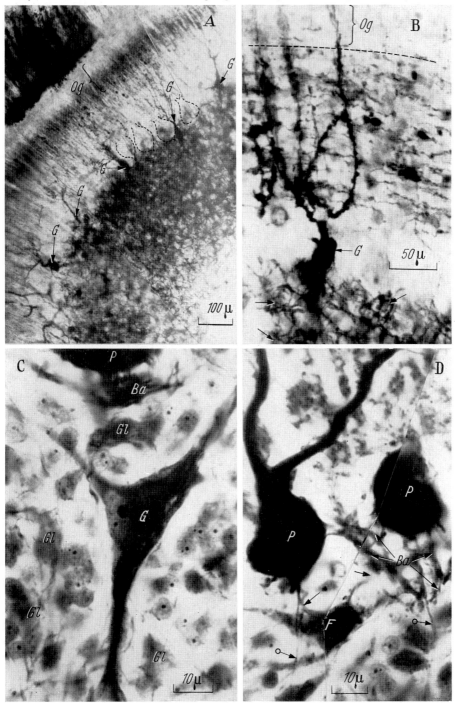

Fig. 15 A—D.

the deep Golgi cells, from which few if any dendrites ascend to the molecular layer, however, CAJAL (1911, Fig. 32 B) gives a beautiful illustration of a deep Golgi cell that has two ascending dendrites, which upon reaching the molecular

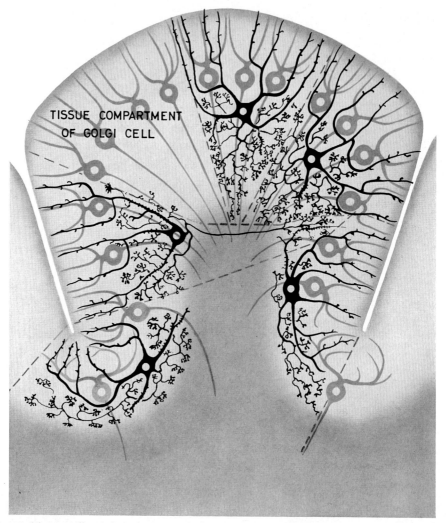

Fig. 16. Diagram illustrating arrangement of Golgi cells (drawn in full black) in relatively in-dependent space compartments — i. e. without major overlap of their processes — of the cerebellar cortex. Tissue compartments are separated by dashed lines. Some of the compartments can reach over, either by axonal or dendritic branches, through the medullary lamina into the other side of the folium (synarmotical cells of LANDAU)

layer arborize in the same manner as the ascending branches of the typical cell. The descending dendrites of Golgi cells appear to be involved in the glomeruli of the granular layer (Figs. 14, 72).

The axon of the typical Golgi neuron arises generally from the base of the cell body, or from a descending dendrite, and immediately begins to arborize in the fashion of Golgi type II axons. The terminal arborization pattern of the axon was clearly recognized by CAJAL (1911, Figs. 30, 31 and p. 46) as indicating that it must be involved in the glomeruli. The arborization of the axon covers the entire depth of the granular layer, with an expansion in tangential directions at least as wide as that of the dendritic tree (Fig. 13).

Considering the number ratio — roughly 10 : 1 — of Purkinje cells to Golgi cells — as well as the wider span and expansion in all directions of the dendritic tree of the Golgi cells, one would arrive at the assumption that there ought to be neither any major overlap between the dendritic trees of neighbouring Golgi cells, nor large gaps in the molecular layer between the dendrites of neighbouring Golgi cells (Fig. 15 A). This fits rather nicely with observations both of CAJAL (1911, Fig. 29) and JAKOB (1928, Fig. 132). The same considerations are applicable also to the axonal ramifications of the Golgi cells, which leads to the assumption of a similar separation of the axonal territories of neighbouring cells with relatively little overlap, and hence relatively little if any convergence in their synaptic actions in the glomeruli. As diagrammatically shown in Fig. 16, each Golgi cell occupies a tissue compartment of its own both with its dendritic and axonal arborization. These tissue compartments have the shapes of irregular truncated pyramids. In the unfolded cortex they could be considered ideally as hexagonal prisms (see Fig. 116), which reach generally through the entire depth of the cortex and sometimes even may extend into the other side of the folium.

These considerations apply specifically to the Golgi cells having a typical location of the cell bodies in the superficial region of the granular layer and with typical dendritic and axonal ramifications. It also applies approximately to those Golgi cells displaced towards the depth of the granular layer with at least some of their ascending dendrites entering the molecular layer. There are, however, some other types of large or medium sized cells both in the granular and the ganglionic layers and even some in the molecular layer and in the subjacent white matter, which usually are classified also as Golgi cells. At least they have been classified by most authors into a major group of large stellate neurons of the submolecular layer, from which the typical Golgi cells are considered, in general, only as a subgroup. This view is confusing because some of these cells have long axons and, therefore, cannot be considered as Golgi II type neurons. On account of their scarcity and irregular distribution they can be of little concern in this monograph, since it is unlikely that they should participate in any significant manner in the physiological observations to be presented. However, in order to complete the anatomical treatment brief descriptions will be given.

a) Fusiform Cells. These large cells have three main locations: They may be oriented tangentially beneath the ganglionic layer (Fig. 15 D). Rarely they are in the depth of the granular layer, and more frequently again in the white lamina of the folia. Their dendrites originate from the opposite poles of the cell body and have a considerable span of sometimes over 10 Purkinje cells and finally enter into the molecular layer. The dendrites of the deeper fusiform cells terminate in the granule layer. Their axons originate either from the cell body or one of the main dendrites, and after giving rise to a large number of initial collaterals, can be traced according to CAJAL (1911) to the white matter. — A somewhat similar description is given by FOX and BERTRAM (1954) of the cell bodies of the so called "intermediate cells" of LUGARO (1894), but with an entirely different course of the axon, which ascends to the molecular layer and behaves like the parallel fibers. Our own experience with these cells is limited to observations in reduced silver preparations, and indicate their rarity, being in the cat less than 1 % of the Purkinje cells. Strangely, most of these cells are surrounded by the endings of basket axons. This has been mentioned repeatedly by earlier authors as being the case with Golgi cells in general. But according to our own material this does not occur with the typical Golgi cells, which are completely devoid of basket contacts (Fig. 15 C). It is exclusively the fusiform cell, which has these basket contacts. One might therefore speculate whether these cells might not be modified and displaced Purkinje cells.

b) Intercalated Cells of PENSA. This is a row of medium sized stellate cells which are described in the cat as almost exactly alternating with Purkinje cell bodies (PENSA, 1931). The dendrites mainly ascend in the molecular layer in Golgi cell like fashion, but with predominant orientation in the transversal plane of the folium. The descriptions of the descending dendrites and axon arborizations are obscured by the reticularist views of this author. Stellate cells with this position of cell body have been observed very occasionally in our own material. However, it is our impression that they may be either basket cells displaced downwards or Golgi cells displaced upwards (particularly in young animals, Fig. 15, A and B). The observations and pictures of PENSA (1931) could be explained as a misinterpretation in relatively thick and obliquely cut preparations of either the deepest row of basket cell bodies or of typical Golgi cell bodies projecting into the ganglionic layer. Another explanation would be that the large Bergmann glial cells, having exactly this position, were mistaken for neurons in consequence of the incomplete staining of their processes.

c) Deep Golgi II and Long Axon Stellate Cells. The larger Golgi cells with at least some dendrites reaching the molecular layer are not incorporated into this group. Most of these deep stellate cells are considerably smaller than the typical Golgi cells, although much larger than the granule cells, even than the larger granule cells, which are mostly situated in the depth of the granular layer and give rise to the coarser deep parallel fibers as described above. These deep stellate cells are occasionally referred to, without justification, as a peculiar type of granule cell. Their dendritic tree is confined to the granular layer. If situated in the medullary lamina they may send their dendrites to the granular layer of both sides of the folium. These cells have been called by LANDAU (1928, 32, 33) "synarmotic cells". According to our own Golgi observations the dendrites undoubtedly are engaged in the cerebellar glomeruli. The axons may be either true Golgi II type arborizations, or may enter the white matter. Even in this case it is not certain that they are not a peculiar kind of Golgi II type cell, since there is the observation of CAJAL (1911) that typical Golgi axons enter the medullary lamina for a while and emerge on the other side of the folium to arborize in the granular layer in a typical Golgi II manner (Fig. 19).

The typical Golgi cells can be recognized easily under the EM because their cell bodies differ grossly from those of the granule cells. They have characteristic relatively light plasma structure (Figs. 17, 18). The cell body surface is covered by numerous synaptic terminals, which will be discussed later in Chapter IV. The larger dendrites can be seen to originate from the cell body (Fig. 17) and they have a unique structural property, that can be used as a criterion for their recognition. The dendritic surface has short finger-like processes of about 0.1—0.4 μ diameter and 1—1.5 μ length which protrude into a somewhat wider intercellular space that surrounds the Golgi dendrites at the sites of the processes. These processes are considerably smaller than the usual dendritic spines and also they have no synaptic contacts. The Golgi dendrites become synaptically involved in the glomeruli of the cerebellar isles, as will be dealt with in detail in Chapter VII. Unfortunately

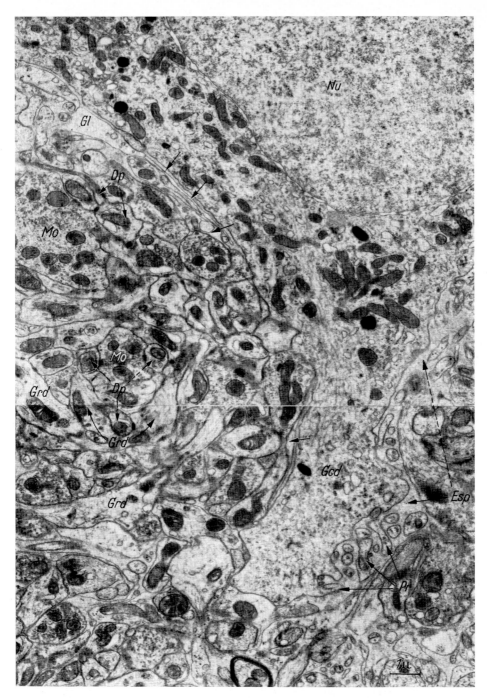

Fig. 17. EM photograph of Golgi cell, grossly differing from granule cells (see Fig. 67 in Chapter VII) both in size and plasma structure. Nucleus (*Nu*) is seen above, dendrite (*Gcd*) descending towards the depth of the granule layer has characteristic finger-like protrusions (*Pr*) embedded into a relatively wide extracellular space (*Esp*). At left of photograph cerebellar isle or glomerulus is seen with centrally localized mossy fiber profiles (*Mo*) surrounded by the terminal protrusions (*Dp*) or bulbs of granule cell dendrites (*Grd*) that do not have immediate contacts with mossy fiber rosettes. The glomerulus is surrounded by a thin sheet of glial processes (*Gl* and blank arrows). (Detailed description of the glomerulus is in Chapter VII)

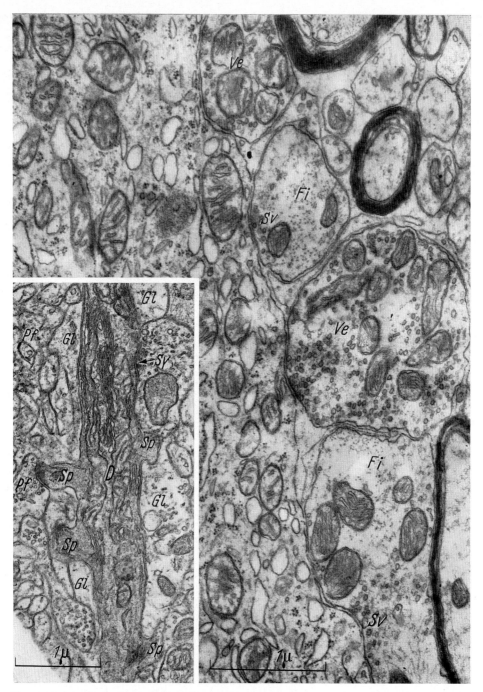

Fig. 18. Golgi cell plasma structure (left) and synaptic terminals in contact with cell body surface (right). Two kinds of synapses can be found regularly: those of neurofilamentous (*Fi*) character having but few synaptic vesicles (*Sv*) at the sites of immediate contact and those of vesicular (*Ve*) structure (SZENTÁGOTHAI, 1965a). The first type has been identified (HÁMORI and SZENTÁGOTHAI, 1966) as the ending of the climbing fiber collaterals (SCHEIBEL and SCHEIBEL, 1954). Small myelinated fibers correspond to the infraganglionic plexus of recurrent Purkinje axon collaterals (see

in the cat the ascending dendrites have not been as yet identified under the EM. Occasionally there are dendritic profiles oriented vertically in the Purkinje cell body layer. Since the Golgi dendrites are the only ones that run through the Purkinje cell layer, these strange beaded dendritic profiles with their abundance of synaptic knobs might well be the ascending Golgi cell dendrites, but this is still uncertain. In human material some dendrites could be identified (Fig. 18), which, on the basis of their rather sparse short and stiff spines could correspond very well to ascending Golgi dendrites (see also Fig. 27 F).

Chapter IX). Adult cat. — Inset: Dendrite (D) that with some probability can be identified as being from Golgi cell, with short stiff spines (Sp) contacting parallel fibers (Pf). There is one axo-dendritic synaptic contact (Sy) with large axonal profile, that may be a thickened part of a parallel fiber, but could be also a stellate or ascending basket axon. The greater part of the dendrite surface is covered by glial (Gl) processes. From human adult

Chapter II

Termination of Afferent Fibers

Extracortical afferent systems terminate in the cerebellar cortex by two different kinds of terminal arborizations and endings: 1. the mossy and 2. the climbing
fibers. Very little of significance was added to the description by CAJAL (1911) of
the mossy fibers until it became possible to analyse their origin by the use of secondary degeneration (MISKOLCZY, 1931), and until further investigation could be
undertaken by the aid of the electron microscope (GRAY, 1961). With the climbing
fibers it was different: reinvestigation by SCHEIBEL and SCHEIBEL (1954) have
changed to a considerable extent the classical views concerning their connexions.
Some but not all of their conclusions have been recently substantiated under the EM
(HÁMORI and SZENTÁGOTHAI, 1966 a).

A. The Mossy Fibers

The afferents terminating in mossy fibers are rather coarse myelinated fibers
that ascend to the cerebellar cortex through the white matter. They are seen to
give off collaterals along their entire course through the white matter, and not only
in the medullary lamina of that folium in which they largely terminate. Many
mossy afferents have been observed by CAJAL (1911) to bifurcate and to enter two
neighbouring folia (Fig. 19). Moreover the numerous branches given by the afferent
fibers in deeper parts of the white matter indicate that mossy terminals of the
same afferent fiber may reach more than two folia and probably not exclusively the
closely neighboring ones. But it may indicate, too, that the afferent tract fibers that
terminate in mossy fibers give collaterals to the cerebellar nuclei. (Chapter XIII.)
Upon entering the folium the mossy afferent fibers run along the medullary
lamina and give off numerous collaterals to both sides of the granular layer. In the
granular layer the collaterals branch once or twice and develop presynaptic expansions and sinuous convolutions which either are the fiber terminals or are of
"de passage" character. In these presynaptic zones there are grape-like groups of
bulbs which are connected with the fiber by short stout stalks. Each of these presynaptic loci of the mossy fibers is situated in one of the so called "cerebellar isles"
or glomeruli and they are generally referred to as the mossy fiber "rosettes".
Inside a single folium a mossy afferent fiber might have 20—30 such presynaptic
sites (Fig. 19), which enter into contact mainly with the dendritic ends of granule
neurons. Based on information received from SCHEIBEL and SCHEIBEL[1], BRODAL
(1958) has put forward the view that this classical concept of the mossy fiber
synapse may have to be given up in favour of the assumption that axo-somatic
contacts are established between mossy fibers and granule cell bodies. However,

---

[1] Personal communications and figures given to BRODAL (see 1958).

electron microscopy has fully corroborated CAJAL's view of terminal dendritic synapses. This important question will be analyzed in detail when giving a full account of the ultrastructure of the mossy fibers and of the cerebellar glomeruli in Chapter VII.

The first reliable information on the origin of mossy fibers from a particular afferent system was the observation of MISKOLCZY (1931), who employed experi-

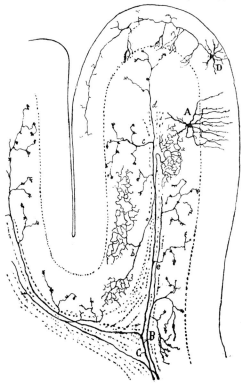

Fig. 19. Mossy afferents (B and C) terminating in two neighboring folia. (From CAJAL, 1911, Fig. 41). A basket cell (D) and Golgi cell (A) are also shown in this figure, the latter having two sites of axonal ramification in both sides of the folium

mental axonal and terminal degeneration to prove that the spinocerebellar fibers terminated as mossy fibers. With the aid of the same technique the termination of ponto-cerebellar fibers by means of mossy fibers was shown by SNIDER (1936). There was some evidence in the same study of vestibulo-cerebellar fibers giving rise also to mossy fibers. More recently with the aid of the Nauta procedure it has been shown that the reticulo-cerebellar fibers (SZENTÁGOTHAI, 1962) and the fibers from the external cuneate nucleus (GRANT, 1962) terminate as mossy fibers.

It would be far beyond the scope of this monograph to go into any details of the projection of afferent systems upon various regions of the cerebellar cortex. The reader is, therefore, referred to the excellent treatments of this subject by JANSEN and BRODAL (1954 and 1958).

From the early branching of mossy afferents in the depth of the white matter and the termination of mossy fibers in two or more adjacent folia it is obvious that there can be no sharp projection of "point to point" character in any system that terminates by mossy fibers. In spite of that, however, there are very definite differences in the degree of branching and especially in the spread of the branches in the cortex of fibers belonging to different afferent systems. Thus the dorsal spino-cerebellar tract (DSCT) fibers terminate in rather small areas (LUNDBERG and OSCARSSON, 1960) and the ventral spinocerebellar tract (VSCT) fibers in large areas (LUNDBERG and OSCARSSON, 1962).

The problem of somatotopic organization of afferent cerebellar pathways has given rise to lengthy discussions[2]. Undoubtedly the diffuse termination of many systems ending by mossy fibers would be clearly unfavourable for any precise somatotopic projection. On the other hand the mode of relay between primary afferents and the cerebellar afferent system — as for example in CLARKE's column (SZENTÁGOTHAI, 1961) — is singularly unfavourable for anatomical studies of exact somatotopic projections. This is essentially so in many other afferent systems of the cerebellum too. In spite of that there is a quite clear all-over somatotopic projection of the most caudal segments to the most anterior folia of the anterior lobe and then of the following segments in correct sequence within successive lobuli. The hindlimb projection by the DSCT and VSCT is rather sharply separated from the forelimb area, as far as this is conveyed over the external cuneo-cerebellar tract (CCT) the boundary being at the border between lobules IV and V (OSCARSSON, 1965).

The diffuse termination of mossy fibers raises another important question: that of the convergence of afferents from various sources at any given site of the cerebellar cortex. There is a very large convergence of the projections of the various afferent systems that are known to terminate by mossy fibers, as has been so thoroughly elaborated by the Oslo group (summarised in JANSEN and BRODAL, 1954 and 1958). From the general arborization patterns of mossy fibers, in Golgi preparations, it could be surmised that there is a simple random overlap of the converging pathways. However, the convergence is not necessarily of random character, but may show specific patterns, as can be seen in the overlap between the spinocerebellar tracts on the one hand and on the other the reticulo-cerebellar tract, originating from the lateral reticular nucleus of the medulla oblongata. Both systems have projections to the same folia of the anterior lobe, although the latter are shifted considerably towards Lobule V. There is the strange difference, that the DSCT favours cortical regions around the base of the lobuli, i.e. in the depth of the sulci, whereas the reticulo-cerebellar terminals are more abundant in cortical regions situated at the free surface of the cerebellum. In addition there is an interesting difference in respect of the depth at which the two systems preferentially terminate. After transection of the DSCT in midthoracic level, the degeneration fragments accumulate in the deeper strata of the granular layer, whereas the upper third of this layer is almost free from degeneration (Fig. 20 A). Consideration of the ascending course of the mossy fibers leads to the expectation of a larger density of degeneration fragments in the deeper layer because the fibers terminating in the

---

[2] For detailed information the reader is referred to JANSEN and BRODAL (1954, 1958).

most superficial layer have also to traverse the deeper layers. However, this explanation does not account for the virtual absence of any degeneration fragments in the upper layer. In the same folia there is a reverse termination of the reticulo-cerebellar fibers originating from the lateral reticular nucleus. The degeneration fragments appear to be concentrated in the superficial zones of the granular layer (Fig. 20 B). In addition to this difference, the degeneration fragments of the spino-

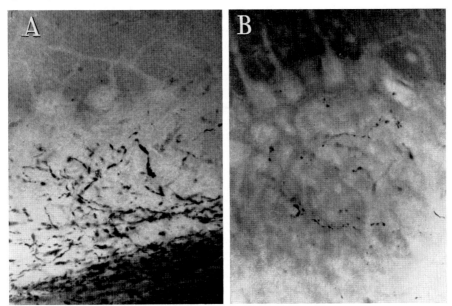

Fig. 20. (A) Degeneration pattern of mossy afferents (in Lob. IV) four days after transection in upper thoracic level of the spino-cerebellar tracts. Very large fragments (large caliber fibers) in lower 2/3 of the granular layer, and almost no fragments in upper third. Purkinje cells can be recognized as negative shadows. Side of folium. — (B) Degeneration pattern in the summit of the same folium after focal lesion placed into the lateral reticular nucleus of the medulla obl. with much smaller fragments predominantly in more superficial strata of the granular layer. — Nauta-Gygax procedure, cat

cerebellar mossy terminals are much larger than those of the reticulo-cerebellar mossy terminals.

Disregarding the differences between the basal and top regions of the folia, the predominant terminations of spinocerebellar afferents in the deeper zone of the granular layer and of the reticulo-cerebellar afferents in the superficial zone indicate a rather interesting mode of convergence of spinocerebellar and reticulo-cerebellar afferents on the same Purkinje cells. The mossy fibers terminating in deeper strata have synaptic contacts only with granule cells localized in the same stratum. The ascending axons of the latter bifurcate in deeper layers and give rise to the coarser deep parallel fibers of the molecular layer, which make synaptic contacts with the deeper dendritic branches of Purkinje cells. Conversely the lateral reticulo-cerebellar mossy fibers, terminating predominantly in the superficial region of the granular layer, would cause discharges of the superficial granule cells and so would influence mainly the more superficial dendrites of Purkinje cells. We do not know as yet whether synaptic stimulation of the Purkinje cells on their upper or lower dendritic sites has any integrative significance, but this simple example does suggest a special type of integration by the specific patterns of overlap between mossy fibers of various afferent systems converging upon the same region of the cerebellar cortex.

B. The Climbing Fibers

The climbing fibers have been described by CAJAL as afferents of extraneous origin that ascend undivided through the white matter of the cerebellum and the

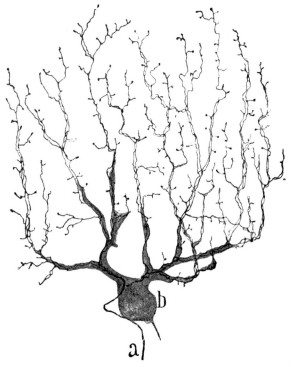

Fig. 21. Terminal arborization of climbing fiber (a) on the dendrites of Purkinje cell (b). (From CAJAL, 1911, Fig. 47)

medullary lamina of the folia, eventually to enter and traverse the granular layer in radial direction and so to reach the Purkinje cell layer. Each climbing fiber then attaches itself to a single Purkinje cell and climbs up on the dendritic tree in an ivy-like fashion (Fig. 21). The course through the granular layer is undivided and straight showing only some sinuosities as it bypasses granule cells or glomeruli. Although a climbing fiber begins to divide at the level of the Purkinje cell body, its arborization is closely attached to the dendritic ramifications of a single Purkinje cell and only very exceptionally can one observe with assurance climbing fibers establishing contact with more than one Purkinje cell. SCHEIBEL and SCHEIBEL (1954) have utilized their vast Golgi material from various laboratory mammals (rat, rabbit, cat, dog, monkey) as well as from chimpanzee and man in order to reinvestigate the synaptic connexions of the climbing fibers. They stress the importance of the side branches of climbing fibers that terminate in boutons. These side branches were already described and illustrated by CAJAL (1911, Fig. 47), but apparently he did not seem to realize that the climbing fiber may in this way establish synaptic contacts with other cells in addition to the dendrites of its own Purkinje cell. Although full credit has to be given to SCHEIBEL and SCHEIBEL (1954) for having pointed out that these side branches have important synaptic contacts with basket and outer stellate neurons, their conclusion that a climbing fiber may have contacts with a number of Purkinje cells has not been confirmed. It is, of course, possible that one or the other of the short side branches terminating in and end-knob might enter into contact with a dendrite of a neighboring Purkinje cell. But this would be a completely insignificant contact when compared with the repeated long synaptic contacts established by the climbing fiber with the dendrites of its P-cell. Its main branches attach themselves to the primary and secondary dendrites, but not to spiny branchlets of the dendritic tree.

Until very recently the origin of climbing fibers has remained obscure. CAJAL (1911) thought that they would originate from ponto- and vestibulo-cerebellar afferent systems, and other authors for various reasons expressed different views. These questions could be decided, of course, only by means of degeneration studies, but all afferent systems investigated in this way gave only degeneration of mossy fibers (MISKOLCZY, 1931, 1934; SNIDER, 1936; ROSIELLO, 1937).

The writer of this chapter had realized already at that time [SCHIMERT (SZENTÁGOTHAI), 1939] that the negative result of these studies with respect to climbing fibers might be the failure of the impregnation procedures to stain degeneration fragments of axons in the molecular layer[3]. He suspected already that the olivo-cerebellar system was the chief source of climbing fibers because after olivary lesions degenerated axons could be traced to the level of the origin of the main dendrites of P-cells; but he became discouraged by the observation that degenerated horizontal or chiefly descending side branches issued from the main fibers at or slightly below the P-cell body level. As this did not fit with the classical description of the undivided course of the climbing fiber, further pursuit of the question was abandoned.

A new turn was given to this story by CARREA, REISSIG and METTLER (1947) who claimed to have found degeneration of climbing fibers after lesions in the cerebellar nuclei. Thus the climbing fibers would have to be considered not as extraneous afferents, but as recurrent collaterals of cerebellar nuclear neurons. Serious doubts against this interpretation were expressed by ULE (1957) on the basis of well preserved climbing fibers in several human cases of near complete cellular degeneration of the cerebellar nuclei.

The study was later resumed by SZENTÁGOTHAI and RAJKOVITS (1959) under more favourable circumstances: firstly, they had at their disposal the more specific Nauta-Gygax staining procedures; and secondly, they were in the possession of the new data by SCHEIBEL and SCHEIBEL (1954) on the descending collaterals of climbing fibers. In spite of the difficulties involved in staining degeneration fragments of

---

[3] See detailed treatment of this problem by SZENTÁGOTHAI (1965 a).

climbing fibers in the molecular layer, it became now possible to identify the climbing fibers as originating from the inferior olive and the accessory olives (Fig. 22). This could have been guessed already from the observation of BRODAL (1940) on the unusual sharpness of topographical projection from the olive to the cerebellar cortex, which is difficult to reconcile with the diffuse termination of mossy fibers. Whether or not there are other afferent systems that terminate in climbing fibers is not known. SZENTÁGOTHAI and RAJKOVITS (1959) have seen degeneration patterns resembling those of climbing fibers in the contralateral flocculus after a lesion in the brachium conjunctivum. Another source that could yield climbing fibers is the dorsomedial nucleus of the pons (the Bechterew nucleus). Taking into consideration the difficulties of staining the degeneration fragments of climbing fibers in the molecular layer, where the nature of the fiber becomes first apparent, it seems extremely difficult to obtain convincing data of any system that has no precise topographic projection and that gives only a few scattered climbing fibers to any region.

The observations of degeneration climbing fibers have also led to the discovery that the descending collaterals described first by SCHEIBEL and SCHEIBEL (1954) do not terminate on granule neurons, as the authors presumed, but on the cell bodies and initial parts of dendrites of Golgi neurons (SZENTÁGOTHAI and RAJ-KOVITS, 1959). This could be later substantiated also in electron microscope studies combined with experimental degeneration (HÁMORI and SZENTÁGOTHAI, 1966a). The important conclusion reached by the SCHEIBELS that the synaptic relations of the climbing fiber are not limited to a single Purkinje cell have thus been confirmed to a certain degree. The study of experimental degeneration is ill suited for the investigation of neuron connexions in the molecular layer by means of light microscopy. However, this question will now be discussed in relation to electronmicroscopic investigations.

The climbing fiber can be identified under the EM with fair assurance on the bases both of its close attachment to the larger smooth dendrites of Purkinje cells (Figs. 23, 24), and its strongly filamentous structure with only relatively small groups of synaptic vesicles accumulated at the sites of synaptic contact with the Purkinje dendrites (HÁMORI and SZENTÁGOTHAI, 1966a). These synapses are mainly of "de passage" character. Whenever both the climbing fiber and the Purkinje dendrite are cut longitudinally, one can see that the fiber does not terminate at the site of the synaptic contact but continues its course. The identity of these axons with the climbing fibers has been established by HÁMORI and SZENTÁGOTHAI (1966a) by means of secondary degeneration. They disappear completely in chronically isolated folia, whereas surviving under these circumstances are numerous vesicular synaptic terminals that are of local origin and that have mainly terminals of "end-knob" type in contact with the large Purkinje cell dendrites (Fig. 57).

Using the same criteria for recognition of climbing fibers under the EM, i.e. the filamentous character and the disappearance in chronically isolated folia, it was possible to confirm the conclusion reached by SCHEIBEL and SCHEIBEL (1954) in Golgi studies that climbing fibers make synaptic contacts with basket cells (Fig. 35), and there was some support in the case of the postulated similar synapses on stellate neurons. There is, however, no electronmicroscopic evidence of axo-dendritic synapses between climbing fibers and basket dendrites, which seem to have largely

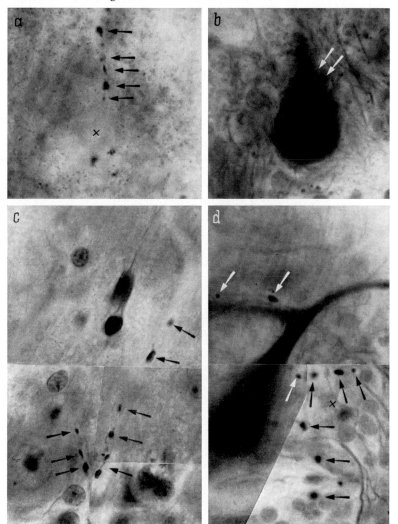

Fig. 22. Degeneration of climbing fibers 4 days after a focal lesion in the inferior olive, in Nauta-Gygax stain (*a* and *c*) and Gros-Bielschowsky stain (*b* and *d*). Degeneration fragments (arrows) can be traced only along the primary dendrites of Purkinje cells (arrows). (*X*) in photomicrograph (*a*) indicates tangentially cut cell body of Purkinje cell. In (*d*) horizontal collateral (descending coll. of SCHEIBEL and SCHEIBEL, 1954) can be seen above (*x*) to branch off directed towards Golgi cell bodies. (From SZENTÁGOTHAI and RAJKOVITS, 1959)

axo-spine synapses with parallel fibers. In the case of the outer stellate cells this is not clear, because their bodies have extremely few synaptic contacts and their dendrites have synapses both directly on their surface and on their long spines.

All EM evidence available, however, appears to be against the claims of SCHEIBEL and SCHEIBEL (1954) that climbing fibers have axo-axonic synapses with

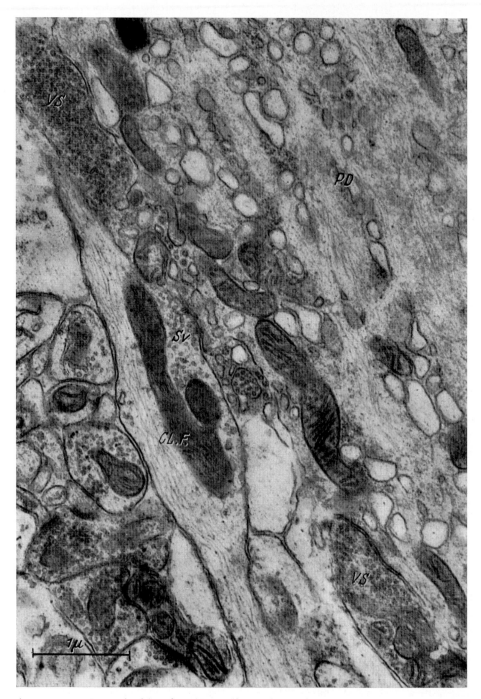

Fig. 23. Large primary dendrite of Purkinje cell (*PD*) having synaptic contact "de passage" with large terminal axon, containing coarse neurofilaments and identified as climbing fiber (*Cl.F*). Only few synaptic vesicles (*SV*) accumulate at the sites of contact. Other vesicular synaptic profiles (*VS*) have more the character of terminal synaptic endings. (From HÁMORI and SZENTÁGOTHAI, 1966a)

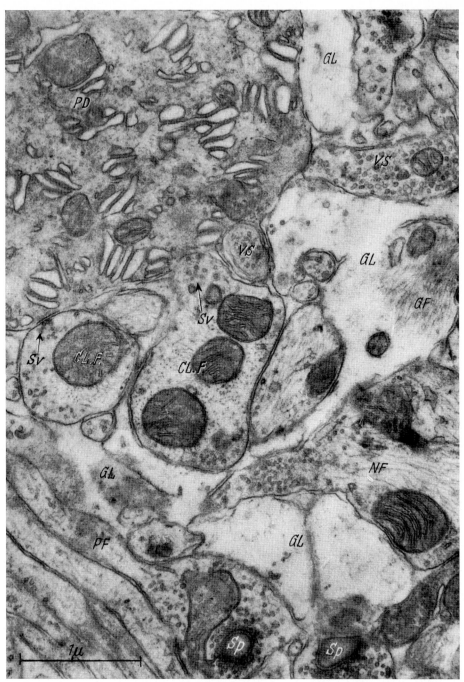

Fig. 24. Secondary Purkinje cell dendrite (*PD*) with several axonal and terminal profiles attached. Profiles packed with neurofilaments can be identified as climbing fibers (*CLF*), having small accumulations of synaptic vesicles (*SV*) mainly at sites of close attachment to the dendrite surface. Vesicular synaptic profiles (*VS*) are poor in neurofilaments. Most part of the dendritic surface is covered by glial processes (*GL*), some of them containing bundles of glial filaments (*GF*). Irregular axonal profile at right containing coarse neurofilaments (*NF*) is ambiguous: it could be either a climbing fiber or a basket axon, which is also rich in neurofilaments. At bottom two dendritic spines (*Sp*) can be seen embedded and synapsing with thickened parts of parallel fibers (*PF*). (From HÁMORI and SZENTÁGOTHAI, 1966a)

parallel fibers as well as basket and stellate cell axons. It is obvious that, due to the dense packing of elements, especially in the molecular layer, close appositions between various kinds of axons (parallel fibers, climbing fibers, stellate, basket and recurrent Purkinje axons) are frequent, but all these appositions are completely devoid of the usual synaptic differentiations, i.e. accumulations of synaptic vesicles at the assumed presynaptic sites and membrane thickenings on the opposite post-synaptic sites, widening of the synaptic cleft, etc. All of these structural details have been observed in the real axo-axonic synapses that have been described hitherto by various authors in many regions: spinal grey matter (GRAY, 1962); lateral geniculate body (SZENTÁGOTHAI, 1962a; COLONNIER and GUILLERY, 1964); thalamus (MAJOROSSY et al., 1965; PAPPAS et al., 1965). Unmyelinated preterminal axons rarely if ever appear to be protected from getting into close contact with one another. Conversely the dendrites are very often carefully wrapped by glial elements and appear to be protected against contacts by axonal elements with the exception of their specific synaptic sites. Since this structural principle is particularly conspicuous in the cerebellar cortex, this aspect of its structure will be considered in more detail in Chapter XI.

Chapter III

The Parallel Fibers

Before attempting to develop ideas on the mode of operation of neuronal circuits in the cerebellar cortex, it is necessary to attempt to understand both the structural-functional correlations of component elements and the mode of operation of the synapses between these elements. In this way we will derive simple levels of understanding which can be assembled together, rather as in a jig-saw puzzle, to form more integrated levels of understanding. It is convenient to begin this structure-functional correlation in this Chapter with the parallel fibers, then with the inter-neurones of the cerebellar cortex (Chapter IV) and the Purkinje cells (Chapter V).

A. Structure of the Parallel Fibers and their Synapses

The axons of the granule neurons ascend to the molecular layer, where they form a T-junction in giving rise to the two branches of the parallel fibers. As already described, there is a very definite geometric relation between the position of the granule cell body in the granular layer and that of its parallel fiber in the molecular: deeper granule neurons give rise to deep parallel fibers and superficial

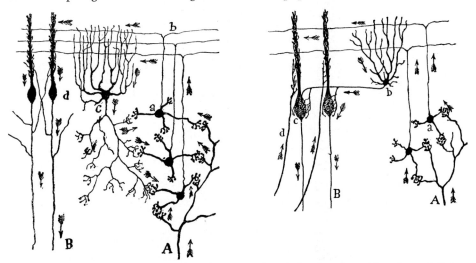

Fig. 25. Two diagrams of CAJAL (1911, Figs. 103 and 104) showing that, although not fully appreciating the significance in this contact of the dendritic spines, he correctly understood the principle of the "crossing over" synaptic system between the unmyelinated parallel fibers and the various kinds of dendrites in the molecular layer. Diagram at left shows arrangement with Golgi cell (c) and at right with basket cell (b). Legends in left diagram: A=mossy fiber, a=granule neuron, b=parallel fiber, c=Golgi cell, d=Purkinje cells, B=Purkinje axons. Right diagram: A=mossy fiber, a=granule neuron, b=basket cell, B=Purkinje axon, c=Purkinje cells, d=climbing fibers. Arrows indicate direction of impulse flow

43

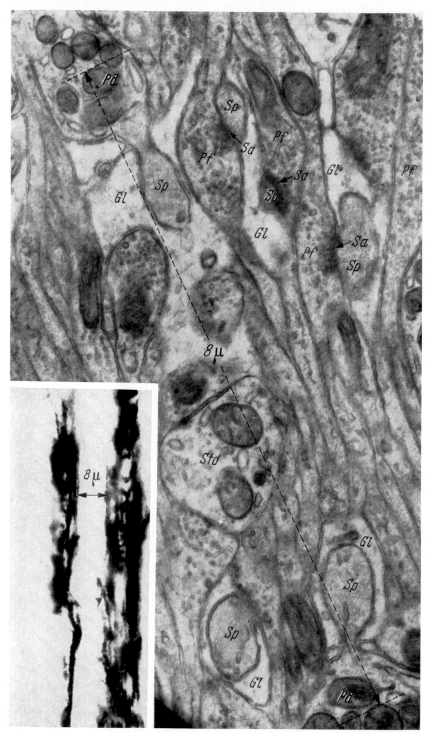

Fig. 26. Tangential plane of sectioning reveals the principal mode of synaptic articulation (*Sa*) between fusiform thickenings of parallel fibers (*Pf*) and dendritic spines (*Sp*). The two transversally cut dendrites (*Pd*) at upper left and lower right belong obviously to the dendritic sheets

neurons to superficial fibers. In addition, the caliber of the deep parallel fibers is much larger than that of the superficial ones — 1.0 micron versus 0.2 micron according to Fox and Barnard (1957) and Fox, Siegesmund and Dutta (1964). One might expect that the deeper granule cells giving rise to the larger deep parallel fibers ought to be larger. The differences between the sizes of granule cell bodies in different depths are not conspicuous, but exact measurements of nuclear size might reveal differences. Although we do not have direct quantitative information, one has the impression that deeper granule cells have more and longer dendrites than the superficial ones. Since, other things being equal, longer axons are more likely to be thicker than shorter ones, one might expect that the deeper parallel fibers are longer than those running more close to the surface.

Cajal (1911) has correctly interpreted the peculiar synaptic relation of the parallel fibers mainly with the Purkinje cell dendrites, but also with all other dendrites in the molecular layer; two of his diagrams (Figs. 103 and 104) being reproduced in Fig. 25. Strangely, Cajal could not make up his mind with respect to the significance in this synapse of the dendritic spines. The decisive role of the spines as postsynaptic structures was first correctly interpreted in the cerebellum by Fox and Barnard (1957) on the basis of Golgi studies and of ingenious indirect reasoning in which the quantitative relations were taken into consideration.

The concept that the spines must be the main postsynaptic structures of the dendrites was substantiated by the EM studies of Gray, first in the cerebral cortex (1959), and later (1961) in the cerebellar cortex, and he gave a detailed description of the axon-spine synapses. Further EM studies made independently by Fox, Siegesmund and Dutta (1964) and by Hámori and Szentágothai (1964) helped to clarify the remarkable structural arrangement between dendritic spines and parallel fibers. There are but minor discrepancies between the two descriptions: Fox stresses the significance of the so called "warty rosettes" or hook-like side branches of parallel fibers as the main presynaptic sites; whereas Hámori and Szentá-gothai, using sections carefully oriented in planes parallel to the parallel fibers, laid emphasis on the fusiform thickenings of the parallel fibers at the synaptic sites (Fig. 26). The presynaptic sites are thus considered not to be endings but sites of "de passage" character and the synapse has been designated a "crossing over" synapse. In contrast to the description given and the nomenclature used originally by Gray (1959, 1961), Hámori and Szentágothai (1964) consider that most axon-spine synapses are synapses of contact by overcrossing without the necessity of having separate presynaptic endings, although of course such may occur as short side-hooks or warty rosettes at the light microscope level. Since the dendrites of all cells engaged in the molecular layer have spines (Fig. 27), and since axon-spine

of two neighbouring Purkinje cells with a distance (indicated by dotted line) of 8 microns. This corresponds to the distance between two dendritic sheets seen in the Golgi picture (inset left below) of Purkinje cells in a longitudinal section of the folium. (Actually the distance here between Purkinje dendrites is exceptionally large — see discussion of quantitative aspects in Chapter XI.) Another dendrite, most probably of a stellate neuron (*Std*), can be seen in the center, occupying the space between Purkinje dendrites and having direct synapses as in Fig. 12 B. Glial processes (*Gl*) surround particularly dendrites and their spines

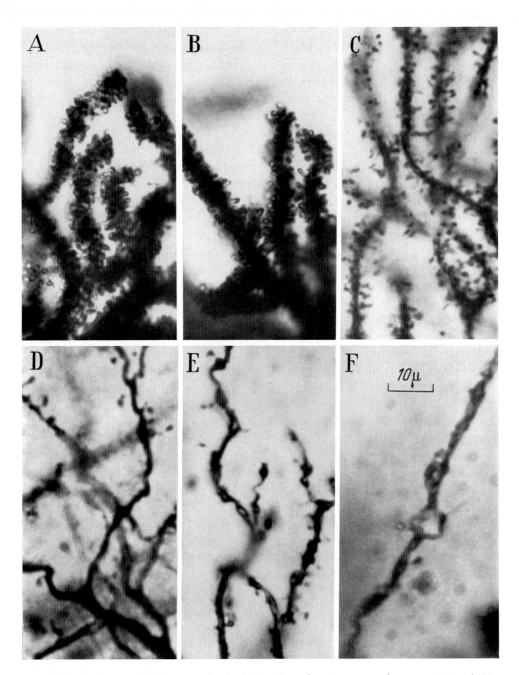

Fig. 27 A—F. A comparison between the dendritic spines of various types of neurons: (A) and (B) from Purkinje cells of the cat. Perfusion Kopsch procedure; and (C) Purkinje cell in human adult. Strong staining of the drum-stick heads of the spines made counting easy and reliable in this material. Rapid Golgi procedure. (D) Stellate neuron of the cat, rapid Golgi. (E) Basket neurons and (F) Golgi neuron in the cat, both from perfusion Kopsch preparations. Spines are quite numerous, although irregularly arranged, thin and often hooked in the stellate and basket neurons, they are very sparse, short and stiff in the Golgi neuron

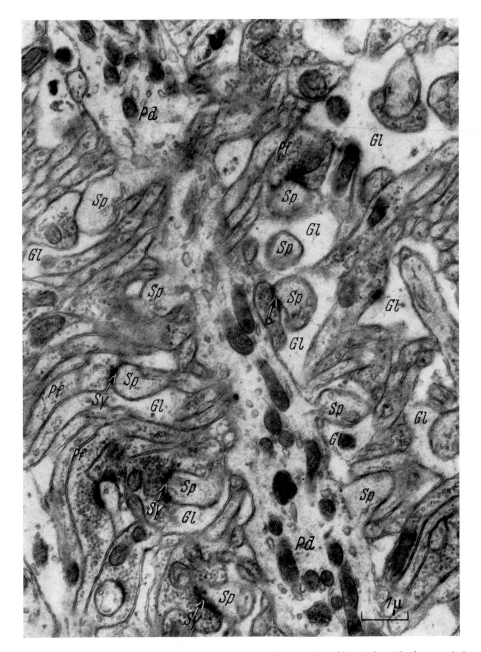

Fig. 28. EM picture of longitudinally cut Purkinje cell spiny branchlet (*Pd*) with characteristic plasma structure seen to emerge in the tertiary branchlet in Fig. 6 B. Regularly spaced, short and rather stout spines (*Sp*), with well marked drum-stick heads are engaged in synaptic contacts (*Sy*) with thickened parts of parallel fibers (*Pf*). The dendrite and particularly the spines, with the exception of the synaptic contacts are well isolated from their environment by glial (*Gl*) processes. Direct axo-dendritic synaptic contacts are rare in Purkinje cell spiny branchlets. Even if the parallel fiber has an intimate contact with the dendrite, its true synaptic contact is with reclining spine at the site marked by the ringed arrow. (From Hámori and Szentágothai, 1964)

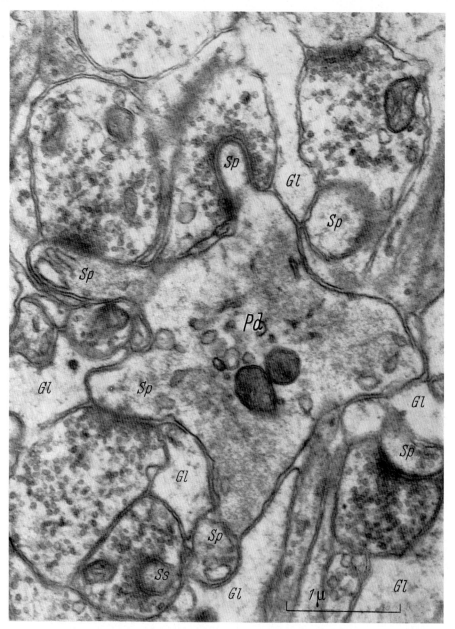

Fig. 29. Transverse section of Purkinje cell spiny branchlet (*Pd*) having as many as 6 spines (*Sp*) in the same plane. One of these spines (upwards) is invaginated into a parallel fiber profile, others being only attached. The spine after having established at its base a synapse with one parallel fiber (lower spine to the left) may go on and have another synapse (not seen in this plane) at its head region. Spine directed downwards has a secondary spine head (*Ss*) protruding into invagination of a parallel fiber. The drumstick head of this spine probably has its main synapse with a parallel fiber in the plane above or below. Spineheads generally contain a few wide endoplasmic vesicles that are connected with the endoplasmic vesicle system of the dendrite with delicate channels. (From HÁMORI and SZENTÁGOTHAI, 1964)

synapses appear under the EM to be effected with parallel fibers, the conclusion is close at hand that these fibers establish synaptic relations with Purkinje, basket, outer stellate as well as typical Golgi cells. The parallel fibers on the other hand appear strictly to avoid (Fig. 28) synaptic contacts at dendritic or cell body surfaces that are not spines.

HÁMORI and SZENTÁGOTHAI emphasized that the net result of this system of crossing-over synapses is the very large divergence and the enormous convergence which was stressed already by FOX and BARNARD (1957). This immense connectivity is achieved by a minimum of arborization or of other structural complications on the presynaptic side. In most cases this is not easy to demonstrate because of the irregularity of structure, but it is relatively easy in longitudinal sections with respect to the folium axis of the cerebellar cortex.

HÁMORI and SZENTÁGOTHAI (1964) have tried also to identify under the EM the spiny branchlets of various cells using criteria gathered from light microscopy of Golgi pictures (Fig. 27), such as the density and regularity of arrangement and the length of the spines, as well as by trying to trace them from identified cell bodies and more recently (unpublished) using the different character of mitochondria. On the basis of these criteria the Purkinje cell spiny branchlets (Figs. 28, 29) can be identified as relatively pale dendrites having small elongated mitochondria and the vacuolar system already described (Fig. 6). The spines are short and stout and very regularly arranged (Figs. 28, 29), as is well shown in Golgi pictures (Fig. 27 A—C).

The spines of the basket dendrites are long, and may be curved or hooked (Fig. 27 E), and they are regularly invaginated into the parallel fibers (Fig. 30). The discrepancy between the figures of FOX et al. (1964) and of HÁMORI and SZENTÁGOTHAI (1964) may be due to differences in preparative techniques and in the animals used. In man (Figs. 9 B and 31) the differences between the Purkinje and basket cell spiny branchlets are less conspicuous, although in the same direction as in the cat, so that in man and monkey the spectacular differences described by HÁMORI and SZENTÁGOTHAI (1964) for the cat may be not so distinct, and overlapping types may occur. Nevertheless, if the criterion of the specificity of mitochondria is applied, erroneous identifications may be avoided. The stellate dendrites have also long hooked spines (Fig. 27 D), and we think that they can be differentiated from the equally light Purkinje spiny branchlets on the basis of their large mitochondria (Fig. 12 B), and the frequent occurrence of direct (non-spine) axodendritic synapses. The identification is still more difficult in the case of Golgi cell dendrites. By using the rare and stiff, rather short spines, as well as the rarity of such dendrites as criteria, a fair probability of identification can be achieved in the human cerebellar cortex (Fig. 18 B). Whether or not our attempt at identification is correct, this does not alter the fundamental concept of alternating dendritic sheets that first was shown and interpreted by HÁMORI and SZENTÁGOTHAI (1964); and that is reproduced in Fig. 32 with slight modifications (cf. Chapter XI).

The quantitative relations were first appreciated and exploited in an ingenious manner by FOX and BARNARD (1957). Later FOX, SIEGESMUND and DUTTA (1964) suggested that the numbers of spines, as determined earlier per 10 µ length of the

Golgi pictures of spiny branchlets, are too low in relation to calculations from EM pictures. Combining the numbers of spines seen in longitudinal and in transverse

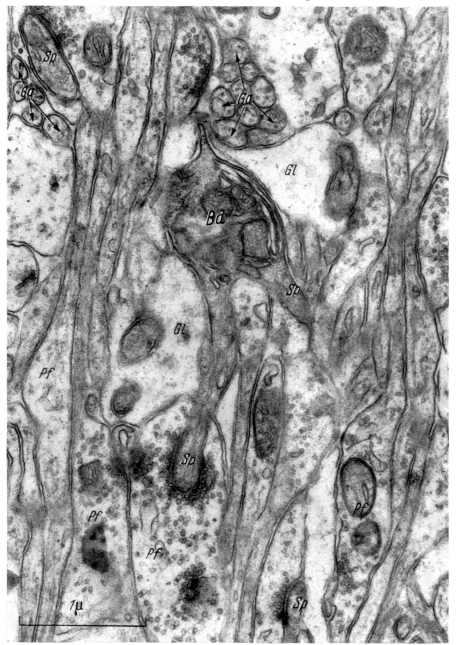

Fig. 30. Basket cell dendrite (*Bd*) cut transversally, with characteristic dark plasma structure. Compare this with longitudinally cut basket dendrite in Fig. 9. Note long slender spines (*Sp*) establishing synaptic and partly invaginated contacts with fusiform thickenings of parallel fibers (*Pf*). Dendrite and basal parts of spines are surrounded by glial (*Gl*) processes. As this section is from the depth of the molecular layer and parallel with surface, groups of ascending granule axons (*Ga*) can be seen cut transversally. (From HÁMORI and SZENTÁGOTHAI, 1964.)

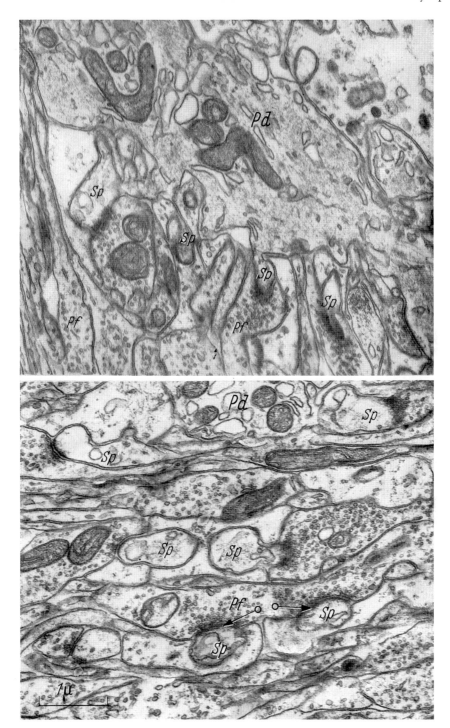

Fig. 31. Purkinje cell spiny branchlets of adult human cerebellar cortex, showing essentially the same features, plasma structure and spines as are seen in the cat (Figs. 28, 29). Above: longitudinally cut dendrite (*Pd*) with regularly spaced spines (*Sp*) at lower side that are somewhat thinner than in the cat (Fig. 27 A, B and C). Below: Oblique cut through Purkinje spiny branchlet (*Pd*) showing that spines (*Sp*), obviously from the same branchlet, may contact (ringed arrows) the same parallel fiber (*Pf*). (BENKE and HÁMORI, 1964)

sections of Purkinje spiny branchlets in the cat, we arrive at numbers at least double those given originally by Fox and Barnard (1957) using the light microscope. When looking among many Golgi series made with various modifications

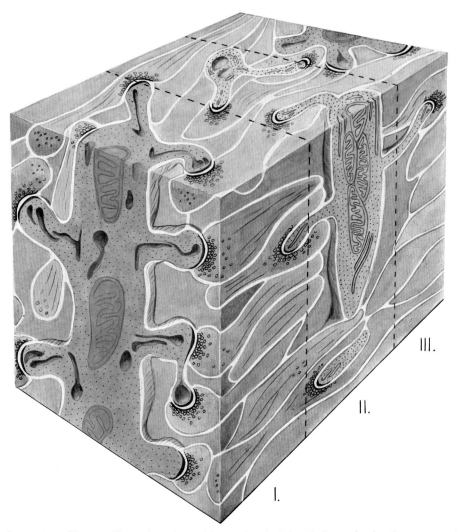

Fig. 32. Stereodiagram illustrating the architectural principle of the molecular layer synaptic system. Parallel fibers (red) are crossing alternating sheets of dendrite arborizations of (I) Purkinje cells (grey), (II) of basket [or stellate, or more irregularly of Golgi] neurons (blue), III again Purkinje cells, etc. While crossing, their fusiform thickenings engage in synaptic contacts with dendritic spines. Direct synapses (yellow) can be made with Purkinje dendrites — albeit more often with larger ones — by stellate and ascending basket axons. Synaptic sites of the dendrite and particularly spine surfaces are sealed from environment by glial processes (green). (HÁMORI and SZENTÁGOTHAI, 1964)

for pictures showing the largest numbers of spines, we found both in man (Fig. 27 C) and in the cat (Fig. 27 A, B) specimens with even higher numbers. In man the thinned "shafts" and stronger "heads" of the spines make counting easier, and the count is 44 spines per 10 μ of the spiny branchlets. In the cat Purkinje cell only one side could be counted and that gave numbers up to 30, so that the whole number must be similar or even perhaps higher than in man. In addition many spines of Purkinje cell dendrites give rise to smaller secondary spines, which establish synaptic contacts with parallel fibers other than those with which the main spine articulates (HÁMORI and SZENTÁGOTHAI, 1964).

The number of parallel axons crossing the dendritic area of the average P-cell has been calculated by Fox and BARNARD (1957) to be between 278,000 and 208,000 in the monkey. This fits nicely with our own calculations, based on EM pictures of about 209,000 parallel axons crossing the dendritic tree of a Purkinje cell in the cat. In man and also in the monkey the number may be somewhat larger due to the larger extension of the Purkinje dendritic arborization, so that 250,000 would be a fair estimate. As the number of spines per 10 μ of spiny branchlet length is close to 45, the original number of spines per Purkinje neuron is about 180,000 if the total length of spiny branchlets in man is assumed to be 40 mm, which is the value for the monkey (FOX and BARNARD, 1957). In the cat the spiny branchlet length may be somewhat smaller on account of the smaller size of the dendritic arborization. It is impossible to judge the quantitative significance of the secondary spines. Our original estimate was that because of secondary spines and of spines making dual contacts with parallel fibers, the number of parallel fibers contacted by any Purkinje cell might be double the number of its spines, but this estimate is too high. At any rate one arrives at the conclusion that probably few parallel fibers can cross the dendritic sheet of a Purkinje cell without having one contact with a spine. This shows how effective an arrangement the Purkinje cell dendritic arborization is, for it may be regarded as a sieve through which each parallel fiber gives, as it penetrates, just about one synaptic contact. The mechanism of coupling is thus not only effective, but on the other hand one of the strictest economy in the use of nervous living matter. The numerical relations between spines and parallel fibers contacted are modified somewhat by the observation that two spines of the same branchlet may contact the same parallel fiber (Fig. 31 B), probably this rarely happens. If 3 mm is the average length of a parallel fiber, and if 450 Purkinje cells are distributed along this distance (FOX and BARNARD, 1957), each parallel fiber will make contact with at least 300 Purkinje cells, i.e. the divergence factor is probably in excess of 300.

In consequence of their more sparse dendritic arborizations in the molecular layer, all other kinds of neurons probably have contacts with a considerably lower proportion of the parallel axons crossing their arborization areas. In the human cerebellum, however, the basket cell dendrites have quite considerable numbers of rather long spines, which probably ensures the establishment of synaptic relations with parallel axons crossing at larger distances than are possible with the spiny branchlets of Purkinje cells (Fig. 9 B). This may compensate for the lower density of dendritic branches, if not with respect to proportions of parallel axons contacted, at least by ensuring that the parallel fibers contacted are more uniformly distributed than would be the case if the dendritic spines were as short as those of Purkinje cells. In the Golgi cell, as already mentioned, the synapses from parallel fibers onto the sparse dendritic tree with its scanty spines are increased in number because of the spread of the dendrites also in the longitudinal direction of the folium.

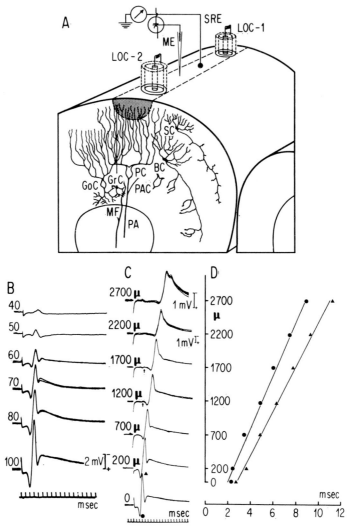

Fig. 33 A—D. *Parallel fibre impulses.* A. Diagram of section of a folium of the cerebellar cortex showing the location of the concentric stimulating electrodes on the surface (the local or LOC electrodes). Also shown is the surface recording electrode (*SRE*) and the microelectrode (*ME*) in position for penetration. Purkinje cell (*PC*) shown with axon (*PA*) and axon collateral (*PAC*). Also shown are outer stellate (*SC*), basket (*BC*) and Golgi (*GoC*) and granule (*GrC*) cells. The broken line shows the boundaries of a beam of parallel fibres excited by a weak LOC stimulus. B. Extracellular potentials evoked by graded LOC stimulations at the indicated strengths in arbitrary units and recorded by a microelectrode that had just penetrated into the molecular layer. C. LOC stimulation at strength 100 and recording of parallel fibre volley at just below surface at the indicated distances from the recording position closest to the LOC electrode. All records at same amplification except that at 2700 μ. D. Plotting of conduction distances against the latencies measured for the peaks of initial positivity and negativity as indicated in the lowest record of C. (ECCLES, LLINÁS and SASAKI, 1966 b)

B. The Responses evoked by Parallel Fiber Stimulation

1. Impulse Propagation in Parallel Fibers

When the parallel fibers are stimulated by a current applied through the concentric LOC electrode on the surface of a folium, as in Fig. 33 A, the very restricted distribution of the applied current would be expected to result in the excitation of a narrow band or beam of parallel fibers (ANDERSEN, ECCLES and VOORHOEVE, 1964; ECCLES, LLINÁS and SASAKI, 1966 b), because these parallel fibers run in the molecular layer with an orientation strictly longitudinal to the folium (Figs. 25, 32, 76). An appropriately located microelectrode should therefore record the conducted action potential in the parallel fibers, as is illustrated in Fig. 33 B. A stimulus about three times threshold strength (100 in lowest trace) evokes a brief triphasic potential followed by a slow negative wave, and with progressive reduction of the stimulus strength (80 to 40 in B) the triphasic potential is correspondingly diminished, but not otherwise altered. The triphasic configuration is, of course, characteristic for a fairly well synchronized volley of impulses propagating in a bundle of nerve fibers immersed in a volume conductor, as is the case for the parallel fibers. The sizes of the triphasic potentials evoked by the graded stimuli in Fig. 33 B signify approximately the numbers of parallel fibers excited by the stimulus.

For the series of Fig. 33 C, a stimulating current of three times threshold is applied through a LOC electrode in a fixed position on the folium. As shown in Fig. 33 A, the action potentials with a negative spike-like configuration can be recorded only in a narrow band running longitudinally along the folium. The potentials along this band (Fig. 33 C) are arranged from above downwards in their order of recording, the distances being expressed relative to the position of closest apposition of the recording electrode to the concentric stimulating electrode. A conduction distance of rather more than 500 μ should be added to the distances indicated in Fig. 33 C in order to obtain the actual conduction distances from the site of stimulation. From the progressively increasing conduction times, a conduction velocity can be calculated, as shown in the approximately linear relationship for the plotted points of Fig. 33 D. Measurements from the bottom of the initial positive wave (filled circles) give a velocity of about 0.39 m/sec for the fastest impulses of the volley, while a velocity of about 0.33 m/sec is given for the crests of the negative potentials (filled triangles). The mean value so obtained in 5 experiments (0.3 m/sec) is in good agreement with the value of 0.3 to 0.5 m/sec obtained by Dow (1949) using a similar technique, and is in accord with the diameters of the largest of the superficial parallel fibers, which is 0.2 to 0.3 μ (FOX, SIEGESMUND and DUTTA, 1964; HÁMORI and SZENTÁGOTHAI, 1964).

Besides the progressively longer latent period, the action potentials of Fig. 33 C show several other features that are in accord with their postulated derivation from conducted impulses. There is firstly the progressive decrease in height and increase in duration, which would be expected for a volley of impulses becoming more dispersed in time during conduction. Since, as stated above, the total length of the parallel fibers may be no more than 3 mm, the diminution of spike size will also arise on account of the termination of many of the excited fibers at various distances from the stimulating electrode. This termination of impulses after various distances of conduction is also indicated in Fig. 33 C by the progressive decline, and the eventual extinction beyond 700 μ, of the third phase of the triphasic spike potential. This terminal positive phase is, of course, dependent on the propagation of the impulses well beyond the recording electrode (LORENTE DE NÓ, 1947).

2. Experiments on the Refractoriness following a Parallel Fiber Volley

In Fig. 34, as shown schematically in the diagram, when two stimuli of identical strength are applied through the same LOC electrode, the second stimulus evokes a full-sized spike potential with stimulus intervals down to the 3.4 msec. Moreover

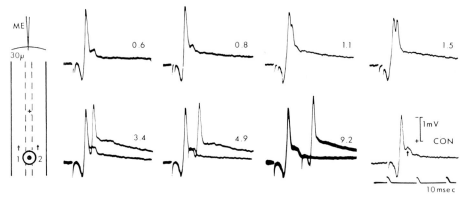

Fig. 34. *Extracellular potentials evoked by double stimulation through the same LOC electrode.* Diagram shows folium with LOC electrode in plan and with the excited beam of parallel fibres outlined. Microelectrode (ME, 30 μ depth) penetration was at the cross. CON shows control response to second LOC stimulation alone, and with arrow indicating a possible Purkinje spike potential. Stimulus intervals indicated on each record in msec, and at 3.4, 4.9 and 9.2 msec the double response was superimposed on the response to the first LOC stimulus alone. (ECCLES, LLINÁS and SASAKI, 1966 b).

the second volley adds a large slow negative wave to the potential generated by the first volley. With shortening of the stimulus interval to 1.5 msec or less, the spike potential is greatly reduced in size until at 0.6 msec the second stimulus is quite ineffective. It is thus possible to demonstrate that the spike potentials of Figs. 33 and 34 have an associated refractory state, exactly as would be expected for spike potentials produced by impulses propagating in the parallel fibers.

An alternative method of demonstrating the refractoriness associated with the propagated spike potentials in the molecular layer is shown in the schematic diagram of Fig. 35. Stimulation is applied through two LOC electrodes that are carefully adjusted in the longitudinal axis of the folium so that they excite the same band of parallel fibers (cf. LOC-1 and LOC-2 in Fig. 33 A). The recording microelectrode is inserted at a depth of 30 μ into this excited band at approximately the midpoint (cross in diagram of Fig. 35) between the two LOC electrodes. At the longest stimulating interval (11.2 msec) the second stimulus evokes a full-sized spike and a large later negative wave, just as in Fig. 34 at intervals of 3.4 to 9.2 msec. As the stimulus interval is shortened from 11.2 to 5.7 msec, there is progressive decrease in the spike. The added negative wave is negligible at 7.3 msec; and there is actually a reverse (positive) slow potential at 5.7 msec. At the still shorter stimulus intervals, there is no appreciable change in the spike; and, so far as can be judged in the absence of superimposed traces, the after-potential added by the second stimulus is but little changed.

A satisfactory explanation is readily provided in terms of the refractoriness following an impulse and of the annihilation of impulses by collision. Stimulation through electrode, LOC-2, can be fully effective in evoking a parallel fiber volley (as at 11.2 msec in Fig. 35) only at the end of the refractoriness which follows the impulses that travel from LOC-1 to LOC-2. This depression is incomplete because,

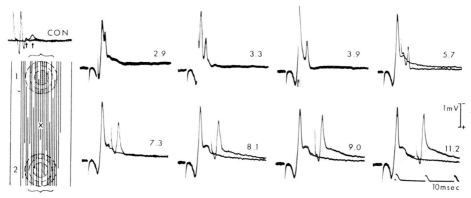

Fig. 35. *Interaction by collision of two parallel fibre volleys.* As shown in diagrammatic plan two LOC electrodes (1 and 2) were placed on a folium in accurate longitudinal alignment. The longitudinal lines show diagrammatically the parallel fibers that could be excited by one or both electrodes and recorded from by the microelectrode inserted at the cross. CON shows the control response to the second LOC stimulus alone superimposed on a base line and with arrows indicating possible Purkinje spike potentials. In all other traces the first LOC stimulus preceded the second at the indicated intervals in msec. There was superposition on the control response to the first LOC stimulus for intervals from 5.7 to 11.2 msec. (ECCLES, LLINÁS and SASAKI, 1966 b).

as indicated in the diagram, many of the parallel fibers excited by LOC-2 do not extend beyond the recording electrode to LOC-1. Such parallel fibers cannot be excited by the initial stimulation at LOC-1, and so are available for excitation by LOC-2 at all test intervals.

Chapter IV

The Neuronal Pathways forming Synapses on Outer Stellate, Basket and Golgi Cells

It is convenient to consider these cells before the Purkinje cells, because the first two types exert a powerful inhibitory influence on Purkinje cells (ANDERSEN, ECCLES and VOORHOEVE, 1964; ECCLES, LLINÁS and SASAKI, 1966 b, 1966 e; ECCLES, SASAKI and STRATA, 1966, 1967 b). The general structural features of these three types of interneurones have been described in Chapter I. Since these interneurones are all excited by the same presynaptic channels, the parallel fibers and to a very much less extent the climbing fibers, they will be considered together. Firstly, there will be an account of the presynaptic pathways, then of the responses generated thereby.

A. Outer Stellate Cell Connexions

The outer stellates are a relatively dense population of cells occupying the outer two thirds (or half) of the thin spaces left free in the longitudinal direction of the folium between two neighboring Purkinje cell dendritic arborizations. Their dendrites have both spine and direct surface synapses with parallel fibers (Fig. 12 B). Although most of these synapses can be recognized as being made by parallel fibers, it is nevertheless possible that some of the presynaptic contacts are either from outer stellate axons, or from ascending basket axon collaterals. However, this is improbable because the terminal branches of most outer stellate axons as well as of ascending basket axon collaterals have a vertical course, so that they should be easily distinguisable from parallel fibers. A few axo-somatic terminals are found on the characteristic smooth spherical cell body of the outer stellate cell. They are certainly not from parallel axons, because frequently the parallel axons can be seen curving around in immediate contact with the cell body surface, without the slightest indication of specific synaptic regions. These axo-somatic synapses are established by terminal branches of irregular direction, which probably are either collaterals from climbing fibers (SCHEIBEL and SCHEIBEL, 1954; HÁMORI and SZENTÁGOTHAI, 1966 a) or branches of the supraganglionic plexus of the Purkinje axon collaterals. Alternatively, some of them could originate from outer stellate or basket axons, but this is less probable because they seem to be absent in chronically isolated folia.

B. Basket Cell Connexions

The basket neurons are a population of cells with a similar dendritic arborization pattern as the outer stellate neurons, albeit with a larger spread and a similar density. From EM pictures in which the basket dendrites can be recognized without difficulty on the basis of their unusually dense structure, it becomes evident that

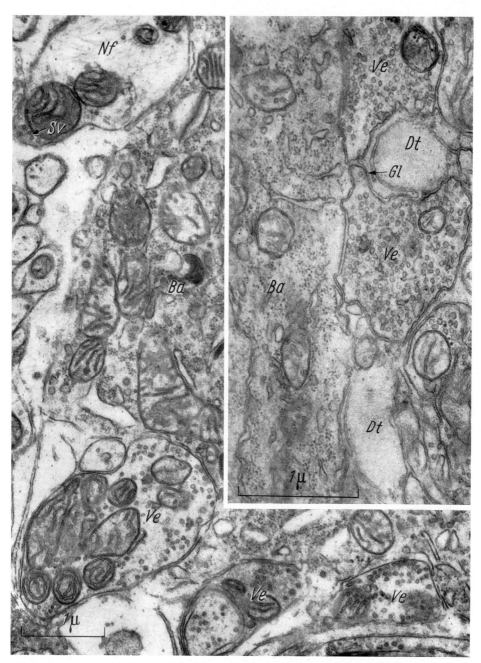

Fig. 36. Two kinds of axons establish synaptic contacts with basket cell bodies (left): one is of neuro-filamentous (*Nf*), the other of vesicular (*Ve*) character. In the chronically isolated folium (right) only vesicular terminals persist (*Ve*), while the original sites of the degenerated filamentous terminals are still visible (*Dt*). Some of their original space has been taken over by glial (*Gl*) profiles. This shows that the filamentous terminals are climbing fiber collaterals, whereas the vesicular ones are from other sources, which presumably are mainly from recurrent Purkinje axon collaterals (see Chapter IX, Fig. 102). (From Hámori and Szentágothai, 1966 a)

they form mainly spine synapses with parallel fibers (Fig. 30). The basket den-drites are particularly conspicuous in the human cerebellar cortex, but their struc-ture is essentially similar to the cat. Since practically no axo-dendritic synapses can be seen on the surface proper of these dendrites, it may be inferred that the basket dendrites are excited almost exclusively by parallel fibers.

One of the two different kinds of axo-somatic endings on basket cells originates from the climbing fibers (SCHEIBEL and SCHEIBEL, 1954). These climbing fiber synapses have been identified under the EM with the filamentous type of ending (HÁMORI and SZENTÁGOTHAI, 1966a; Fig. 36). The other type of rather vesicu-lar character could correspond to three different local connexions: (i) outer stellate axon endings; (ii) ascending basket axon endings; (iii) recurrent Purkinje axon collaterals. They are certainly of local origin because they persist in the chronically isolated folium (Fig. 36B; HÁMORI and SZENTÁGOTHAI, 1966a). On the basis of indirect reasoning, these authors have discarded postulates (i) and (ii) as improbable from the functional point of view, especially with respect to the inhibitory charac-ter of both types of neurons receiving virtually the same input. Quite recently direct evidence in favour of postulate (iii) has turned up (Fig. 103) and it will be discussed in Chapter IX.

C. Golgi Cell Connexions

The Golgi cells are a thin population of neurons, which by their widespread processes fill in the space available — both in the molecular and in the granular layer — without significant overlap, but also without major gaps between the dendritic, and, with somewhat less regularity, also the axonal ramifications. This can be gathered from Golgi pictures[1] (Fig. 15 A), and also from calculations based on the ratio of Golgi cells to Purkinje cells and the average spread of the dendritic trees and the axonal ramifications of Golgi cells (Chapter I). The number of typi-cally located Golgi cells is somewhat above 10% of Purkinje cells; hence in order to fill the molecular space completely, the upper dendritic tree of the Golgi cells ought to occupy a cylinder or more exactly a hexagonal prism with a diameter somewhat larger, both in the longitudinal and the transverse direction of the folium, than the distance occupied by three Purkinje cell bodies. This fits quite well with Golgi pictures.

By this spatial arrangement the parallel fibers in all parts of the molecular layer synaptically excite the relatively sparsely distributed Golgi dendrites. Because of this sparse distribution, it is still not possible to identify with certainty the Golgi dendrites in the molecular layer by the EM technique. Consequently there is no direct information with respect to their synaptic contacts. From the facts that the Golgi dendrites have sparsely distributed irregular stiff spines and that axon-spine synapses in the molecular layer are established almost exclusively with parallel fibers, one may infer that they have contacts mainly with parallel fibers. In the human cerebellum rather characteristic dendrites have been found recently by HÁMORI (unpublished observation), which on the basis of their stiff straight course

[1] See characteristic drawing by CAJAL (1911; Fig. 29) or by JAKOB (1928; reproduced in JANSEN and BRODAL, 1958, as Fig. 123).

could very well be Golgi dendrites. They certainly do not look like Purkinje or basket dendrites, neither could they be dendrites of outer stellate cells (Fig. 18). Their few short blunt spines are in synaptic contact with parallel fibers. It is conceivable that outer stellate axons and ascending branches of basket axons or even recurrent Purkinje axons also have synapses with dendrites of Golgi cells.

By means of its descending dendrites the Golgi cell has also direct synaptic contacts with the mossy fibers (HÁMORI and SZENTÁGOTHAI, 1966 b). Some at least of these contacts have a considerable area (Fig. 72) so that this synaptic articulation may be quite powerful. On the other hand the descending dendrites arborize rather sparsely in the granular layer and with less spread than the ascending dendrites. This means that they can be excited only from a much more limited field of active mossy fibers than are the upper dendrites that traverse a broad beam of parallel fibers which originate from granule cells influenced by the mossy terminals in a field of about 3 mm length.

The Golgi cell is additionally impinged upon by two different kinds of presynaptic fibers having synapses on the cell body. As shown by SZENTÁGOTHAI and RAJKOVITS (1959), one type of these axo-somatic synapses is formed by the recurrent collaterals of the climbing fibers described by SCHEIBEL and SCHEIBEL (1954). The axo-somatic endings of these collaterals on the Golgi cell have been identified under the EM as the filamentous terminals (Figs. 18 A, 103; HÁMORI and SZENTÁGOTHAI, 1966 a).

The other kind of axo-somatic endings, the vesicular ones, are of local origin, since they persist in the chronically isolated folium (HÁMORI and SZENTÁGOTHAI, 1966 a). According to Golgi analysis there is no local axonal element in the granular layer other than recurrent Purkinje axon collaterals and Golgi cell axons: hence the conclusion is that the vesicular terminals (Figs. 18, 103) most probably are formed by the Purkinje axon collaterals. This is all the more probable because the PURKINJE recurrent collaterals are known since CAJAL's description (1911) to participate in two tangential plexuses, one immediately beneath the Purkinje cell body layer and one above (Fig. 101). The so-called infra-ganglionic plexus is situated exactly at the level where the bodies of the typical Golgi cells are located. This would not, of course, preclude the possibility that Golgi axons themselves establish contacts with other Golgi cell bodies. But this would be inconsistent with the fact that the few Golgi cell bodies that have been encountered under the EM deep in the granular layer are devoid of axo-somatic contacts (HÁMORI, unpublished). This finding is readily explicable if these synapses were entirely from climbing fiber collaterals and/or Purkinje collaterals, because these fibers do not terminate in deeper strata of the granular layer. If even a small fraction of the synapses were from Golgi axon endings, they should not be lacking in the deeper Golgi cells, which are of course embedded in an abundance of Golgi axon arborizations.

D. The Responses of Outer Stellate, Basket and Golgi Cells to Parallel Fiber Volleys and other Afferent Inputs

Since, as shown above, the parallel fibers make "crossing-over" synapses with the dendritic spines of three types of cells in addition to the Purkinje cells, it would be expected that these synapses on the dendritic spines of the basket, outer stellate and Golgi cells would be similar in action to the excitatory synapses made by

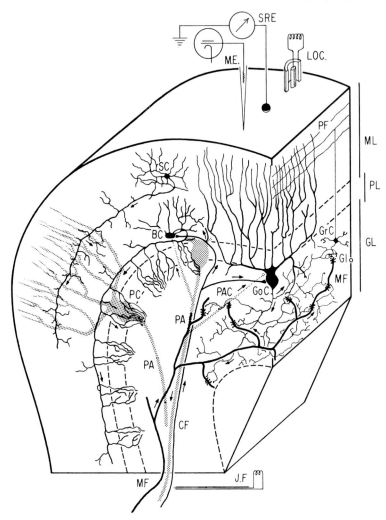

Fig. 37. *Perspective drawing of a cerebellar folium to show the anatomical relationships of the inhibitory interneurones and the experimental arrangements with respect to stimulating and recording electrodes.* The cerebellar cortex is seen to be divided into three layers, the molecular layer (*ML*), the Purkinje cell layer (*PL*) and the granular layer (*GL*). The input to the cortex is by two types of fiber, the mossy fiber (*MF*) and the climbing fiber (*CF*). Single examples are shown of four types of interneurones, granule cells (*GrC*), Golgi cells (*GoC*), basket cells (*BC*) and outer stellate cells (*SC*). Also shown are two Purkinje cells, one (*PC*) with its dendritic ramifications, and both axons (*PA*), one with two collaterals (*PAC*) ending on the Golgi cell and the basket cell. The mossy fiber is shown with numerous branches and thickenings at the sites of its synapses on granule cell dendrites, so forming the glomeruli (*Glo*). Collaterals of the climbing fiber (*CF*) are shown making synapses on the Golgi cell and the basket cell. The axons of the granule cells bifurcate to give rise to the parallel fibers (*PF*) in the molecular layer. The electrode arrangements are as in Fig. 33. Arrows show directions of normal propagation in the mossy fiber, the climbing fiber and its collaterals, in the Purkinje axons and collaterals, and in the axons of the interneurones *BC*, *SC* and *GoC*. (ECCLES, LLINÁS and SASAKI, 1966 a)

these same parallel fibers on the dendritic spines of Purkinje cells (ANDERSEN, ECCLES and VOORHOEVE, 1964; ECCLES, LLINÁS and SASAKI, 1966 a, 1966 b, 1966 e, 1966 f; ECCLES, SASAKI and STRATA, 1966).

Under present experimental conditions, the only criterion for discriminating between the three types of interneurones is provided by the depth below the surface of the cortex at which the sharply localized spike potentials can be recorded, it being assumed that this gives the approximate level of the respective somata.

Table 1. *Properties of 14 inhibitory interneurones that were accurately located in depth below the surface of the cerebellar cortex. The horizontal spaces suggest their subdivision according to depths into superficial stellate, basket and Golgi cells. (ECCLES, LLINÁS and SASAKI, 1966 a)*

Depth (μ)	Loc. Stim.			J. F. Stim.		Inferior olive stimulation	
	Range of latency (msec)	Maximal duration of discharges (msec)	Maximal frequency (impulse/ sec)	Latency (msec)	Spike number	Latency (msec)	Spike number
170	5.0—7.3	23	445	5.0	1	11.2	1
180	2.9—7.0	11	770	1,9	1	6.0	1
200	3.0—5.5	14	715	3.7	1	4.7	1
260	4.3—7.1	25	700	2.1	1	3.6	1
270	2.2—7.8	17	455	1.7	2	7.2	1
300	3.0—7.7	30	1,000	1.5—4.0	2—3	3.5	1
300	1.9—2.5	20	500	1.3	1	4.0	0—1
300	2.5—4.0	20	1,000	3.0	1	—	
320	1.5—4.1	20	500	1.0—3.7	1—2	3.2—4.4	1
350	2.3—3.5	20	500	1.5—3.2	1	5.0—8.0	1
350	1.5—5.5	30	500	2,4	1	—	—
400	3.0—5.5	27	400	2.1—2.7		8.0	0—1
500	2.7—9.0	35	1,000	1.2—3.0	2—3	9.0	1—2
500	3.0—4.0	30	1,000	2.0—3.0	3	4.0—7.0	0—1

According to anatomical evidence that has already been presented (cf. Fig. 37) the somata of the Golgi cells are almost always situated just deeper than the layer of Purkinje cell bodies, i. e. at about 400 to 500 μ, while just superficial thereto are the basket cell somata, i. e. at about 250 to 350 μ. The somata of the outer stellate cells are still more superficial. A classification of the investigated cells according to the depth criterion (Table 1) reveals that no other criterion for discrimination is immediately obvious in their responses to the synaptic inputs here employed (ECCLES, LLINÁS and SASAKI, 1966 a).

A typical series of responses of an interneurone of the cerebellar cortex is illustrated in Fig. 38. The large extracellulary recorded spike potentials are always diphasic with an initial positivity, which is the typical configuration when an electrode is in very close proximity to a neurone. A weak stimulus applied to the parallel fibers evokes a single response with a latency of 5.5 msec (A), and with progressively stronger stimulation there is an increase in the number of spike discharges and a shortening of latency, which is only 1.5 msec with the strongest stimulations (D to G). The spike discharges are as close as 2 msec apart in F and G and the total duration of the discharge is in excess of 30 msec. The lower traces are recorded by a surface electrode (cf. SRE in Fig. 33 A), and, as in Fig. 33, are produced by the propagated action potentials in the parallel fibers (ECCLES, LLINÁS and SASAKI, 1966 b).

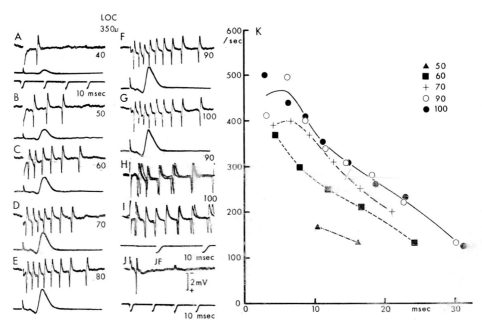

Fig. 38 A—K. *Extracellular recording of responses of presumed inhibitory interneurone at a depth of 350* μ. A volley of impulses was generated in the parallel fibers by a stimulus of progressively increasing strength (given in arbitrary units) that was applied through a surface electrode (LOC in Fig. 37) within 1 mm of the recording microelectrode. The lower trace of each record shows the mass spike potential produced by this parallel fiber volley and recorded by a surface electrode about 2 mm from the stimulating electrode, i.e. more than 1 mm beyond the recording microelectrode. All electrodes were placed in accurate alignment along the length of the folium. The superimposed traces of H and I were similarly produced in the same interneurone but at a faster sweep speed. J shows the single spike potential (latent period, 2.4 msec) produced by a juxtafastigial (*JF*) stimulus. The same voltage scale obtains throughout and the same time scale for A—G and J. In K the reciprocal of each cycle of the rhythmic responses B—D and F, G has been plotted as frequency against as abscissae the time between the stimulus and the end of that cycle. A single curve has been drawn through the points derived from F and G. (ECCLES, LLINÁS and SASAKI, 1966 a)

With Purkinje cells there is usually only one spike discharge, even in response to a large parallel fiber volley (Fig. 47), because the discharge is curtailed by the inhibitory action of the basket (ANDERSEN, ECCLES and VOORHOEVE, 1964) and outer stellate cells (ECCLES, LLINÁS and SASAKI, 1966 b, 1966 e; ECCLES, SASAKI and STRATA, 1966). This explanation is corroborated by recent experiments by LLINÁS and BLOEDEL, (1967) on the frog cerebellum, which lacks basket cells. A parallel fiber volley evokes a repetitive discharge of Purkinje cells resembling the responses of inhibitory interneurones in Figs. 38—40.

The response of inhibitory interneurones to juxta-fastigial stimulation also gives a clear-cut discrimination from Purkinje cells. Instead of the antidromic spike potential with a latency usually of 0.6 to 1.0 msec (Fig. 42; ECCLES, LLINÁS and SASAKI, 1966e), there is in Fig. 38 J a more delayed spike potential, the latency being 2.4 msec. Its production by synaptic activation of the cell is demonstrated by the variability in its latency (cf. Table 1) and by its failure to follow high stimulus frequencies, the following of stimulus frequency being often no higher than 10/sec.

Close inspection of the rhythmic responses of Fig. 38 D—G reveals that, with the stronger stimulations, the second cycle may be briefer than the first. During the high frequency response there is a reduction in size of the spike potentials. Undoubtedly refractoriness contributes to this reduction; but to a considerable extent it must be accountable to the continued severe depolarization that generates the high frequency discharge, just as has been observed with the synaptic excitatory action of climbing fibers on Purkinje cells (Figs. 91, 92, 93; GRANIT and PHILLIPS, 1956; ECCLES, LLINÁS and SASAKI, 1966 d).

The regularly repeatable character of the discharge evoked by a given parallel fiber volley is illustrated by the superimposed tracings of Fig. 38 H and I. As a first approximation it can be postulated that at any instant the reciprocal of the rhythmic cycle (the frequency of the discharge) is a measure of the intensity of the excitatory synaptic transmitter action. In Fig. 38 K the frequency so calcaulated is plotted against time after the stimulus so as to give an approximate time course of the excitatory transmitter action. Presumably the effect of stronger stimulation in shortening the latency in Fig. 38 A—D is in part due to the steeper rise of the summed transmitter action, though doubtless the shortening of neural conduction time by the spread of stimulation along the parallel fibers is a contributory factor. Measurements of the latencies of the parallel fiber spike potentials in the lower tracings of Fig. 38 A—D reveal that this effect is quite small, there being less than 1 msec shortening of neural conduction time from the weakest to the strongest stimulation.

In Fig. 39 A—F there are the responses evoked by graded sizes of parallel fiber volleys from a cell at a depth of 350 μ. The weakest stimulus (A) evokes a discharge with variable latency and with stronger stimulation (B—E) there is a shortening of latency and an increase in the number of discharges; but even the strong stimulation evokes only 7 discharges (F). As in Fig. 38 J the identification of this cell as an interneurone and not a Purkinje cell is confirmed by the long latency (2.1 to 4.4 msec) of its response to juxta-fastigial stimulation.

Fig. 39 G—K illustrates the responses of a much more superficially located cell (depth 180 μ) to graded parallel fiber stimulation. Again, increase in size of the parallel fiber volley shortens the latency and increases both the frequency (up to 770/sec) and number of the discharges, there being a curious partial spike at the strongest stimulation (K). The response (L) to juxta-fastigial stimulation with a latent period of 1.9 msec provides further evidence that this cell is not a Purkinje cell.

The extremely powerful synaptic action of a parallel fiber volley on a deep interneurone (500 μ) is illustrated in Fig. 39 N—Q. Differentiation from a Purkinje cell is aided by the juxta-fastigial response (M) with a latent period of 2.6 msec, and in N—Q there is progressive increase of the parallel fiber stimulus from just above threshold (N) to more than three times threshold (Q). In the largest response (Q) the synaptic depolarization is so severe that there is disorganization of spike

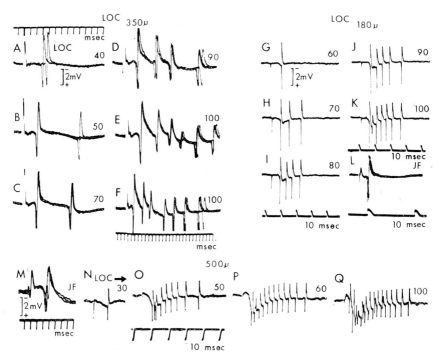

Fig. 39 A—Q. *Extracellular recording of responses of presumed inhibitory interneurones at depths of 350 μ (A—F), 180 μ (G—L) and 500 μ (M—Q). Just as in Fig. 38 A—G, the responses A—E were evoked by parallel fiber volleys of progressively increasing strength (given in arbitrary units), but from another interneurone. F was at the same strength as E, but at a slower sweep speed. G—K are a similar series of responses to progressively increasing parallel fiber volleys in a more superficial interneurone, L giving the response to juxta-fastigial stimulation (1.9 msec latent period) at a faster sweep speed. N—Q gives also a similar series of responses, but of a deeper interneurone, M showing its response (2.6 msec latent period) to juxta-fastigial stimulation at a faster sweep.* (ECCLES, LLINÁS and SASAKI, 1966 a)

production and a fragmentation of spikes, which presumably is related to the process of spike depression or suppression that is seen after the third spike in Fig. 39 E, F. This disorganization of spike generation is a common feature with the more powerful synaptic excitations of interneurones of the cerebellar cortex, and can also be seen in the conditioning responses of Fig. 40 A—E and J, and in the strongly facilitated responses of Fig. 40 A, B, I, J.

In Fig. 40 A—E a strong conditioning stimulation of the parallel fibers is followed at various intervals by a weaker testing stimulus applied through the same electrode. The control response to this testing stimulus is shown in F at a faster

by climbing fibers and mossy fibers, which in the normal cerebellum would be excited by the J. F. stimulus along with the Purkinje cell axons. In Fig. 42 G—J the initial antidromic spike potential shows a slight inflexion on the initial positive wave, which indicates a delay in invasion, and which presumably corresponds to that recorded intracellularly in Fig. 42 B, C. The extracellular responses to the second J. F. stimulation (Fig. 42 G—J) also correspond to the intracellular (D—F) in showing an increased delay at the presumed IS—SD inflexion (arrows), but again at the shortest response interval there is no blockage between the IS and SD components.

It would be expected that there would be a relatively low safety factor for propagation of an antidromic impulse into the enormously expanded surface membrane of the soma and dendrites of a Purkinje cell; hence an explanation is provided for the failure of antidromic propagation during the relatively refractory period (Fig. 42 G), and for the greater prominence of the IS—SD inflexion in D and G—J.

2. Field Potentials Produced in the Cerebellar Cortex by Antidromic Activation of Purkinje Cells

When the mossy and climbing fibers of the cerebellum are eliminated by the degeneration resulting from bilateral pedunculotomy, J. F. stimulation in each of the nine chronically deafferented cerebella produces the greatly simplified potentials illustrated in Fig. 43 A. The triphasic spike potential at 800 µ is attributable to the recording in volume of the propagating impulses in the Purkinje cell axons. At depths from 400 µ to 150 µ there is an initial diphasic wave (positive-negative) and it is followed by a slow positive wave having a total duration of about 15 msec. The diphasic wave is due to the antidromic propagation of impulses up the axons and into the somata and dendrites of Purkinje cells, as may be seen with selective recording from a single Purkinje cell in Fig. 42 G—J. In chronically deafferented cerebella no structures other than the axons of Purkinje cells would be available for conducting impulses from the site of stimulation in the J. F. region up to the cerebellar cortex. The manner of production of the slow positive waves of Fig. 43 A will be considered later in relation to Fig. 46.

The very fast records from another deafferented cerebellum (Fig. 43 B) give opportunity for studying in detail the temporal relations of the extracellular spike potentials throughout the whole thickness of the cerebellar cortex. As shown in Fig. 43 C (filled circles), the plotted measurements of the spike summits in B are synchronous within the limits of measurement at all depths from 700 µ up 250 µ, and synchronism is also observed for the antidromic spike potentials (crosses in C) set up by another J.F. stimulating electrode in this same experiment. However, this synchronism does not obtain for the rising phases of the spike potentials, which are progressively delayed along the antidromic pathway from 700 µ to 250 µ depth, as may be seen by the vertical broken line in Fig. 43 B at 0.35 msec latency and by the plotted points for the latencies in attaining a negative potential of —0.15 mV at the various depths (C, open circles). Thus the early rising phase of the spike potential exhibits a conduction velocity indicative of the progressive invasion of propagating impulses at approximately 5 to 10 m/sec. These findings

73

of a progressively delayed rising phase and of a synchronized summit in the deafferented cerebellum exactly match those obtained on the normal cerebellum, but superimposed on the antidromic spike potential there are spike potentials of mossy and climbing fibers that would also be stimulated by the J. F. stimulus (ECCLES, SASAKI and STRATA, 1967a), and, immediately following the initial spike, are the potentials generated by the synaptic actions of the impulses in the mossy and climbing fibers.

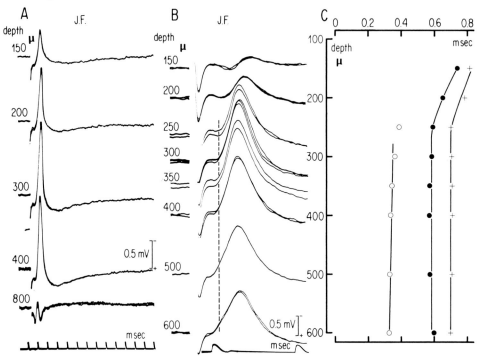

Fig. 43 A—C. *Field potentials produced in the chronically deafferented cerebellar cortex by an antidromic volley in Purkinje cell axons.* A. Potentials at the indicated depths below the cortical surface showing the typical positive-negative spike and the slow positive wave at depths of 150 μ to 400 μ. B. Spike potentials in another experiment at very fast sweep speed in order to allow accurate comparison of the rising phases and summits at the different depths. The vertical line at a latency of 0.35 msec shows the progressively delayed onset of the negative spike at more superficial levels. C. Measurements from B are plotted to show no significant difference in time to summit (filled circles) from depths of 600 μ to 250 μ, and the progressive increase more superficially. On the other hand (open circles) there was a progressively longer latency from 600 μ to the surface when it was measured to a fixed voltage (a negative deflection of 0.15 mV) on the rising phase. The crosses also show the constant latency of the antidromic spike sumit when set up by another J. F. stimulus in this same experiment. (ECCLES, LLINÁS and SASAKI, 1966e)

Fig. 43 B, C shows that more superficially than 250 μ the antidromic spike potential declines rapidly in size and is progressively more delayed both in its rising phase and summit. In some experiments there is actually a complete reversal of potential at the most superficial levels, the negative spike being changed to positivity, and being followed by a slow negative wave (Fig. 50 C). The explanation of this mirror reversal will be given later.

3. Conditioning of the Antidromic Potential Complex by a Preceding Antidromic Volley

In the normal cerebellum it is almost impossible to set up an antidromic volley in the Purkinje cell axons without at the same time exciting mossy fibers and climb-

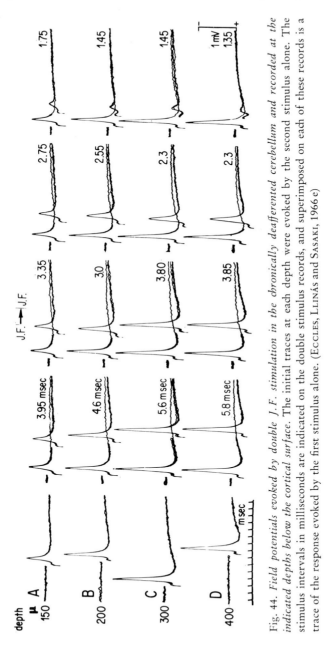

Fig. 44. Field potentials evoked by double J. F. stimulation in the chronically deafferented cerebellum and recorded at the indicated depths below the cortical surface. The initial traces at each depth were evoked by the second stimulus alone. The stimulus intervals in milliseconds are indicated on the double stimulus records, and superimposed on each of these records is a trace of the response evoked by the first stimulus alone. (ECCLES, LLINÁS and SASAKI, 1966 e)

ing fibers, which themselves have profound influences on the excitability of Purkinje cells, as will be described later. On the other hand the chronically deafferented cerebellum is ideal for this investigation because, as we have seen, the conditioning

J. F. stimulus influences the Purkinje cells under examination solely by the anti-dromic impulses in their axons and axon collaterals.

In Fig. 44 the testing J. F. stimulus typically evokes the antidromic potential complex at levels of 400, 300, 200 and 150 μ. At the two longest testing intervals the testing J. F. stimulus adds on to the conditioning response a potential complex closely resembling the control. With testing intervals from 2.3 to 2.75 msec there is at all depths a diminution of the negative spike and the later slow positive wave. Since the two stimuli are of similar strength and are applied through the same

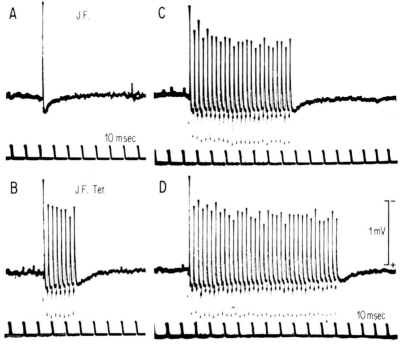

Fig. 45 A—D. *Field potentials evoked in the chronically deafferented cerebellar cortex by repetitive J. F. stimulation.* A shows control response recorded at a depth of 500 μ and in B—D there was progressively longer tetanic stimulation at a frequency of 310/sec. (ECCLES, LLINÁS and SASAKI, 1966 e)

electrode, relative refractoriness of the Purkinje axons would be expected to di-minish the response to two stimuli at intervals of less than 3 msec. Finally at the briefest intervals (1.35 to 1.45 msec) there is only the same very small negative spike at all depths from 400 to 200 μ. These changes signify that at such brief intervals the antidromic impulses are very ineffectively transmitted into the cere-bellar cortex. Presumably there is blockage of many impulses that normally invade the somata and dendrites of Purkinje cells.

It is essential to recognize that in Fig. 44 the field potentials evoked by the antidromic impulses are produced by the summed responses of many Purkinje cells. The failure of antidromic invasion at a test interval of 1.7 msec is illustrated for a single Purkinje cell in Fig. 42 G for the extracellularly recorded antidromic spike potential. However, account has also to be taken of an additional pathway for the antidromic impulses, namely along the collaterals of the Purkinje axons, that have been described in Chapter I as forming a fairly dense meshwork both deep and superficial (Fig. 101) to the layer of the Purkinje cell somata. Possibly propagation along these collaterals is solely responsible for the small spike potentials in Fig. 44 at such test intervals as 1.35 and 1.45 msec in the records at 400, 300 and 200 μ depth. This interpretation is supported by a detailed examination of the responses evoked by the second antidromic volley when the stimulus interval is very finely adjusted over the range between failure of response and the least interval for a full-sized response (ECCLES, LLINÁS and SASAKI, 1966e).

4. Repititive Antidromic Activation of Purkinje Cells

As explained in the preceding section, this investigation can be performed in the chronically deafferented cerebellum. In this preparation antidromic propagation of impulses continues to produce during a tetanus the large negative spike potential characteristic of soma-dendritic invasion. For example in Fig. 45 B—D at a frequency of 310/sec there is a small reduction in the height of the first few responses, but thereafter a fairly steady level is maintained for the terminal 25 spikes of the longest tetanus (35 impulses). In all tetani (B—D) each negative spike declines to a positive potential comparable with that following a single response (A). There is little or no increase in this background positive potential during the whole tetanus, and on cessation of the tetanus in B—D the slow positive wave is not noticeably larger or longer than after a single stimulus. Certainly there is very little cumulative effect during an antidromic tetanus. The significance of this observation will become apparent in relation to Fig. 46.

5. Interpretation of Laminated Potential Fields produced by Antidromic Invasion of Purkinje Cells

Fig. 46 A shows diagrammatically the flow of current at about 0.3 msec after the J. F. stimulation, when the somata and adjacent dendrites of the Purkinje cells would be acting as sources in the external circuits for the sinks at the regions of the axonal impulses. Since the circuit loops are so extensive vertically relative to the transverse dimensions of the surface folium under investigation, the circuits correspond to the well-known features for parallel core-conductors immersed in a conducting medium. At depths well below the superficial cortical layer (Fig. 43 A, 800 μ), the typical triphasic spike potential is sometimes observed as the volley of antidromic impulses passes by the tip of the recording electrode. At the more superficial levels there is similarly an initial positive potential, and the time courses of these potentials are almost identical at depths of 400 to 150 μ (Fig. 44), which would correspond to the somata and major dendrites. However, as stated above, careful measurement of fast records (Fig. 43 B, C) discloses that the origin of the negative wave becomes progressively later at more superficial levels. This is of course due to the current that flows as the Purkinje dendrites are being depolarized by electrotonic spread from the regions already invaded by the antidromic impulses.

The negative antidromic spike usually is well maintained in size up to 200 to 250 μ depth (Figs. 43 B, 44 B, 50 A, 51 C). More superficially the size rapidly declines and the summit is progressively more delayed (Fig. 43 B, C). The laminated potential field at the time of the summits of the antidromic spike potentials (Figs. 43 B, 51 C, E) suggests that the flow of current in the cerebellar cortex is as shown in Fig. 46 B. Since the spike potentials are of almost the same voltage at

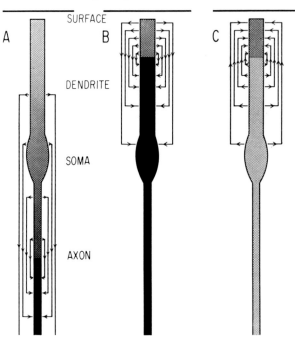

Fig. 46 A—C. *Diagrams to show field potentials generated by the antidromic propagation of an impulse into a Purkinje cell.* The grey shading indicates depolarization, the darker the grey, the more intense the depolarization. The zones occupied by the impulse are shown black. A single Purkinje cell only is shown in A, B and C, but the lines of extracellular current flow are drawn confined to the immediate surround, as they would be in the situation where all Purkinje cells in an area are being simultaneously invaded. In A the antidromic impulse is propagating up the axon and there is a graded electrotonic depolarization of the soma and dendrites. In B the impulse has invaded the soma and dendrites to the maximum extent, there being a terminal dendritic zone not invaded, but merely deeply depolarized by the electrotonic currents as shown. In C the axon, soma and the invaded part of the dendrites have almost completely recovered from the impulse, with the consequence that those regions are less depolarized than the uninvaded dendritic zone; hence the reversed current flow. Further description in text. (ECCLES, LLINÁS and SASAKI, 1966 e)

depths from 500 μ to 250 μ, there is only a slight potential gradient at that time, hence there is little vertical current flow. On the other hand, from 250 μ to the surface the steep extracellular potential gradient shows that there is a large current flowing from sources near the surface to sinks as deep as 250 μ, but not so much to still deeper sinks, as is roughly indicated by the density of vertical current lines in Fig. 46 B.

Despite the slightly later onset at more superficial levels, there is a virtually synchronous attainment of the peak negativity at depths 600 μ to 250 μ (Fig. 43 B, C);

hence, it can be envisaged that the whole complex of soma plus large dendrites of a Purkinje cell tends to fire almost synchronously, presumably on account of so-called "trigger zones" which are located at strategic sites on the dendrites — perhaps at main branching sites — and which generate impulses at a lower threshold of depolarization, as has been postulated for example for hippocampal pyramidal cells (SPENCER and KANDEL, 1961). These trigger zones may arise on account of background synaptic activation on the Purkinje cell dendrites, for it must be appreciated that Purkinje cells usually are firing repetitively at a frequency of about 30 to 60/sec (Chapter X).

The small and later spike potential at levels of 150 and 200 μ (Fig. 43 A, B) shows that there is at least some antidromic invasion after the virtually instantaneous invasion up to about 250 μ, but the rapidly diminishing spike indicates that for the most part impulse invasion fails for dendrites at such levels, and there can be but little invasion more superficially than the 100 μ level. If the fine superficial dendrites are in this way merely passively depolarized without spike initiation, as indicated by the shading in Fig. 46 B, it can be presumed that the small Purkinje dendrites that are densely packed between the larger dendrites at deeper levels are also not invaded antidromically.

Over a wide range of levels (100 μ to 600 μ) in the chronically deafferented cerebellum the sharp negative potential signalling antidromic invasion of the Purkinje somata and dendrites is always followed by a slower positive wave (Figs. 43 A, 44, 45) of 10 to 20 msec duration. At more superficial levels than 200 μ this positive wave declines in parallel with the initial spike potential. There may even be reversal at the surface, which again parallels the reversal of the initial spike (Fig. 50 C). The laminar profile for this slow positive wave thus shows that, as in Fig. 46 C, the generating extracellular current corresponds to an exact reversal of that during the negative spike. Since most experimental procedures link these two potentials together (cf. Fig. 44), a common mechanism of generation seems likely at least for part of the positive wave. It has been postulated (ECCLES, LLINÁS and SASAKI, 1966 e) that it arises because of the much slower recovery of those dendritic regions that are depolarized but not invaded antidromically, there being as a consequence a much slower recovery of this depolarization and the reversal of extracellular current flow as indicated in Fig. 46 C. This reversal of current would of course generate the slow positive wave. This postulated diphasic current flow between the activated and passive components of a single core-conductor element has been demonstrated in the spinal motoneurone when the antidromic impulse in the initial segment fails to invade the soma-dendrite membrane (COOMBS, CURTIS and ECCLES, 1957, Fig. 8). It was also demonstrated by TERZUOLO and ARAKI (1961) and by NELSON and FRANK (1964), and was theoretically discussed by RALL (1962).

It will be recognized that a very great simplification has been introduced into this theoretical discussion by assuming that the small dendrites (the spiny branchlets) are concentrated in a layer superficial to the large invaded dendrites. Actually these small dendrites are also inextricably mixed up with the larger Purkinje dendrites at all the deeper levels of the molecular layer (Figs. 2, 4). However, the currents flowing in this mixed zone will be completely randomized, and so will not contribute to the general field potential. On the other hand, more superficially than 200 μ the large dendrites will be rapidly terminating by profuse branching; consequently there will be a progressive preponderance of small dendrites; hence there will be a laminated arrangement in the integral of the currents generated by the individual elements, which gives justification for the construction of the diagrams in Fig. 46 A—C.

B. The Excitatory Responses evoked in Purkinje Cells and the Generation of Spike-Potentials

On account of the wealth of synapses that parallel fibers make with Purkinje cells (Chapter III, Figs. 26—29), it would be expected that the volley of parallel fiber impulses set up by surface stimulation, as in Figs. 33, 34, 35, would powerfully excite Purkinje cells. In the lower traces of the intracellular records of Fig. 47 A, B this LOC stimulation (cf. Fig. 42 A) evokes a spike potential with a latency of 3.5 msec and a voltage of about 65 mV. In the more highly amplified upper traces the spikes are seen to arise from slowly developing depolarizations with onsets approximately indicated by the arrows. It will be recognized that in A and B there is a slowly rising background depolarization, which distorts the potentials subsequent to the spike potentials. As is usual with Purkinje cells in fairly good condition, there is a spontaneous background discharge, which is responsible for this disturbed base line. Nevertheless, it would appear in A and B that the spike potentials are followed by prolonged hyperpolarizations.

In Fig. 47 C, D the J. F. stimulus fails to excite the axon of the impaled Purkinje cell, but evokes a later complex of spike potentials, an initial spike rising from a slowly developing depolarization, and about 1.5 msec later the spike potential complex that is produced by the climbing fiber innervating that Purkinje cell (Figs. 91, 92, 93; ECCLES, LLINÁS and SASAKI, 1966 d). The earlier slowly rising depolarization with the single superimposed spike must be produced as a consequence of the excitation of the mossy fibers, for these are the only afferent fibers, other than the climbing fibers, that pass from the region of the J. F. electrode to the cerebellar cortex, where they excite the discharge of impulses from granule cells along their axons, the parallel fibers (ECCLES, LLINÁS and SASAKI, 1966 c; ECCLES, SASAKI and STRATA, 1967 a). It therefore seems that the initial responses in C and D are produced by the synaptic excitatory action of parallel fiber impulses on the Purkinje cell, just as are the responses of A and B. There is a general similarity of these responses, the only difference being that in the J. F.-evoked responses the spike arises from a much larger synaptic depolarization than in those evoked by the LOC stimulation.

Fig. 47 E and F are recorded from a Purkinje cell immediately after a particularly good impalement by the microelectrode, the resting membrane potential being —60 mV, and the spike potentials of 98 mV being the largest that we have observed. The J. F.-evoked spike (F) arises from a small slowly developing depolarization resembling that in C and D, but rather smaller. By contrast in E there is only a trace of a slow depolarization preceding the LOC-evoked spike. Both spike potentials are followed by a prolonged hyperpolarization. Evidently, the J. F. stimulus excites neither the axon nor the climbing fiber of the impaled Purkinje cell, the whole potential complex of F being attributable to mossy fibers.

In response to LOC stimulation, extracellular recording also displays spike potentials with a latency that would be expected if they were produced by the

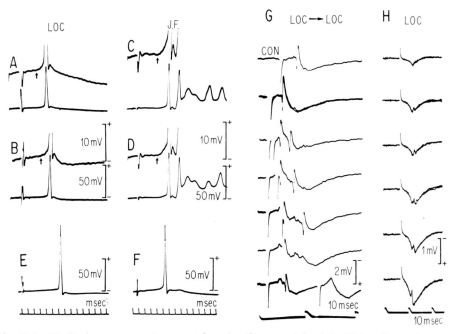

Fig. 47 A—H. *Excitatory synaptic potentials and spike potentials of Purkinje cells.* A—D. Intracellular recording from a Purkinje cell at a depth of 700 μ and with a resting potential of —50 mV. A and B show two responses to LOC stimulation, there being with each an upper high amplification trace simultaneously with the lower trace. C and D are likewise the responses to J. F. stimulation. Arrows mark the onsets of the EPSPs in the high amplification traces. In E and F the resting potential of the Purkinje cell was —60 mV, E being the response to LOC and F to J. F. stimulation. (ECCLES, LLINÁS and SASAKI, 1966f). The upper trace of G shows the control extracellular response evoked by the second LOC stimulus and recorded at 250 μ depth. Below are the responses to two similar LOC stimuli at progressively longer intervals, the second stimulus failing to evoke a spike potential at the shortest interval (0.6 msec). H. Responses of a chronically deafferented cerebellum (9 days) at a depth of 250 μ to single LOC stimuli of progressively increasing strength. (ECCLES, LLINÁS and SASAKI, 1966b)

direct excitatory action of the parallel fiber volley on the Purkinje cells. For example in Fig. 47 G stimulation by the LOC electrode evokes a single spike potential recorded at a depth of 250 μ, the latency ranging from 2.5 to 3.7 msec. A second similar LOC stimulus also evokes a spike potential when the stimulus interval is between 0.9 and 2.8 msec. At longer intervals up to 10.3 msec in Fig. 47 G the second volley always fails to evoke a discharge, and slower recording gives 50 msec as the upper duration for this suppression.

The unitary response in Fig. 47 G indubitably is produced by a Purkinje cell. The only other cells at that level (250 μ depth) of the molecular layer would be basket and outer stellate cells. In both of these types a repetitive discharge is evoked by a single parallel fiber volley, unless it is just above threshold (Figs. 38 A—I and 39); and with two volleys in succession there is a potentiation of the response to the second with an increased number of discharges (Fig. 40; ECCLES, LLINÁS and SASAKI, 1966 a), not the inhibition here observed. This inhibition is characteristic of Purkinje cells and is attributable to the postsynaptic inhibitory action of the basket and outer stellate cells that are directly excited by the conditioning parallel fiber volley (Chapter VI; ANDERSEN, ECCLES and VOORHOEVE, 1964; ECCLES, LLINÁS and SASAKI, 1966 a, 1966 e; ECCLES, SASAKI and STRATA, 1966, 1967 b). Presumably it is the early onset of this inhibition that precludes the repetitive discharge of Purkinje cells despite the long duration of the synaptic excitatory action evoked by a single parallel fiber volley (cf. Fig. 53 B; ECCLES, LLINÁS and SASAKI, 1966 e). In Fig. 47 G 7.0 msec is the longest time after the conditioning stimulus at which the second volley evokes a discharge; despite the potentiation of the excitatory synaptic action produced by the second volley and its summation with the residual action produced by the first volley, the inhibition of spike discharge to the second volley is completely effective in this experiment with stimulus intervals from 3.3 msec to 50 msec.

Fig. 47 H gives an example of the generation of a Purkinje cell discharge by a parallel fiber volley in a chronically deafferented cerebellum. Except with the weakest stimulus in the upper trace, the spike potentials occur near the summit of the positive wave. Their configuration suggests that at least two Purkinje cells are responding to the stronger stimuli, and that the latencies of the responses are shortened by strengthening the stimulation.

C. Excitatory and Inhibitory Postsynaptic Potentials of Purkinje Cells

In Fig. 48 A—F are the intracellularly recorded responses of a Purkinje cell to a progressively increasing LOC stimulus, the intensities being indicated in arbitrary units. The field potential recorded after withdrawal of the microelectrode to a just extracellular position is given in F immediately below the corresponding intracellular response. Subtraction of these two potential records shows that in F the parallel fiber volley evokes an initial membrane depolarization (an EPSP) of 3.6 mV followed by a hyperpolarization (an IPSP) that develops slowly to attain a maximum of —3.0 mV towards the end of the trace. With the stimulus strengths of 60, 70 and 80 there is also a brief initial EPSP preceding the IPSP. The latent periods of the EPSPs in C to F are about 3.2 msec, while presumably the latencies of the IPSPs can be measured at the points of the sudden downward deflections that terminate the summits of the EPSPs. As so measured, the IPSP latencies shorten from 4.5 msec in C to 4.2 msec in E and F, and are thus at least 1.0 msec longer than the EPSP latencies (cf. ANDERSEN, ECCLES and VOORHOEVE, 1964).

A more usual series of intracellular responses to graded LOC stimulation is illustrated in Fig. 48 G—K together with the corresponding field potentials just outside that Purkinje cell. Subtraction of these extracellular potentials shows that there is no detectable phase of initial membrane depolarization as in Fig. 48 C—F, the hyperpolarization having a latency of about 6 msec. Nevertheless, the series of L to P reveals that there is a large EPSP that begins with a latency of about 5 msec. By applying a steady hyperpolarizing current through the recording microelectrode, the IPSP is decreased and the EPSP increased (cf. ECCLES, LLINÁS and SASAKI, 1966 d, 1966 f) with the consequence that, with the progressively larger currents applied in M to P, the EPSP-IPSP balance normally obtaining (L) is biassed in M to P correspondingly further in favour of the EPSP. Fig. 48 Q—T gives

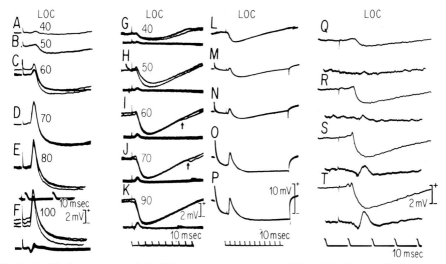

Fig. 48 A—T. *Excitatory and inhibitory postsynaptic potentials of Purkinje cells.* A—F, intracellular recording at a depth of 200 μ from a Purkinje cell, probably from a large dendrite, graded strengths of LOC stimulation being applied at strengths indicated on the records. Below the intracellular trace of F there is the just-extracellular recording elicited by the same strength of LOC stimulation. G—P. Intracellular recording from a Purkinje cell at a depth of 360 μ by a 12 MΩ potassium citrate microelectrode. With G—K there was graded LOC stimulation at the indicated strengths, there being a corresponding just-extracellular recording below each trace. L—P. The LOC-evoked IPSP of L was elicited in M—P during a progressively stronger hyperpolarizing current applied through the microelectrode. The onset and cessation of the current can be seen at the beginning and end of the traces. Q—T. Upper traces are IPSPs generated in a Purkinje cell (depth, 350 μ) as in G to K by progressively increasing LOC stimulation, but in a chronically deafferented (6 days) cerebellum. The lower traces are the corresponding surface recordings of the parallel fibre volleys. (ECCLES, LLINÁS and SASAKI, 1966 f)

a series with graded LOC stimulation as in G—K, but in a chronically deafferented cerebellum. Note that below each intracellular response there is the monitored record of the parallel fiber volley recorded by a more distal surface electrode.

Comment

With the LOC stimulation by a concentric electrode there is only a superficial band of excited parallel fibers (ECCLES, LLINÁS and SASAKI, 1966 b); hence the excitatory synaptic action is restricted to the superficially located Purkinje dendrites and is remote from a recording electrode in the soma. The unusually large initial EPSP in Fig. 48 D—F may be correlated with the very superficial location of the intracellular electrode — at about 200 μ depth. At such a depth the electrode probably is inserted into one of the large dendrites and hence is much more favorably placed for recording the EPSPs evoked by the parallel fiber volley on the Purkinje cell dendrites than is the case with Fig. 48 G—K, at a depth of 360 µ, where the electrode presumably is in the soma. In Fig. 47 A, B, E the electrode is also inserted deep to the superficial layer of excited dendrites, hence the very low level of EPSP from which the spike appears to arise. It can be presumed that under such conditions the spike is generated in the dendrites close to the zone of excited synapses. Evidence has been given above (Fig. 43; cf. ECCLES, LLINÁS and SASAKI, 1966 e) that, at least up to 200 µ, spike propagation can occur in dendrites, and hence presumably that synaptic excitation can initiate impulses at such a locus in the dendrites. In Fig. 47 A—F the impaled Purkinje cells are in such good condition that they respond by large spike potentials when there is an adequate initial depolarization by the EPSP.

When a LOC stimulation generated both an EPSP and an IPSP of a Purkinje cell, the latency of the former is always briefer — usually by 1 to 2 msec, as in Figs. 48 and 49. The present observations are in accord with the previous report of ANDERSEN, ECCLES and VOORHOEVE (1964) and with their postulate that this differential is attributable to an interneurone in the inhibitory pathway. As already suggested, the EPSP would be produced by the direct excitatory action of the parallel fiber impulses at the crossing-over synapses on the spiny branchlets of the Purkinje cells, whereas the inhibitory pathway for parallel fiber impulses would lead through either basket cells or outer stellate cells and so to the inhibitory synapses on Purkinje cells, as will be fully described in Chapter VI.

The location of the intracellular microelectrode makes it a biassed recorder of IPSPs generated by the basket cells with their synapses concentrated on the axonal pole of the soma (Figs. 8, 37, 55, 56). Evidence for the mediation of outer stellate cells in the inhibitory action of parallel fiber volleys is provided solely by recording extracellularly the potential profiles in the molecular layer and the inhibitory action on antidromic propagation along the Purkinje cell dendrites, as will be described in Section E of this Chapter and in Chapter VI. By electrotonic spread, inhibitory synaptic action on the dendrites would contribute to the IPSP recorded intracellularly from a Purkinje cell soma, but it is not possible to distinguish this subsidiary component from that produced by the much more favorably located inhibitory synapses on the soma.

D. Excitatory and Inhibitory Postsynaptic Potentials evoked by a Second Parallel Fiber Volley

In the simplest experimental situation there is intracellular recording from a Purkinje cell in a chronically deafferented cerebellum (Fig. 49 A—I), the graded strength series of Fig. 48 Q—T being from the same cell. As already stated, under these circumstances the stimulus through the LOC electrode will excite only parallel fibers, and the inadvertent complication of mossy and climbing fiber stimulation is avoided. At long stimulus intervals (Fig. 49 H, I) the second stimulus evokes a full-sized IPSP with a time course comparable with the first response, but, with shortening of the interval from G to B, the additional IPSP is depressed so that the summed IPSP results in a hyperpolarization no larger than that produced by the first alone, i.e. there appears to be an occlusion of the IPSP. Correspondingly, there is in B—E a large uncovering of the EPSP produced by the LOC stimulation, just as is effected by a background hyperpolarization in Fig. 48 L to P.

A comparable series in a normal cerebellum is seen in Fig. 49 J—O, where the second LOC stimulus is a little stronger than the first, as is shown by the larger IPSP in the control response (O). There is a considerable depression (50—65 %) of the added IPSP even at the long intervals (M, N), and at the briefest interval

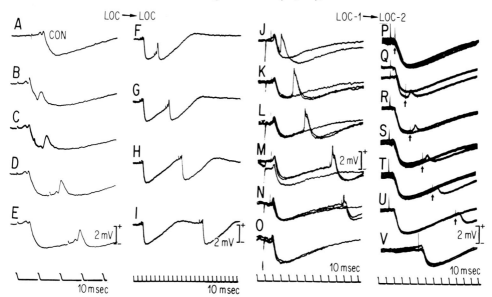

Fig. 49 A—V. *Intracellular recording from a Purkinje cell of the effect of a LOC stimulation on the response of a later similar LOC stimulation. A—I are recorded in a chronically deafferented cerebellum and from the same Purkinje cell as in Fig. 48 Q—T. Note separate time scales for A—E and F—I, but same voltage scale throughout. In J—O a potassium citrate electrode recorded from a Purkinje cell at 300 μ depth. In J—N there was double LOC stimulation, there being superimposed control traces of the first response alone. O is the control IPSP to the second LOC stimulation. P—V is a similar series recorded from a Purkinje cell at a depth of 360 μ, arrows indicating the second stimulus. V gives response to second LOC stimulation.* (ECCLES, LLINÁS and SASAKI, 1966 f)

(J) the second IPSP does not reach a more hyperpolarized level than the control response in O (cf. ANDERSEN, ECCLES and VOORHOEVE, 1964, Fig. 3 B). The series P—V is produced by stimulation through two different LOC electrodes in close proximity, but the control IPSP evoked by the second stimulus (V) is smaller than the first. There is a severe depression of the IPSP added at the long intervals of T and U, and at briefer intervals (Q—S) an almost complete suppression of the IPSP uncovers a small EPSP, while at the briefest interval (P) there is only a small additional IPSP during the declining phase.

Complex problems are involved in attempting to account for the varied degrees of depression exerted by a conditioning LOC stimulus on the IPSP produced by a later testing stimulus. In Fig. 49 P—V there is a very severe depression, which is almost total at the shorter stimulus intervals of P—S, whereas there is much less depression in another Purkinje cell from the same experiment (J—O). Yet under such conditions there is always a considerable potentiation of the basket cell discharge evoked by the second volley (Fig. 40; Eccles, Llinás and Sasaki, 1966 a). Three explanations may be given for the depression of the IPSPs despite the potentiation of basket cell responses, which is observed in the chronically deafferented as well as in the normal cerebellum: depletion of transmitter in the synaptic terminals of the basket cells; desensitization of the sites of action of the synaptic transmitter; approximation of the membrane potential of the conditioning IPSP to the equilibrium potential for the inhibitory synaptic currents of the test response.

E. Conditioning by a Parallel Fiber Volley of the Response of Purkinje Cells to an Antidromic Volley

Fig. 50 A gives the profile of an antidromic invasion into the cortex of a chronically deafferented cerebellum, and, as in Fig. 43 A, the antidromic potential complex becomes progressively smaller towards the surface. In Fig. 50 B parallel fiber stimulation produces in the chronically deafferented cerebellum a slow positive wave having a potential profile in depth resembling that in a normal cerebellum (Fig. 58 C; Andersen, Eccles and Voorhoeve, 1964; Eccles, Llinás and Sasaki, 1966 b). In Fig. 50 B the parallel fiber volley has the usual inhibitory effect at depths from 600 to 200 μ, both on the negative spike and the subsequent slow positive wave. By contrast, the much smaller antidromic spike complex from 100 μ to the surface actually is facilitated by the parallel fiber volley. This facilitation at superficial levels is also displayed in the normal cerebellum. In both the normal (Fig. 61; Eccles, Sasaki and Strata, 1966) and the chronically deafferented cerebellum the facilitation is observed only when the recording is in proximity to the beam of excited parallel fibers, being present in Fig. 61 E, F and not in G, H and I.

Fig. 50 C is a series comparable with that of Fig. 50 A, and in another experiment on a chronically deafferented cerebellum. However, it differs in that the negative antidromic spike potential declines rapidly at a depth of 400 μ to 300 μ, and from 250 μ to 50 μ it appears as a small positive deflection. There is an accompanying transformation by the slow positive wave, so that the wave-form at 150 to 50 μ is virtually a mirror image of that below 250 μ. For depths below 250 μ in Fig. 50 D the parallel fiber volley has the usual inhibitory effect on the antidromic spike potential: the negative spike is depressed by the preceding parallel fiber volley and the later slow positive wave suffers a larger depression. In addition, D shows that the parallel fiber volley effects a re-reversal of the antidromic potential at all depths from 250 μ up to 50 μ. A similar re-reversal is observed in experiments on the normal cerebellum. As will be appreciated from reference to Fig. 50 B, this re-reversal occurs because of the facilitated antidromic propagation further up the Purkinje dendrites, so that there would be a more superficial extension of the black zone in the diagram of Fig. 46 B.

Fig. 51 C gives a typical depth profile of the action of a parallel fiber volley on the antidromic spike potential, specimen records being shown in A and B for the normal series and the series with the stronger inhibition (filled triangles in C). The antidromic spike potential for this normal cerebellum resembles in general that for the deafferented cerebellum in Fig. 43 A, but the specimen records show the complex potentials that immediately follow the antidromic spike and that will be considered later (Chapter VII). The depth profile (open circles) in Fig. 51 C shows typically that there is not a large decrement of the uninhibited antidromic spike until it is

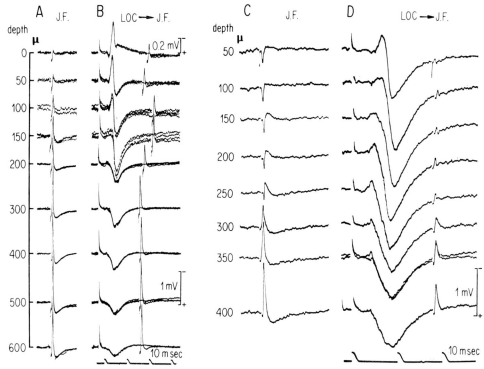

Fig. 50 A—D. *Inhibitory and facilitatory influences of a parallel fiber volley set up by LOC stimulation on the antidromic spike potentials in a chronically deafferented cerebellum.* A shows potential fields set up by a J.F. stimulus at the indicated depths below the cortical surface (cf. Fig. 43A), and in B conditioning by a preceding LOC stimulation, the stimulus interval varying from 18 to 24 msec. Note the higher amplification in both A and B for traces at 150 μ and more superficially. C and D were obtained in another chronically deafferented cerebellum with experimental conditions as in A and B, but with 18 msec stimulus interval. Note in C the inversion of antidromic potentials at superficial levels. (ECCLES, LLINÁS and SASAKI, 1966 e)

more superficial than 200 μ. On the other hand the inhibited spikes (filled circles and triangles) are quite small at 200 μ, there being a continuous severe decrement in spike size from the deepest level. The depth profiles of the inhibitory diminution of the antidromic spikes (Fig. 51 D) show typically that, from a relatively small amount of inhibition at the deepest level, there is a progressive increase to a maximum at 250 to 200 μ depth.

For the most part the rapid decrement in the amount of inhibition more superficially than 200 μ is attributable to the rapid decrease in size of the uninhibited response (Fig. 51 C), but a contributory factor would also be the replacement of inhibition by facilitation at the most superficial levels, as illustrated in Fig. 50 B, D.

The depth profiles of the uninhibited and inhibited spikes for the experiment illustrated in Fig. 50 A, B are plotted in Fig. 51 E for a testing interval of 25 msec, and in Fig. 51 F is the depth profile for the actual changes in the spike heights. In general this latter curve resembles those of Fig. 51 D, but differs in that there is the clear facilitatory phase superficial to 150 μ.

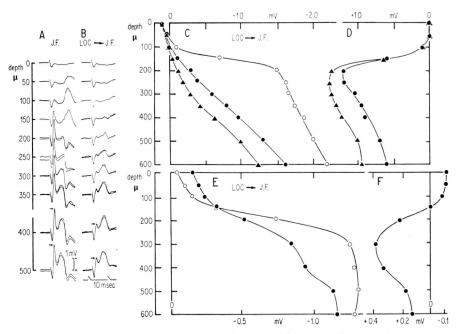

Fig. 51 A—F. *Depth profiles of the field potential generated by an antidromic volley in Purkinje axons.* In A a J. F. stimulus evoked a complex potential wave at the indicated depths below the cortical surface. The initial diphasic (positive-negative) component is the antidromic spike potential of Purkinje cells (cf. Fig. 43 A) plus the spike potentials in the directly stimulated mossy and climbing fibers. The observations of B were produced concurrently with those of A by the same J. F. stimulus, but were conditioned by a parallel fiber volley 18 msec earlier, just as in Fig. 50 B and D. In C the heights of the negative components of the antidromic spike potentials are plotted against the depths for the series of A (open circles) and B (filled triangles) and also (filled circles) for a series similar to B, but with conditioning by a parallel fiber volley evoked by a weaker stimulus (half strength). In D there are similar depth profile plots for the amount of inhibition by these two sizes of parallel fiber volley, which is expressed as the difference between the control and the inhibited responses. In E there is a similar plot for the depth profile of the control and the inhibited antidromic spike potentials as in C, and in F is plotted the amount of inhibition as in D for a similar investigation on a chronically deafferented cerebellum. Specimen records are illustrated in Fig. 50 A and B. (ECCLES, LLINÁS and SASAKI, 1966 e)

The actions of a parallel fiber volley are tested in Figs. 50 and 51 at intervals of about 20 msec, which is approximately the time of the maxima both of inhibition and facilitation. In Fig. 52 are a series of specimen records of an antidromic spike potential at a depth of 400 μ in a normal cerebellar cortex (A) and at various intervals after a conditioning parallel fiber volley (B—F). At the two briefest testing intervals (B, C) there is no detectable inhibition, and in D to F the inhibition increases progressively with increasing test intervals. The full time course of the

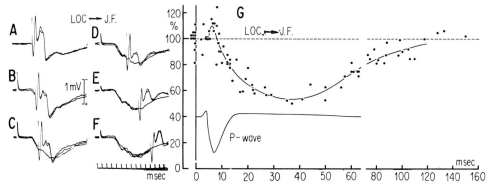

Fig. 52 A—G. *Time course of the action exerted by a parallel fiber volley on the antidromic spike potential in the cerebellar cortex.* A shows the typical complex potential produced by a J. F. stimulus in a normal cerebellum and recorded at a depth of 500 μ. In B—F this response was conditioned by a parallel fiber volley at various stimulus intervals, there being superimposed in C—F a trace of the response to the conditioning volley alone in order to aid measurements of the size of the negative component of the antidromic spike. The sizes of similar potentials in another experiment are expressed as percentages of the mean control responses and are plotted against the stimulus intervals in G. Note the change in abscissal scaling at the interruption of the base line at 70 msec. In G there is also a tracing showing on the same time scale the P wave that was produced by the conditioning parallel fiber volley as in C to F. (Eccles, Llinás and Sasaki, 1966 e)

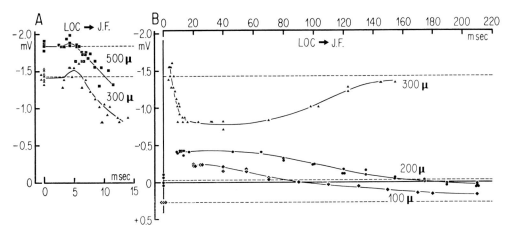

Fig. 53 A and B. *Time courses of the facilitatory and inhibitory actions exerted by a parallel fiber volley on the antidromic spike potentials at various levels of a chronically deafferented cerebellar cortex.* The antidromic spike potentials were similar to those of Fig. 50 C, D in that the dominant negative phase of the antidromic spike potential reversed to a positive spike potential at superficial levels such as 100 μ, the 200 μ depth being transitional, but the experiment was on another chronically deafferented cerebellum. In A the sizes of the conditioned antidromic spike are plotted as in Fig. 52 G against stimulus intervals of up to 14 msec for depths of 500 μ (filled squares) and 300 μ (filled triangles). In B there is a similar plotting of the conditioned antidromic spike potential for intervals up to 210 msec and for depths of 300 μ (filled triangles), 200 μ (filled circles) and 100 μ (filled squares). Note that the mean control potentials in B were about zero at 200 μ and positive at 100 μ. Note also that at 100 μ the facilitatory influence converts the positive spike to a negative spike, from below to above the zero line, as is illustrated at the superficial levels of Fig. 50 D. (Eccles, Llinás and Sasaki, 1966 e)

conditioning action of a parallel fiber volley is plotted in Fig. 52 G from a comparable series of observations in another experiment. The inhibition is maximum at test intervals of 20 to 50 msec and full recovery does not occur until about 120 msec. Furthermore, Fig. 52 G gives an indication of a slight and transient facilitation at about 7 msec test interval.

There is a similar brief and slight facilitation in several other experiments, and it may be correlated with the intracellularly recorded potentials from Purkinje cells, which sometimes show an EPSP and even a spike potential just preceding the onset of the IPSP generated by a parallel fiber volley (Figs. 48, 49). The prolonged time course of these IPSPs matches the time course of the inhibition of the antidromic spike potentials in Fig. 52 G.

The curve in Fig. 52 G gives the time course of inhibition at the depth of 500 μ. In Fig. 53 A there are plotted the early parts of the inhibitory curves at depths of 500 and 300 μ in a chronically deafferented cerebellum. Just as in Fig. 52 G there is probably at 300 μ a small initial facilitation at 4 to 6 msec intervals, and there may even be a trace in the 500 μ depth series. However, at depths of 200 and 100 μ there is facilitation (Fig. 53 B) resembling that illustrated in Figs. 50 B, D and 51 E, for testing intervals of about 20 msec. In Fig. 53 B this facilitation has a time course as prolonged as the inhibitory time courses at 300 μ depth in Fig. 53 B and at 500 μ depth in Fig. 52 G. In Fig. 53 B it can be seen that the inhibitory (at 300 μ) and facilitatory curves (at 200 and 100 μ) have a mirror-image relationship.

Though intracellular recording from Purkinje cells, particularly in the large dendrites (Fig. 48 A—F), demonstrates the production of EPSPs by the action of parallel fiber volleys, it does not provide satisfactory evidence on the time course of these EPSPs. A parallel fiber volley always evokes also an IPSP that rapidly reverses the initial depolarization of the EPSP. The time course of the EPSP can therefore be determined only if the IPSP is neutralized by application of a steady hyperpolarizing DC current of suitable strength. Fig. 48 M—P gives an example of how this technique uncovers an EPSP having a duration of at least 20 msec, but a reliable determination of time course requires a much more carefully controlled experiment, with of course in addition the superimposition of control curves for the potential changes produced by the applied currents alone. A duration of almost 50 msec is seen in Figs. 84 A, F and 86 P, where the hyperpolarization of the IPSP is greatly reduced by the raised intracellular chloride, so uncovering the EPSP (cf. COOMBS, ECCLES and FATT, 1955 a). However even this duration is much shorter than the facilitation of Fig. 53 B.

F. Interpretation of the Inhibitory and Excitatory Synaptic Actions on Antidromic Impulse Conduction

When the inhibitory action of a parallel fiber volley on the antidromic spike potential is at a moderate level, as in Figs. 50 and 51, it provides information on the range of depths in the cerebellar cortex at which the inhibitory synapses are effectively acting on the Purkinje cells. It is an almost invariable finding of such experiments that the depth profile of the spike diminution reaches a maximum at the 200 to 300 μ level (Figs. 50 and 51 D, F). The inhibition is considerably less at

$400\,\mu$ and is progressively less at deeper levels. This inhibitory action exhibits a time course with a maximum at 20 to 40 msec and a total duration of about 140 msec (Figs. 52 G, 53 B, 87 D; Eccles, Sasaki and Strata, 1967 b), which corresponds to the time course of the intracellular IPSP that is recorded in the Purkinje cell soma (Figs. 48, 49, 85). This IPSP is attributed to the inhibitory action of the basket cell synapses (Chapters I and VI) on the Purkinje cell somata (Andersen, Eccles and Voorhoeve, 1964; Eccles, Llinás and Sasaki, 1966 f). Such an IPSP would be expected to block the propagation of antidromic impulses into all those somata where the safety factor is low, and so to cause the observed depression of the antidromic spike potential. It can be concluded that in normal Purkinje cells the inhibitory synaptic action is effected by the hyperpolarization of the IPSP, and that this inhibitory hyperpolarization of the IPSP is not an artefact arising because of the depolarized state of Purkinje cells impaled by the microelectrode.

If the blockage were due solely to an inhibitory action concentrated on the somata, it would be expected that there would be a rapid diminution in the number of antidromically propagated impulses at and more superficially than the soma level, i.e. at and above $350\,\mu$. Furthermore, if the impulses were able to propagate through such an inhibitory barrage at the soma level, it would be expected that they would continue to propagate in a normal manner up the dendritic trees. However, the depth profile of the antidromic spike potential indicates that the inhibition increases considerably in effectiveness during this phase of dendritic propagation, and in some cases there is even a distinct second zone of effective inhibition at a depth of 250 to $200\,\mu$. There will be discussion in Chapter VI of the hypothesis (cf. Eccles, Llinás and Sasaki, 1966 b, 1966 e; Eccles, Sasaki and Strata, 1966) that this dendritic inhibition is due to the inhibitory action of the synapses that the outer stellate cells apply to the Purkinje dendrites (Fig. 57; Hámori and Szentágothai, 1966 a).

In addition to this depressant action on the antidromic propagation of impulses, parallel fiber stimulation provides two demonstrations of facilitation of antidromic propagation. At depths of about 200 to $400\,\mu$ a small transient facilitation sometimes occurs at test intervals of about 6 msec (Figs. 52 G, 53 A), which is just before the onset of the inhibition; at superficial levels ($200\,\mu$ to surface) there is often a facilitation or a re-reversal of the small antidromic spike (Figs. 50 B, D; 53 B; 61 B, E, F). Both of these facilitation phenomena appear to be explicable by the direct excitatory action of parallel fibers on the Purkinje dendrites; and, as would be expected, they are observed (Fig. 61) only when the recording electrode is in or close to the beam of excited parallel fibers. So far as has been investigated (Fig. 53 B), the time course of the antidromic spike facilitation at superficial levels resembles that for inhibition at deeper levels. At these levels the slightly earlier onset of the monosynaptic excitatory action gives it a brief initial advantage over the disynaptic inhibition (Figs. 52 G and 53 A), and presumably it continues as a submerged background during the dominant inhibition.

Fig. 53 B shows that, despite the inhibitory depression of the antidromic spike at deeper levels and its facilitation superficially, there continues at all times to be a progressive decrement of this spike potential towards the surface, as is shown by the curve through the filled circles in Figs. 51 E and 61 E, F. Inhibition accentuates the decrement at deeper levels (Fig. 51 C, E), and the superficial excitatory action of the parallel fibers merely slows down the rate of the decrement at that level (Fig. 51 E). These observations can be interpreted as due to the opposed actions of synaptic inhibition and excitation on antidromic propagation in the Purkinje dendrites: the net inhibition at deeper levels lowers the safety factor and causes blockage; at the more superficial levels the net excitation raises the safety factor above normal and so enhances the dendritic propagation of the surviving impulses, as in Fig. 50 B, D.

It will be appreciated that the method of setting up a parallel fiber volley by weak surface stimulation through a LOC electrode results in a superficial beam of excited fibers, and all the observations described in Chapters III, IV, V and VI have been obtained in this way. There has as yet been no investigation of the action of volleys set up in the deep parallel fibers by a stimulating electrode inserted deep in the molecular layer. It can be expected that selective activation of the deep parallel fibers would have a much more effective synaptic excitatory action on Purkinje cells than that exerted by the superficial parallel fibers as here reported. For example the action on the depth profile of antidromic propagation presumably would be quite different from those plotted in Fig. 51 C and E. The excitatory synapses perhaps even may dominate the inhibitory and so give facilitation of antidromic invasion at depths of 300 to 400 μ, or at least much less inhibition than with the superficial volley of Fig. 51.

Chapter VI

Topography of the Potential Fields produced by Action of a Parallel Fiber Volley on Purkinje Cells

This topographical analysis is designed in order to discover the functional meaning of the known connexions onto Purkinje cells. By means of the crossing-over synapses on the dendritic spines, a narrow beam of excited parallel fibers would act directly only on those Purkinje cells whose dendrites lay in its path. By contrast there would be an extensive transverse spread, for as far as 1000 μ from the beam, of the influence exerted on Purkinje cells indirectly through the basket and stellate cells. In an attempt to give a meaningful interpretation of this pattern of action on Purkinje cells, SZENTÁGOTHAI (1963, 1965 a) postulated that the crossing-over synapses on the dendritic spines are excitatory and that the basket cell synapses are inhibitory, so giving a wide zone of inhibition on each side of the excited zone on-beam. An independent physiological investigation corroborated this postulate of an inhibitory action of basket cells on Purkinje cells (ANDERSEN, ECCLES and VOORHOEVE, 1964), and there is more recent evidence that the outer stellate cells also inhibit Purkinje cells (ECCLES, LLINÁS and SASAKI, 1966b, 1966e; ECCLES, SASAKI and STRATA, 1966).

In Chapter I there is a general account of the synaptic distribution of the axonal endings of basket cells and outer stellate cells, and in Chapter IV there is a full account of the synaptic endings on these cells and of the physiological responses induced thereby. The first part of this Chapter (Section A) is devoted to a more detailed and specific account of the distribution of the axonal endings of outer stellate and basket cells and of the synapses that they form on Purkinje cells. Section B will be an account of experiments designed to reveal the different topographical distributions of the excitatory and inhibitory actions that are exerted on Purkinje cells by a narrow beam of excited parallel fibers. Then in Section C there will be an attempt to interpret the physiological findings in the light of the known structures. Section D will present further experimental investigations on the field potentials produced by parallel fiber volleys and their interpretation. Finally, there will be the development of a kind of contour map of the zones of excitation and inhibition of Purkinje cells that would be evoked by a beam of parallel fiber impulses, narrow transversely, but extending through the whole depth of the molecular layer.

A. Distribution of the Axons of the Inhibitory Interneurones, the Basket and Outer Stellate Cells

1. The Axonal Terminals of Basket Cells

As stated in Chapter I, the axon of the basket cell is remarkable both with respect to its characteristic course, which is strictly parallel to the surface and within the transverse plane of the folium, and with respect to its highly specific terminal ramification. The axons are relatively short. According to Fox and BARNARD (1957) they can be traced as far as the 18th Purkinje cell in the monkey. Our own observations on the cat have been based both on Golgi pictures and on degeneration studies either on isolated folia or after a longitudinal cut through the entire depth of the molecular layer (SZENTÁGOTHAI, 1965 a), and have given a rather smaller

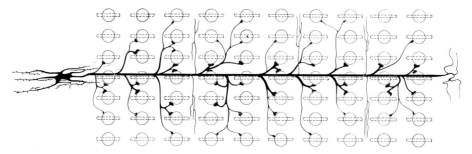

Fig. 54. Matrix of Purkinje cells — indicated by circle and overlying bar as if viewed from above — potentially reached by the descending branches of single basket axon. The basket cell is seen at left. The longitudinal axis of the folium is vertical in this figure. (SZENTÁGOTHAI, 1965 a)

distance, to about 10 Purkinje cells. As seen, however, from tangential Golgi sections both of normal material and of chronically isolated folia (ESTABLE, 1923), the descending branches of the basket axons also spread at right angles to the transverse plane, that is along the folium. The transverse spread of basket axon collaterals is thought by Fox to reach as far as six Purkinje cells in both directions, so giving a distribution to twelve cells, which would mean that a single basket axon could contact as many as $12 \times 18 = 216$ Purkinje cells. Our own estimate is based on degeneration and Golgi studies on isolated folia (SZENTÁGOTHAI, 1965 a) and yields more moderate numbers in the cat: 7×10, i.e. a field containing seventy Purkinje neurons in the baskets of which the branches of a given basket axon potentially can participate (Fig. 54). But this is, of course, only a potential matrix, because especially near the beginning and end of the axon there are fewer descending and transverse branches, so the Purkinje cells actually reached by descending branches of one basket cell axon may be no more than fifty.

At the level of the "bottle neck" of the Purkinje cell, there is usually only one descending axon branch from any particular basket cell, and at the upper level of the cell body or even somewhat earlier, it breaks up in a brush-like manner into several terminal branches. Taking advantage of this, by counting in Bielschowsky preparations the number of descending axons seen at the level of the "bottle neck", the convergence of basket axons upon the Purkinje cell bodies could be determined as being about 20—30 (SZENTÁGOTHAI, 1965 a). Considering that the basket cells are somewhat more numerous, by about 10—20 %, than Purkinje cells, this convergence does not agree well with the divergence of around 50 Purkinje cell bodies reached by the branches of the average basket axon. Taking, however, into account the inaccuracies of the procedures by which these estimates are being made, especially in the counting of fibers and cells in Golgi and neurofibrillar preparations, the discrepancy is not unexpected. Certainly it shows that the calculated divergence of 50 is too high rather than too low.

The Purkinje cell baskets are a synaptic system of almost unique architectural design. An EM analysis (HÁMORI and SZENTÁGOTHAI, 1965) shows that there is no contact between the descending basket axon collaterals and the upper part of the Purkinje cell body, which is sealed from its environment by an envelope of the Bergmann-glia. The basket axons can be recognized on the basis of their numerous neurofilaments, although at the upper level of the Purkinje cell body they cannot be differentiated with certainty from the single climbing fiber that is ascending here and that is also very rich in neurofilaments. A useful criterion in the differentiation of the basket axon preterminal branches is provided by the transverse membrane structures (Ms in Figs. 10 and 55 C). But this difficulty in differentiation is immaterial since, out of the 20—30 presumed preterminal basket axon profiles clustering around a Purkinje cell body, only one can be, in general, a climbing fiber. At the base of a Purkinje cell the branches of the basket preterminal axon attach themselves to the cell body surface with the usual structural differentiations of synapses. The number of synaptic vesicles is here rather small, but there are clear accumulations at the region of specific contact. There is no widening of the synaptic cleft and also no general thickening of the postsynaptic membrane, hence this synapse belongs to Gray's type 2. A peculiar postsynaptic differentiation is found at many places in the form of dense bars, which at suitable places can be recognized as flat sacs lying immediately beneath and parallel with the postsynaptic membrane (Fig. 55 B).

The basket axon branches do not terminate here, but descend farther along the initial segment of the Purkinje axon, as is clearly seen also with the light microscope (Fig. 55 A). Another group of synaptic contacts with a considerably larger number of synaptic vesicles is found here between the basket axon terminal branches and the initial segment of the Purkinje axon (Figs. 10 and 55 C), which is strictly not a true axon, but an extension of the soma as described in Chapter 1, where the name pre-axon is suggested. The terminal branches of the basket axons have on their outer surface strange finger-shaped processes of about 0.08—0.1 µ diameter, containing few synaptic vesicles. However, they are completely devoid of synaptic contacts and interdigitate with similar fingerlike processes of the Bergmann-glia, which contain dark glycogen bodies. There is an unusual amount of extracellular space between the interdigitating processes. This space has a density considerably higher than that of the glial profiles, so that it appears to contain an intercellular matrix and not to be simply an intercellular space filled with some watery fluid resulting from a fixation artefact. The structure of this strange synaptic system is diagrammatically shown in Fig. 56.

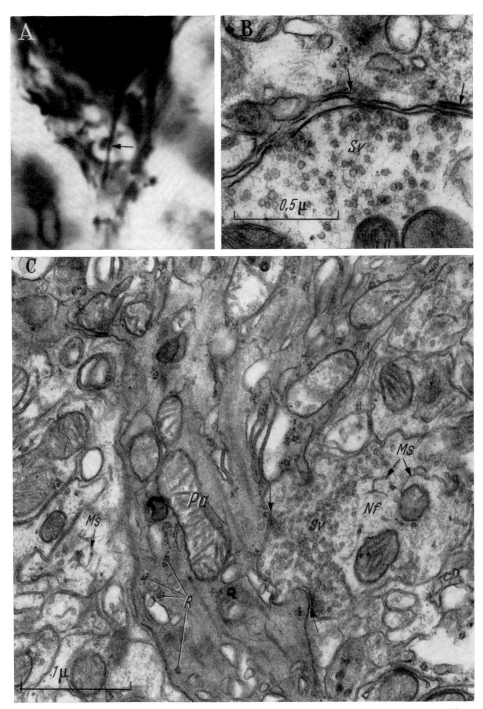

Fig. 55 A—C. Light (A) and electron microscope structure (B and C) of the Purkinje cell basket. — As seen in (A) the axon (arrow) originating from the bottom of Purkinje cell is surrounded by the descending beard-like part of the basket. Dejnek silver stain, cat. — (B) Contact, containing synaptic vesicles (Sv), of basket axon with bottom part of Purkinje cell body. At sites opposite to accumulations of synaptic vesicles there occur postsynaptic differentiations (arrows) that usually

In addition to the descending collaterals contributing to the Purkinje baskets, the basket axons have also ascending collaterals and ascending terminal ramifica-

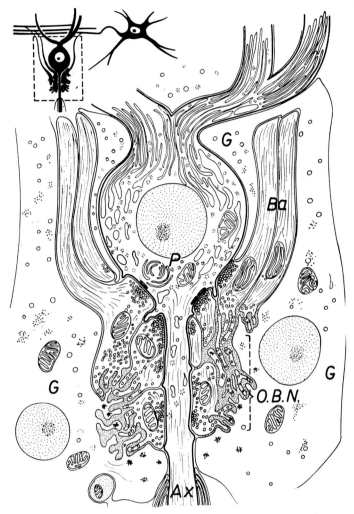

Fig. 56. Diagram illustrating the ultrastructure of the basket synapse. Inset diagram, left above, shows situation on light microscope level. The greater part of the Purkinje cell body (*P*) and dendrite surface is covered by processes of Bergmann glia (*G*). The terminal branches of basket axons (*Ba*) have synaptic contacts with the bottom of the Purkinje cell body and the "pre-axon". The real axon (*Ax*) begins only some 30 microns (or more) deeper and soon becomes myelinated. Finger-shaped processes of basket axon endings and similar processes of the Bergmann glia are entangled in a relatively loose "axon-cap neuropil" or "outer basket neuropil" (*OBN*) which is devoid of synaptic contacts. (HÁMORI and SZENTÁGOTHAI, 1965)

are looking like dense bars, but are actually flat endoplasmic sacs. — (C) The most important synaptic contacts (arrows) are established between the descending basket axons — having neurofilaments (*Nf*) and their characteristic membrane systems (*Ms*) at the far side and synaptic vesicles (*Sv*) at the near side of the contact — and the initial part of the Purkinje axon (*Pa*). With respect to its structure, particularly the numerous ribosomes (*R*), this part of the neuronal process is considered to be not truly axonal, but a pre-axon. (HÁMORI and SZENTÁGOTHAI, 1965) tions. The exact site of termination of these collaterals has been recognized neither under the light nor under the electron microscope. From their vertically ascending course the most probable assumption is that they contact Purkinje cell dendrites. Fig. 8 B shows the terminal knobs of an ascending collateral (Aab) which are

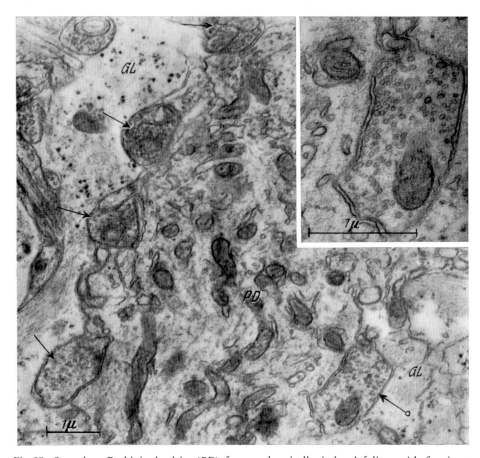

Fig. 57. Secondary Purkinje dendrite (*PD*) from a chronically isolated folium with five intact vesicular synaptic terminals (indicated by arrows), but no axonal profiles containing neurofilaments. Glial profiles (*GL*) are somewhat hypertrophic and are containing dark glycogen bodies. Vesicular profile indicated at right by ringed arrow is shown in upper inset at larger magnification. As these axonal profiles persist in the chronically isolated folium they must belong to local elements, most probably ascending basket axon branches and stellate axons. (HÁMORI and SZENTÁGOTHAI, 1966 a)

situated convincingly on a P-cell dendrite. This is consistent with the persistence in chronically isolated folia of considerable numbers of synaptic terminals on the smooth (non-spiny) surface of large Purkinje dendrites (Fig. 57; HÁMORI and SZENTÁGOTHAI, 1966 a). Since the outer stellate cell dendrites have direct (non-spiny) axo-dendritic synapses that persist in the isolated folium, it is possible that ascending basket axon collaterals also make synaptic contacts with outer stellate cell dendrites. The character, however, of the mitochondria in the axons in synaptic contact with stellate dendrites suggests that they may be parallel fibers.

2. The Axon Terminals of Outer Stellate Cells

As already described in Chapter I, the axons of outer stellate cells have two different kinds of arborizations (Fig. 11). Although both belong to Golgi type II, the axons of some — mainly of the smaller cells — are local or predominantly of descending character (A, B), while those of the larger cells run horizontally in a transverse plane for a distance up to 900 μ (C). During their whole course they give off numerous ascending or descending collaterals. The terminal branches of both axon types are predominantly vertical (Fig. 11); and it was recognized already by JAKOB (1928) that this kind of distribution is most consistent with the assumption that they establish synaptic contacts mainly with the primary and secondary dendrites of the Purkinje cells. When in Golgi preparations Purkinje and outer stellate cells are stained simultaneously, one can quite well observe that the terminal branches of stellate axons enter into particularly close topographical relations to the larger (smooth) Purkinje dendrites. This is consistent with the EM observations that, in chronically isolated folia, many small synapses of vesicular character persist on the surface of the larger Purkinje dendrites (Fig. 57; HÁMORI and SZENTÁGOTHAI, 1966 a). This finding will be further discussed in Chapter IX in connexion with the recurrent Purkinje axon collaterals.

B. Topographical Studies on the Slow Potential Waves produced by a Parallel Fiber Volley

In Figs. 33, 34 and 35 the parallel fiber volleys set up by LOC stimulation evoke slow potential waves in addition to the spike potentials attributable to the impulses in the parallel fibers. Fig. 58 shows diagrammatically the experimental arrangements employed in setting up a narrow beam of excited parallel fibers, and in studying by microelectrode recording the slow potential waves generated thereby at all depths of the cerebellar cortex and in a series of parallel microelectrode tracks evenly spaced across a wide cerebellar folium in a plane orthogonal to the excited beam of parallel fibers.

Microelectrode tracks are indicated in Fig. 58 by vertical broken lines (A—H) penetrating through the molecular layer. The microelectrode is shown in the track labelled C which intersects the excited beam of parallel fibers, and Fig. 58 C shows a series of potentials actually recorded at the indicated depths in this track. At depths of 0, 50 and 100 μ, there is the initial spike potential produced by the parallel fiber volley. It is followed by a slow negative wave at depths of 0 and 50 μ, just as in Fig. 33 B for example, but deeper thereto there is a large slow positive wave which is maximum at 150 μ depth and then declines progressively through to 500 μ. When the microelectrode track is displaced transversely so as to be remote from the excited beam of parallel fibers, as in the track labelled F above, 600 μ from track C, there is of course in Fig. 58 F no trace either of the initial spike potential or of the superficial slow negative wave. However the slow positive wave develops with progressive increase in depth so that at 400 and 500 μ it attains a size of almost half that in track C. Evidently this complex pattern of wave forms is not susceptible to any simple interpretation.

It is important firstly to eliminate by chronic deafferentation possible complications that would arise if the LOC stimulus excited mossy and climbing fibers in addition to parallel fibers. Fig. 59 shows that under such conditions a parallel fiber volley sets up slow potential waves in which the on-beam series of A resembles that of Fig. 58 C, and similarly the 600 µ off-beam series of B resembles that of Fig. 58 F. Complications arising from stimulation of mossy fibers by the LOC

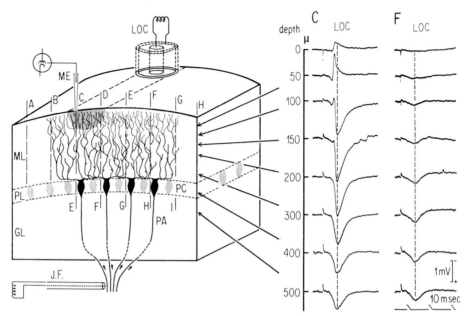

Fig. 58 A—H. *Diagram as in Fig. 33 of experimental arrangements for plotting the depth profiles across the folium of two effects of a parallel fiber volley: the field potentials and the inhibition of Purkinje cells (PC).* The microelectrode ME is shown inserted along track C that passes through the parallel fiber volley set up by the LOC stimulus. A—H show the tracks 200 µ apart. J. F. is the stimulating electrode deep in the white matter that sets up antidromic impulses in Purkinje cells widely distributed across the folium. In C are the potentials evoked by the LOC stimulus and actually recorded in track C at the indicated depths, and similarly for F and track F. The vertical broken lines drawn at a latency of 6.7 msec give the times of the measurements plotted in Fig. 60 C and F respectively. (ECCLES, SASAKI and STRATA, 1966).

stimulus are easily recognized (ECCLES, LLINÁS and SASAKI, 1966 b; ECCLES, SASAKI and STRATA, 1966), and certainly were negligible in the series of Fig. 58 C, F.

In general the potentials of track D in Fig. 59 (200 µ) resemble those of track A, but the initial diphasic spike potential and the associated slow negative wave are smaller and its reversal occurs more superficially (at 50 µ), while the slow positive wave is considerably larger at 300 µ and deeper thereto. In track C (400 µ) this tendency for the positive wave to be larger in depth is further exemplified at 300 µ and deeper thereto. However in track B (600 µ) the positive waves are small at all depths.

Since the declining phases of the slow negative and positive waves have comparable time courses throughout the whole series of Fig. 58 C, F, it is justifiable to compare the sizes by measuring all potentials at the same fixed interval after the LOC stimulus, this chosen interval (6.7 msec) being shown as the vertical broken lines. The measurements give the plotted potential profiles of Fig. 60 C and F respectively. The other depth profiles plotted in Fig. 60 are measurements from series resembling those of Fig. 58 C and F and observed in the microelectrode tracks A—H of Fig. 58, which are spaced 200 μ apart and in the same plane orthogonal to the parallel fiber volley, specimen records at depths of 150 and 500 μ being given in Fig. 60 A—H.

The potential profiles of the two tracks on beam (C and D) are remarkable for the very steep negative to positive potential gradient at depths from 50 μ to 150 μ.

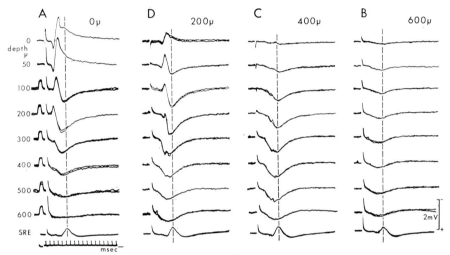

Fig. 59 A—D. *Field potentials produced in a cerebellar folium by a standard LOC stimulus in a chronically (22 day) deafferented cerebellum.* The potentials recorded in four tracks are arranged in four columns at the indicated depth sequences, the lowest trace in each column being the monitored response of the parallel fiber volley recorded by the SRE (Fig. 33 A) at least 1 mm further from the LOC electrode than the microelectrode. The track recordings were made in the sequence A, B, C, D as indicated, A being accurately on the beam of excited parallel fibers, B 600 μ lateral thereto and C, D at lateralities of 400 and 200 μ. All traces were at the same sweep speed and amplification. Perpendicular broken lines indicate point of measurement of all traces at 5.3 msec latency. (ECCLES, LLINÁS and SASAKI, 1966 b)

Evidently, at the time of the measurements (6.7 msec) and thereabouts, a large extracellular current is flowing from sources deeper than 150 μ to superficial sinks. The shaded areas in Fig. 60 C and D give the depth profiles of the negative spike of potentials of the parallel fiber volley, being plotted in C from the negative spike potentials in Fig. 58 C at depths of 0, 50 and 100 μ. It will be seen that the depth profile of the slow potential in Fig. 60 C is in precise accord with the postulate that the excitatory synaptic action of the parallel fiber volley on the Purkinje dendrites is responsible for producing at depths of 0 to 150 μ the active sinks that draw current from passive sources deeper on the Purkinje dendrites, and so produce the observed steep potential gradient at depths of 50 to 150 μ. This postulate will be further developed in relation to Fig. 63.

The series of depth profiles in Fig. 60 A—H shows a profound change in the tracks 200 µ off-beam, there being in B and E not only no superficial negative wave, but also a positive wave that at depths of 200 to 500 µ is as large or even larger than superficially. It is postulated that this positive wave is largely due to active sources produced by the inhibitory actions of basket and stellate cell synapses on the Purkinje cells (ANDERSEN, ECCLES and VOORHOEVE 1964; ECCLES, LLINÁS and SASAKI, 1966 b, 1966 e; ECCLES, SASAKI and STRATA, 1966). With further displacement off-beam (A, F, G, H) there is an over-all decline of the positive wave, and this also occurs in Fig. 59 with the displacement of the track from 400 (C) to

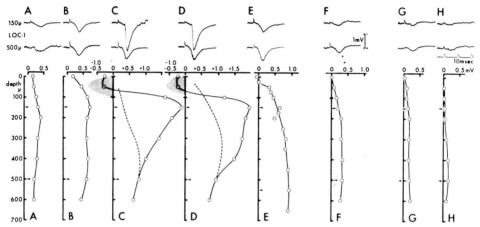

Fig. 60. *Depth profiles of the slow potential waves produced by parallel fiber volleys. Slow potential* waves were generated by the parallel fiber volleys set up by LOC stimuli as in Fig. 58, and were recorded along the 8 microelectrode tracks (A—H) spaced at 200 µ apart and measured at 6.7 msec after the stimulus (indicated by vertical broken lines in Fig. 58 C, F). The potentials were plotted against the depth from the surface, so giving a series of potential profiles at 200 µ intervals, A being the most anterior and H the most posterior. Specimen records at 150 and 500 µ depth are shown above each plot, (550 µ in E), and in Fig. 58 are whole depth spectra of the C and F responses. The shaded areas of negative potential in C, D indicate the depth spectra for the negative spike potentials generated by the parallel fiber volleys and are plotted at half the amplification as shown, these being the only tracks that were on-beam. The broken lines in the plots C, D give the time course calculated for the potential profile produced by the inhibitory synapses. (ECCLES, SASAKI and STRATA, 1966)

600 µ (B) off-beam. The mode of generation of the potential profiles of Figs. 58, 59 and 60 will be considered in relation to the diagrammatic constructions of Fig. 63.

As already described in Chapter V, the excitatory synaptic action of a parallel fiber volley on Purkinje dendrites is revealed by the facilitation of antidromic invasion at superficial levels (Fig. 50). At deeper levels the parallel fiber volley results in an inhibitory action on antidromic invasion of Purkinje cells, which is attributed to the operational sequence: parallel fiber impulses ⟶ excitation of basket and stellate cells ⟶ inhibitory action on the somata and dendrites of Purkinje cells. These postulates have been tested by studying the transverse distribution of the facilitatory and inhibitory actions on antidromic invasion, i.e. in a plane orthogonal to the parallel fiber volley (ECCLES, SASAKI and STRATA, 1966).

As diagrammatically illustrated in Fig. 58, it is sometimes possible to locate the juxta-fastigial electrode (J. F.) so that it excites the axons of Purkinje cells widely distributed across the folium. For example in Fig. 61 there is good antidromic invasion of Purkinje cells with extracellular negative spikes of over 1.5 mV (0 points) for the whole transverse distance from the center of the parallel fiber volley (E) to 800 μ off-beam (I). In Fig. 58 these tracks of Fig. 61 are labelled by the letters E, F, G, H, I in the granular layer. Specimen records of the antidromic potentials evoked by J. F. stimulation are shown in Fig. 61 A and C for tracks E and G respectively. The sizes of the spike potentials are plotted as the open circles in

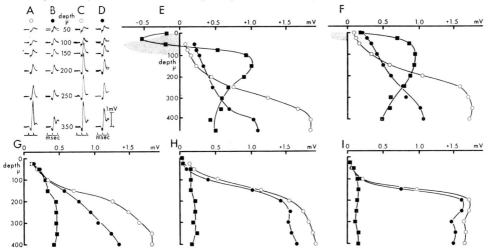

Fig. 61 A—I. *Depth profiles of facilitatory and inhibitory actions on antidromic invasion of Purkinje cells.* A shows antidromic spike responses evoked by a J. F. stimulation and recorded as in Fig. 58 at various depths along a microelectrode track which was on-beam for the parallel fiber volley that caused the conditioned J. F. responses of B, just as with Fig. 51 B. The responses of C were evoked by the same J. F. stimulus as in A, but in a microelectrode track displaced 400 μ transversely (posteriorly) across the folium, and hence well off-beam with respect to the parallel fiber volley that caused the conditioned J. F. responses of D. The sizes of the negative spike potentials in the specimen records of A and B are plotted to give the potential profiles of E. Also plotted as solid squares are the slow potential waves recorded along the same electrode track (cf. Fig. 60). The plotted points of F have the same conventions as in E but were recorded in a track 200 μ posteriorly, and similarly for G which was 400 μ posteriorly, the specimen records being shown in C and D. The microelectrode tracks for H and I were displaced still further posteriorly, being respectively 600 μ and 800 μ from the track for E. Same parallel fiber volley for all tracks. In E and F the shaded areas indicate the depth spectra of the parallel fiber volley as in Fig. 60. Same voltage and time scales for all specimen recording. (ECCLES, SASAKI and STRATA, 1966)

Fig. 61 E and G, just as in Fig. 51 A and C. Corresponding to Fig. 51 B and the filled triangles of Fig. 51 C, the antidromic potentials conditioned by a preceding parallel fiber volley are shown in the specimen records of Fig. 61 B and D and are plotted as filled circles in E and G respectively. Just as in Fig. 51 E, there is in the on-beam records of Fig. 61 inhibition of the antidromic spike in depth, but reversal to facilitation more superficially than about 150 μ, as seen in the specimen records of A and B and the plots of E and F. At 200 μ further from the beam (G) there is still a large inhibition in depth, but the specimen records of D show that, relative to the controls in C, there is virtually no superficial facilitation. With a further 200 μ displacement (H) the inhibition in depth is reduced to half, and is likewise maximal at a depth of 300 to 325 μ. In a still further displacement by 200 μ (I), the inhibition of the antidromic invasion is further reduced to 60% of that in H, and a small inhibition is observed even for the small antidromic spike at 100 μ depth.

The profiles of the slow potentials generated by the parallel fiber volley are also plotted in Fig. 61, just as in Fig. 60, and give opportunity for a correlation between the assumed changes in dendritic polarization on the one hand and the inhibition and facilitation of antidromic invasion on the other. As reported above, the on-beam potential profiles such as those of Fig. 61 E and F have been interpreted as having a dual origin: in part to current flow from deeper passive sources to active sinks on more superficial Purkinje dendrites, this current attaining a maximum during the steepest slope of the potential profile; and in part to a deeper zone of active sources produced by the inhibitory synapses of the outer stellate and basket cells (Eccles, Llinás and Sasaki, 1966b; Eccles, Sasaki and Strata, 1966). Evidently in Fig. 61 E and F there is a close correlation between the potential profile on the one hand, and on the other hand the deep inhibition and the superficial facilitation of the antidromic invasion. In Fig. 61 G to I the potential profile gives evidence that there are deep active sources with little or no superficial active sinks, and correspondingly there is only the deep inhibitory action on antidromic invasion. In the shift from track G to H there is, furthermore, a good correlation between the sizes of the positive waves and of the inhibitions of antidromic invasions, both being approximately halved; and with the still further displaced track (I) both are further reduced approximately to two thirds.

The distribution of inhibition orthogonal to the excited beam of parallel fibers is best displayed by averaging the percentage inhibitions of the antidromic spikes over the range of depths of 300 to 400 μ, as shown in Fig. 61 E to I, and by plotting them as in Fig. 62 A in the transverse plane of the folium. In Fig. 62 A there are two LOC electrodes about 0.5 mm apart on the surface of the folium, not one as in Fig. 58, and the transverse distributions of the excited parallel fiber beams are shown by the shaded areas with appropriate symbols superimposed (open and filled circles). There is good correspondence between the locations of the parallel fiber volleys (shaded rectangles LOC-1 and LOC-2) and the transverse profiles of the respective inhibitions. The maxima of the inhibitions are congruent with the respective beams, and decline on either side therefrom. This decline is surprisingly gradual, approximate measures being a decline to half at 350 μ posterior to LOC-1 and at 700 μ anterior to LOC-2.

In Fig. 62 B there are similarly plotted the sizes of positive waves, which are also means of measurements at 300, 350 and 400 μ depths (cf. Fig. 61). As with the intensities of inhibition in A, the positive waves are maximal at transverse locations corresponding to the respective parallel fiber volleys, and there is the expected good correlation with the respective inhibitory curves. However the rate of lateral decline is considerably steeper, there being a decline to half at 270 μ posterior to LOC-1 and at 260 μ anterior to LOC-2.

Since the parallel fibers run for up to 3 mm in a course strictly parallel to the long axis of the folium (Chapter III), it would be expected that the same distribution of inhibition and of positive waves would occur at any transverse plane of sampling. For example in Fig. 62 C and D the plane is 0.5 mm more remote from the stimulating electrodes than the plane for A and B. Comparison of Fig. 62 C with A reveals similar transverse distributions of inhibitory actions for both parallel fiber volleys, and correspondingly there is also good correlation between the transverse distributions of the positive waves in B and D.

C. Interpretation of the Slow Potential Waves Generated by a Parallel Fiber Volley and of the Associated Inhibition of Purkinje Cells

The initial postulate is that the slow potential waves are produced not by the parallel fiber volley directly, which we have seen to give the initial diphasic or triphasic spike potentials recorded on beam (Figs. 33 B, C; 34; 35; 58 C; 59 A), but as a consequence of the direct and indirect synaptic actions of the parallel fiber volley, as specified below.

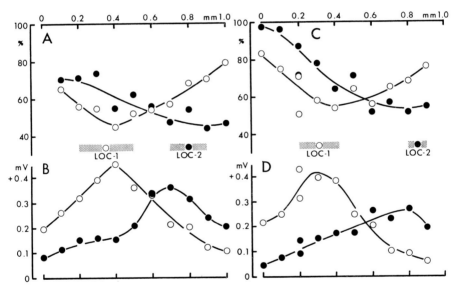

Fig. 62 A—D. *Transverse profiles of inhibitory actions and of the slow positive potential waves produced by parallel fiber volleys.* In A each point is the mean of the percentage sizes of the inhibited responses at 300, 350 and 400 μ depths, as determined from measurements of records such as those of Fig. 61 A—D. The shaded bands show the widths of the parallel fiber volleys evoked by LOC 1 and LOC 2 stimuli and determined by recording of spike potentials at superficial levels as in Figs. 58 C and 59 A. Open and filled circles respectively plot LOC 1 and LOC 2 inhibitions, a similar identification being placed on the shaded bands. In B there is a similar plotting for the mean sizes of the slow positive waves evoked in response to the LOC 1 and LOC 2 stimuli, the potentials at 300, 350 and 400 μ being averaged to give each plotted point. A and B thus give the results for microelectrode tracks at the transverse spacings shown in the scale above, zero being the most anterior track. C and D plot measurements derived as in A and B and for the same parallel volley in that folium, but for microelectrode tracks in a transverse plane at 500 μ more distal from the stimulating electrodes. (ECCLES, SASAKI and STRATA, 1966)

1. An excitatory synaptic action by the parallel fiber volley on the Purkinje cell dendrites by means of the crossing-over synapses on the dendritic spines (Figs. 26, 27, 28, 29, 31, 32). A subsidiary component of this same type would be the excitatory synaptic actions exerted on the other neurones with dendrites in the molecular layer — the basket (Figs. 9, 30, 32), stellate (Fig. 12) and Golgi cells (Fig. 18).

2. Inhibitory synaptic action on the bodies of the Purkinje cells, which is mediated by the pathway: parallel fibers exciting impulse discharge from basket cells, which in turn have an inhibitory synaptic action concentrated on the axonal poles of the somata of Purkinje cells (Figs. 10, 55, 56).

3. Inhibitory synaptic action on the dendrites of Purkinje cells, possibly by synapses such as those of Fig. 57, which is mediated by a path via outer stellate cells, that is analogous to the basket cell pathway.

The long time course — in excess of 100 msec — of the synaptic excitatory action directly exerted by a parallel fiber volley on the Purkinje cell dendrites has been demonstrated by the facilitation of the antidromic invasion of those dendrites that lie within or close to the excited beam of parallel fibers (Figs. 50, 53 B and 61 E, F; ECCLES, LLINÁS and SASAKI, 1966 e). When a relatively weak stimulation is applied through a LOC electrode, as in the present experiments, the excited beam of parallel fibers is concentrated in the superficial zone of the molecular layer. There is always a rapid decrease of the spike potential of the parallel fiber volley at depths below 100 μ (cf. Figs. 58 C and 59, track A). As a consequence of this superficial location, the activated excitatory synapses will be concentrated on the most superficial dendritic branches, which become sinks for extracellular current flow from the passive sources on the deeper dendrites. This current flow provides a satisfactory explanation of the potential profile always observed in tracks through the excited beam of parallel fibers (Figs. 60 C, D and 61 E, F), a positivity deep to the excited beam of parallel fibers steeply grading to the relative negativity at the superficial level of the beam.

Tests utilizing the antidromic invasion of the Purkinje cell somata and dendrites provide a means of demonstrating that, in addition to its superficial excitatory action, a parallel fiber volley results in a prolonged inhibitory action — also in excess of 100 msec — applied not only to the somata, but also to the dendrites of the Purkinje cells. A conditioning parallel fiber volley considerably depresses the antidromic spike potential extracellularly recorded at the level of the Purkinje cell somata, but there is a larger depression more superficially, at the dendritic region, the maximum being attained as superficially as 250 to 300 μ (Figs. 51 D, F and 61 E, F, G; ECCLES, LLINÁS and SASAKI, 1966 e; ECCLES, SASAKI and STRATA, 1966), which is some distance along the dendrites. Evidently there is a very effective synaptic inhibitory action on the dendrites as well as the basket cell inhibition on the soma of a Purkinje cell and this inhibition can be detected as far as 1000 μ laterally from the excited beam of parallel fibers (actually 800 μ in Figs. 61 I and 62 A, C; ECCLES, SASAKI and STRATA, 1966). In line with anatomical evidence it can postulated that this dendritic inhibition is effected by the outer stellate cells, which are the homologues (Chapters I and IV; RAMÓN Y CAJAL, 1911) of the basket cells. The activated inhibitory synapses on the dendrites and somata of the Purkinje cells would cause these regions to be sources of extracellular current flow to passive sinks on the superficial dendritic branches and on the axon and axon collaterals. Hence an explanation is provided for a potential profile (cf. Figs. 59 C

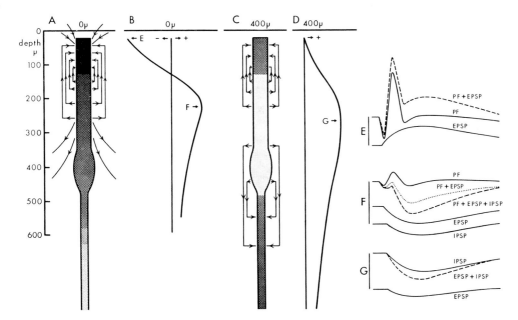

Fig. 63 A—G. *Diagrammatic illustration of the current flow and potential profiles and responses generated in the cerebellar cortex by a parallel fiber volley.* A. Schematic illustrations of a Purkinje cell subjected to synaptic excitatory action by a parallel fiber volley to a depth of about 130 μ. The actively depolarized dendrites are shaded very darkly and the graded lighter shading shows the electrotonic spread of this depolarization produced by the indicated flow of currents. B shows the potential profile produced by this current flow (see text). C. A similar diagram to A, but for the inhibitory action of stellate and basket cells on a Purkinje cell 400 μ lateral to the centre of the beam of excited parallel fibers. The actively hyperpolarized area is very lightly shaded according to the same convention as in A. D shows the potential profile produced by this focus of active hyperpolarization (see text). In E the broken line shows the potential observed at the depth of E in profile B, the component potentials due to parallel fiber impulses and the EPSP being shown by continous lines. Similarly in F and G the broken lines give the actually observed potentials at points F and G in profiles B and D respectively, the various components being indicated by the labelled curves. Further description in text. (ECCLES, LLINÁS and SASAKI, 1966 b)

and 60 A, B, E, F) with a maximum positivity at 200 to 400 μ depth and a lesser positivity (or a relative negativity) superficial and deep thereto.

A stimulus applied through a LOC electrode excites a fairly narrow beam of parallel fibers and has an excitatory synaptic action on those Purkinje cells with dendrites ramifying in this band. Because of the extensive transverse spread of the dendrites of a Purkinje cell, the zone of excited cells will be considerably wider than the band of parallel fibers; nevertheless the transverse spread of the inhibitory synaptic action exerted by basket and outer stellate cells with their transversely directed axons should be much more extensive — at least 1000 μ from each side of the excited beam of parallel fibers (Chapter VI; SZENTÁGOTHAI, 1963, 1965 a; Fox, HILLMAN, SIEGESMUND and DUTTA, 1967). We have now seen that the field potentials and the Purkinje cell inhibition both show this expected spread. No systematic attempt has been made to sample the EPSPs and IPSPs of Purkinje cells at varying transverse displacements from the excited beam of parallel fibers, but our random sampling shows that hundreds of microns "off-beam" the IPSPs may be still very large (cf. Fig. 85 D), whereas EPSPs are not detected.

The conditions obtaining with a schematic Purkinje cell having a superficial dendritic excitation in response to a LOC stimulation are shown in Fig. 63 A on the convention adopted in the treatment of potential profiles produced by anti-dromic invasion (Fig. 46). Since it can be assumed that all the Purkinje cells in an area will be subjected to a similar synaptic excitation, as a first approximation the densest extracellular current flow for each can be regarded as confined to a narrow cylinder private to that cell (cf. Fig. 63 A). The potential profile (B) generated by that current is shown with the steepness of gradient matching the current density, the potential reversing from a superficial negativity to attain the maximum positi-vity considerably deeper than the excited dendritic zone. Deeper to this maximum the positivity is shown to decline slowly, an effect which would be expected for the wider distribution of the less intense current flow that would arise because of the small area of the uniform dendritic excitation relative to these larger vertical depths. As shown in A some extracellular currents would loop widely as with the standard dipole in volume. A further complicating factor is the wide transverse spread (at least 300 μ, Fox and BARNARD, 1957) of dendrites of a Purkinje cell. However the transverse components of the many overlapping dendritic trees would approximately cancel, leaving the dominant vertical components illustrated in Fig. 63 A.

With tracks progressively more lateral to the center of the excited beam of parallel fibers, there would be a rapid decrease in the excitatory synaptic activity on the dendrites, and consequently a rapid decrease in the steepness of the profile. Fig. 63 C shows, with the same convention, the extracellular current flow for a uniform distribution of active inhibitory synapses over the soma and the dendrites up to 150 μ from the surface (cf. ECCLES, LLINÁS and SASAKI, 1966 e). The poten-tial profile (D) so generated is seen to be a relatively gentle slope from the surface to a maximum positivity that would be maintained from about 250 to 400 μ depth, while still deeper there would be a gentle decline. Since the basket and outer stellate cells have axonal distributions running transversely from their dendrite-soma location in and beneath the excited beam of parallel fibers, this potential profile generated by inhibitory synapses would be expected in this lateral position, and it is in fact observed with track C in Fig. 59 C, tracks B and E in Fig. 60 and track G in Fig. 61.

It will be recognized that this theoretical treatment neglects many complicat-ing factors, and hence can provide merely a first approximation in the attempt to explain the production of the slow potential waves. However it does give some justification for attempting to dissect the observed wave forms into their constituents. When attempting this exercise, it is reasonable to assume that there are similar time courses for the currents produced by excitatory and inhibitory synapses because their respective excitatory and inhibitory actions on the invasion of the Purkinje dendrites by antidromic impulses have similar time courses (Fig. 53 B; ECCLES, LLINÁS and SASAKI, 1966 e).

Fig. 63 E gives a diagrammatic illustration of the manner in which the potential observed on-beam and at the surface is compounded of a triphasic spike potential (PF), and a large slow negative wave (EPSP) that begins during the spike (cf. ECCLES, LLINÁS and SASAKI, 1966 b). At 200 μ depth (point F in Fig. 63 B and the plots of Fig. 63 F) the triphasic spike (PF) is much smaller (cf. Fig. 59 A), and the sources for the superficial excitatory synapses (EPSP plot in F) now contribute to the large positive wave as shown in the potential profile (Figs. 60 C, D and 61 E, F), there being also a large contribution from the inhibitory synapses (IPSP plot in F) at that depth. By contrast at 400 μ off-beam (Fig. 63 C, D) no detectable potential would be produced by the parallel fiber impulses and very little by their excitatory synaptic action; and the inhibitory synaptic potential also would be negligible at the surface and small at 100 μ depth, but would give a large positive potential at depths from 200 μ to 400 μ (Fig. 63 D, and IPSP in potential plot in G). More complex problems of dissection are of course involved at intermediate degrees of laterality, but the same general principles obtain.

In the interpretation of the extracellular potential fields set up by LOC stimulation, it is postulated above (Fig. 63 F, G) that a considerable part of the positive potential wave recorded in the depth of the molecular layer and also still deeper (Figs. 59, 60 and 61) is generated by the inhibitory synaptic action of outer stellate and basket cells. The latency of inhibitory action on Purkinje cells is not inconsistent with this interpretation of the extracellular positive wave (cf. ECCLES, LLINÁS and SASAKI, 1966 b, 1966 e). Nevertheless it may appear that the duration of this positive wave (usually 10 to 20 msec, cf. the *P* wave in Fig. 52 G) is far too short for it to be the extracellular counterpart of the IPSP, which has a relatively slow rising phase of 10 to 20 msec and a total duration usually in excess of 100 msec. The records of Figs. 48 G—K and 85 D are very good for this comparison because immediately below the intracellularly recorded IPSPs there are the corresponding extracellular positive field potentials, positivity being upwards. In attempting a reconciliation it is important to recognize that it is the flow of currents generated by the inhibitory synaptic action that produces the extracellular positivity; and, as with other types of synaptic action (ARAKI and TERZUOLO, 1962; ECCLES 1964, pp. 152—155), it is to be expected that the inhibitory current is large only during the rapid rise of the IPSP and tails off to a negligible level during its declining phase, which to a considerable extent is dependent on the electric time constant of the membrane. The residual flow of inhibitory synaptic current during the declining phase of the IPSP may well be so small that there is no appreciable extracellular field, as has been argued for similar observations with hippocampal pyramidal cells (ANDERSEN, ECCLES and LØYNING, 1964). Likewise with Purkinje cells there may be no inconsistency between the durations of the IPSPs and of the extracellular positivities.

D. The Field Potentials produced by a Second Parallel Fiber Volley

In Chapter V there was an account of the EPSPs and IPSPs that a parallel fiber volley evokes in Purkinje cells at various intervals after a conditioning parallel fiber volley. The investigation of the field potentials produced under such conditions should provide a test for the interpretations developed in the preceding section. Intracellular recording suffers from the disadvantage that the microelectrode in the soma or large dendrites of a Purkinje cell cannot "see" effectively the potentials generated on the remote dendrites, which would be the site of action

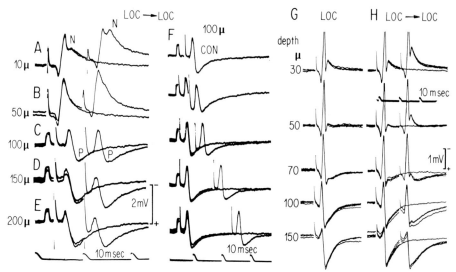

Fig. 64 A—P. *Extracellular responses evoked by double LOC stimulation in chronically deafferented cerebella. A—E* show responses to two identical LOC stimuli at about 7 to 8 msec apart and recorded on-beam to the parallel fiber volley at the indicated depths. Note the superposition on the response to the first LOC stimulus alone. The slow negative and positive waves are labelled N and P. In F the responses at 100 μ (C) are shown for the LOC stimuli at various intervals at a slower speed, but same amplification. G and H are responses to single and double LOC stimuli in another deafferented cerebellum and at the indicated depths. The microelectrode track also was on-beam and there was a very large parallel fiber volley. (ECCLES, LLINÁS and SASAKI, 1966 b)

of a parallel fiber volley generated by a surface stimulation. It is therefore of importance also to examine the extracellular field potentials generated at various depths by a second parallel fiber volley at various intervals. For this purpose the chronically deafferented cerebellum has the great advantage of eliminating complications arising from inadvertent stimulation of mossy and climbing fibers.

In Fig. 64 A the recording microelectrode is very superficial (10 μ depth) and in the excited beam of parallel fibers, as may be seen by the initial positive-negative spike potential. The superimposed trace shows that there is potentiation of the N-wave produced by a second similar stimulus applied through the same LOC electrode at an interval of 8.3 msec. In this series the potentiation is almost to double the control value over a range of intervals of 5 to 15 msec, and there is still a considerable potentiation at 26 msec (ECCLES, LLINÁS and SASAKI, 1966b, Fig. 9). Potentiation has been observed with a test interval as long as 90 msec. Since the initial diphasic spike is slightly subnormal (Fig. 64 A), the potentiation cannot be attributed to an increase in size of the second volley as a consequence of an increased effectiveness in the excitation of parallel fibers by the second stimulus.

At a depth of 50 μ there is also potentiation of the N-wave (Fig. 64 B), but it is much less prominent in the control than at 10 μ. There is reversal of the N-wave to a slow positive wave at just deeper than 50 μ, so that at 100 μ (Fig. 64 C) the positive wave (P) immediately follows the initial spike of the parallel fiber volley and is depressed to about 75 %. In Fig. 64 F this depression of the P-wave is displayed over a range of intervals corresponding to those giving the potentiation of the superficially recorded N-wave. A slight depression is also observed for the second P-wave at depths of 150 μ (D) and 200 μ (E).

Fig. 64 G, H illustrates in another chronically deafferented cerebellum the transitional stages between the superficially recorded N-wave with potentiation in H of the conditioned response evoked by a second LOC stimulus at depths of 30 and 50 μ; and, at depths of 100 and 150 μ, the virtually mirror-image P-wave with a slight depression of the conditioned response. At the intermediate depth of 70 μ there is also potentiation of the N-wave, but it is submerged by the P-wave, and a submerged trace can also be detected at 100 μ depth.

Potentiation of the superficially recorded N-wave is a regular feature of both chronically deafferented and normal cerebella. For example in Fig. 34, at stimulus intervals of 3.4 to 9.2 msec, the second parallel fiber volley adds to the first response an N-wave considerably larger than it evokes in the control response. Similarly, in Fig. 35 the second volley adds a quite large N-wave at stimulus intervals of 9.0 and 11.2 msec, and even at 8.1 msec there is addition of an N-wave, whereas in the control response there are merely two brief negative potentials (at arrows) which probably signal the production of impulse discharges in Purkinje cells.

Comment

The suggested modes of production of the potential fields by a parallel fiber volley in Section C above allow the development of explanations for the diverse results on the conditioning of N- and P-waves by a preceding parallel fiber volley.

1. The potentiation of the N-waves (Figs. 34, 35 and 64 A, H) would be a further example of the potentiated synaptic action produced by repetitive stimulation (CURTIS and ECCLES, 1960; ECCLES, HUBBARD and OSCARSSON, 1961; HUBBARD, 1963; ECCLES, 1964, pp. 83—90). The effectiveness of this potentiation is well displayed by the increased repetitive discharge that a second parallel fiber volley evokes from basket, superficial stellate and Golgi cells (Fig. 40; ECCLES, LLINÁS and SASAKI, 1966 a). With Purkinje cells this potentiation of synaptic excitatory action is not displayed by an increased discharge (Fig. 47 G), presumably because this is prevented by the powerful inhibitory action exerted by the outer stellate and basket cells (Figs. 50, 51, 52, 53, 61).

2. It has been postulated (Fig. 63 F, G) that the P-wave recorded deep to the beam of excited parallel fibers (F) and also at all depths lateral to this beam (G) is in part attributable to the source for the superficial sinks on the synaptically excited dendrites of the Purkinje and the other cells, and in part to the inhibitory

action that is exerted by the outer stellate and basket cells on the dendrites and somata of the Purkinje cells respectively. The diverse affects of conditioning on the size of the P-wave can then be ascribed to various antagonistic effects: for example, to sink-source antagonism within the fields produced by the excitatory synapses as in Fig. 64 H at 70 and 100 µ depth; and also to possible antagonistic effects operating on the inhibitory synaptic action during the conditioning — on the one hand, the increase in the number of impulses discharged by the inhibitory cells (Fig. 40), and on the other a decrease in the effectiveness of the inhibitory synapses during repetitive bombardment (Fig. 49).

E. Conclusions and General Comments

The complexities of the neuronal systems and the virtually simultaneous initiation of excitatory and inhibitory synaptic actions by a parallel fiber volley have

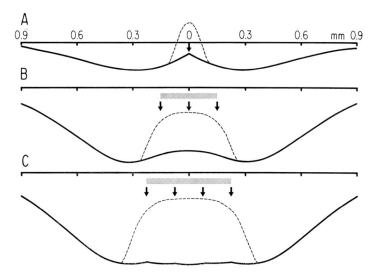

Fig. 65 A—C. *Transverse distributions of inhibitory actions of basket cells on Purkinje cell somata as computed from the distribution determined histologically.* In A the distribution is shown for two basket cells which are located at the arrow, and which send their axons transversely in opposite directions. The maximum inhibitory actions are on the third to the fifth Purkinje cells, the cells being spaced at 50 µ to 100 µ distances. In B it is assumed that the basket cells are excited by a beam of parallel fibers 300 µ across, as shown by the shaded band, and the inhibition is computed for three pairs of basket cells each corresponding to A and located at the three arrows. In C is a similar computation but for a still wider beam. The broken lines give some indication of the superimposed excitatory synaptic action that would be produced in the Purkinje cell somata if the parallel fiber volley was deep in the molecular layer as well as superficial. (ECCLES, SASAKI and STRATA, 1966)

made the interpretation of the laminated field potentials a difficult and perhaps hazardous procedure. Nevertheless, there is general experimental support for the postulated mode of their production as diagrammed in Fig. 63. Of particular significance is the evidence for a powerful inhibitory synaptic action on both the somata and dendrites of the Purkinje cells, actions which have been already indicated by the inhibitory influences on antidromic impulse propagation (Figs. 50, 51, 52, 61). The topographical arrangements of the basket and outer stellate cells conform exactly to the requirements for cells having these respective inhibitory actions, and there are no alternative neuronal pathways for these actions.

The calculated curves of Fig. 65 reveal that there is a good agreement between the experimental observations (cf. Fig. 62 A and C) and the distribution of inhibition predicted on the basis of histological observations on basket cells (Fig. 54 and Chapters I and IV). Curve A is constructed for a pair of central basket cells with axons projecting across the folium in opposite directions, and on the basis of the observed axonal distribution which is slight to the juxtaposed Purkinje cells, maximum at about the third Purkinje cell, and thereafter gradually declining to a negligible level beyond the tenth cell (Fig. 54; SZENTÁGOTHAI, 1963, 1965 a). This idealized situation is expanded in curve B to give the predicted inhibition with the summed inhibitory actions for 3 sites of paired basket cells (at arrows), each pair having axonal projections in opposite directions. Finally, curve C illustrates a similar calculation for a parallel fiber beam 400 μ wide and with 4 pairs of basket cells.

The calculated transverse distributions of inhibition in Fig. 65 B and C are in good general agreement with the distance (700 to 1000 μ from the parallel fiber beam), that is observed for spread of the inhibition, and also in respect of the approximate symmetry of distribution observed for example in Fig. 62 A and C. However there are just as many examples where there is a maximum inhibition at 100 to 200 μ on one side of the parallel fiber beam and from there a continuous decline in the intensity of inhibition across the beam and beyond it (ECCLES, SASAKI and STRATA, 1966, Fig. 7). These asymmetrical variants from the transverse distribution derived from structural investigations (Fig. 65) are perhaps to be expected in an organized structure like the cerebellum that has developed by complex patterns of growth. For example the axon of each basket cell seems to grow out transversely and capture as many Purkinje cell somata as possible (RAMÓN Y CAJAL, 1911, 1959). Under such conditions an asymmetrical distribution of inhibition would be expected if the axonal growth rates were depressed by factors operating in some zones.

As mentioned at the end of Chapter V, the technique of setting up parallel fiber volleys by a surface stimulation results in a dominance of inhibition over excitation when tested by the responses of Purkinje cells to antidromic volleys and also by the observed IPSP relative to the EPSP (Fig. 48). If the beam of excited parallel fibers were narrow transversely, but extended over the whole depth of the molecular layer, there would presumably be much less dominance of inhibition over excitation in respect of the firing of impulses from the soma along the axon, and also in respect of antidromic invasion of the soma from the axon. Evidently the superficial location of the parallel fiber beam accounts for the finding in Figs. 61 and 62 that inhibition is dominant even when testing immediately under the parallel fiber beam. If the beams were at all depths throughout the molecular layer, then the curves of Fig. 62 A would be expected to show a much diminished inhibition in the zone congruent with the beam, and on either side a much larger inhibition would be expected. The broken lines in Fig. 65 are an attempt to represent the way in which the direct excitatory action of the deep parallel fiber synapses would counteract the inhibition indirectly produced through the media-

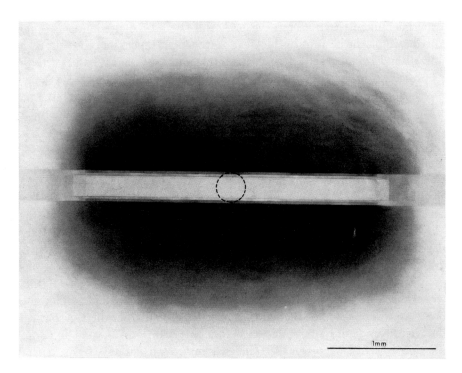

Fig. 66. *Diagram of a cerebellar folium viewed from on top* to show in grey toning the pattern of Purkinje cell excitation and inhibition produced by a parallel fiber volley that is initiated by the discharge of impulses from a focus of granule cells indicated by the central circle. The pattern is idealized because the irregularities and asymmetries as determined by ECCLES, SASAKI and STRATA (1966) have been ignored. It is assumed that there would be a central zone of relative excitation because the parallel fiber volley would be in fibers at all depths of the molecular layer. It is suggested that this pattern of a narrow excited central zone and a wide inhibitory zone on either side is the basic unit of operation of a mossy fiber input into the cerebellum. (Cf. SZENTÁGOTHAI, 1963, 1965 a)

tion of basket cells. Possibly the inhibition may be relatively larger on beam as indicated in B and C, but the net result would be a longitudinal band of fairly excitable Purkinje cells along the whole length of the parallel fiber beam with a deep lateral inhibition extending to about 1000 μ on either side.

Fig. 66 is an attempt to show diagrammatically by depth of shading the excitatory (light) and the inhibitory (dark) effects that a narrow beam of excited parallel fibers exerts on Purkinje cells as viewed from above a folium. It differs from the diagrams of SZENTÁGOTHAI (1963, 1965 a) in that the excitation of Purkinje cells on-beam is shown subdued by the inhibition which certainly is large on-beam (cf. Fig. 62). This diagram can be regarded as giving the operational unit of action of a very restricted mossy fiber input. The way in which these units could interact in integrating responses to diverse mossy fiber inputs will be dealt with in Chapter XII.

Chapter VII

The Mossy Fiber Input into the Cerebellar Cortex and its Inhibitory Control by Golgi Cells

The preceding six chapters have been devoted to the structural and functional features of components of the cerebellar cortex. On the basis of the information assembled and organized in these Chapters, it is possible to consider in detail the responses produced by the afferent inputs into the cerebellum — the mossy fiber input in this Chapter, and the climbing fiber input in Chapter VIII.

The physiological observations described in this Chapter are derived from recent publications (ECCLES, LLINÁS and SASAKI, 1966c; ECCLES, SASAKI and STRATA, 1967a, 1967b; SASAKI and STRATA, 1967). It will appear that they are consistent with the following general postulates of sequential actions that are based on the anatomical arrangements described in Chapters I and II and in the two opening sections of this Chapter. Firstly, there is the brief initial potential produced by the mossy fiber volley itself; secondly, the excitatory postsynaptic potentials produced in granule cells; thirdly, the generation of impulses by granule cells and their propagation along the perpendicular axonal segments and thence along the parallel fibers; fourthly, the production by the parallel fiber impulses of excitatory post-synaptic potentials of Purkinje cell dendrites; fifthly, the generation of impulses by Purkinje cells and their propagation down the axons and through the granular layer. All of these postulates have been subjected to experimental test in the investigations here described. They have stood up well to fairly critical testing, but, in addition to this main pathway, there is the direct action of mossy fiber impulses in exciting Golgi cells to discharge impulses, as has already been described (Fig. 41).

A. The Synapses formed by Mossy Fibers

As seen in Chapter II the average mossy fiber entering an individual folium has about 20 to 30 expansions at synaptic sites scattered over the folium. In consequence of the early branching of mossy fibers in the white matter, it is difficult to estimate the total number of synapses per mossy fiber, but Fox et al. (1967) have counted 44 in a drawing of RAMÓN Y CAJAL that is reproduced in Fig. 19. The spatial arrangement of synaptic sites belonging to the same mossy afferent makes it unlikely that two or more dendrites of the same granule neurone could each have synaptic contact with the same mossy fiber, for the average distance between the synaptic sites of the same afferent is larger than the maximal span of the granule cell dendrites.

Electron-microscopy has established beyond doubt that the mossy fiber has synaptic contacts exclusively in the glomeruli. Although mossy fibers may occasionally have direct apposition to granule cell bodies (Fig. 67), there is not the

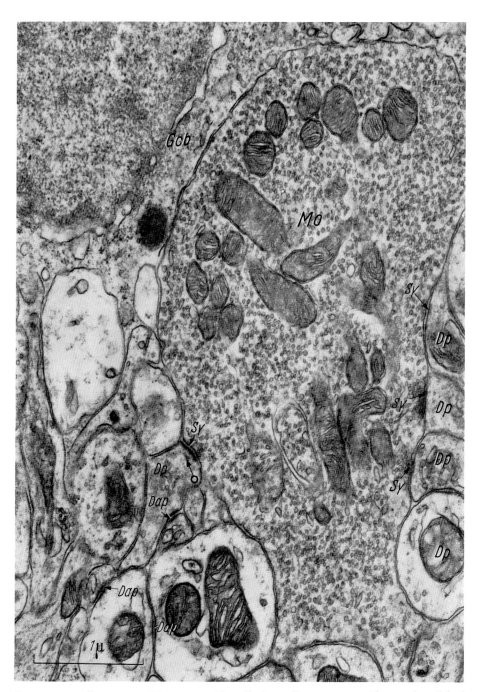

Fig. 67. Mossy fiber rosette (*Mo*) may accidentally have direct contact with granule cell body (*Gcb*), but there is never any synaptic differentiation at this attachment. Synaptic differentiation (*Sy*) is seen everywhere with the spheroid dendritic protrusions (*Dp*) of the granule dendrites. Attachment plaques (*Dap*) of symmetric structure between dendritic ends (or non-terminal parts of dendrites) are frequent. Ringed arrow indicates characteristic postsynaptic differentiation

slightest indication of structural differentiation at these sites. It also frequently occurs that a mossy fiber is closely attached to the outer surface of the Purkinje cell baskets. The baskets themselves are so dense that it seems hardly possible for a mossy fiber to make direct contact with the Purkinje cell surface. Moreover in such situations there is also no structural differentiation of these contacts (HÁMORI and SZENTÁGOTHAI, 1965, Fig. 8), which consequently may be regarded as purely accidental and of no functional significance.

B. The Structure of the Cerebellar Glomerulus

The synaptic glomeruli — or cerebellar islets — are often simply considered as a synapse between the mossy fiber rosettes and granule cell dendrites. This oversimplification does no justice to this highly complex synaptic apparatus, consisting always of one mossy fiber rosette, dendritic ends of numberous granule cells and the terminals of Golgi axons. Many glomeruli are contacted in addition by descending dendrites of Golgi cells, or dendrites in general of deep Golgi cells.

1. Quantitative Relations

There is always only one mossy fiber rosette in a glomerulus, although it may occur that neighboring glomeruli are lumped together into larger complexes, on light microscopic level, but this is apparently purely accidental and has no functional meaning. The glomeruli are considerably less numerous than the granule neurons. In preparations from the vermis of an adult cat, prepared with the Dejnek procedure, in which both granule neurones and glomeruli are quantitatively stained, a count of both elements gives a ratio of roughly 4.5 granule neurones to one glomerulus for a total count of 1,000 granule cells. For granule neurones the average number of dendritic branches terminating in different glomeruli gives almost exactly the same value (4.5) in the vermis of the adult cat. This average is based on over 100 granule cells well isolated with complete Golgi staining and uninjured dendritic trees. This means that about 20 dendrites of granule cells ought to enter the individual glomerulus on the average. This fits nicely with the observation by Fox et al. (1967) that up to 15 granule dendrites could be counted entering the same glomerulus. It will be seen in sub-section 2 of this Section that it is also in accord with EM observations. Since the rosettes of the same mossy fiber are arranged at larger distances than the average span of the dendrites of granule cells, we have seen that it is unlikely that several dendrites of the same granule cell have synapses with rosettes of the same mossy afferent. Consequently the divergence from the mossy fiber could be calculated from the number of rosettes that the average mossy fiber has and the number of dendrites entering the average glomerulus. Using the drawing of CAJAL (1911) reproduced in Fig. 19 in which Fox et al. (1967) counted 44 rosettes on one mossy fiber and the above number of 20 dendrites per glomerulus, one arrives at a total divergence of a single mossy fiber input to 880 granule neurons. As the mossy fiber may have terminal branches in more than two neighbouring folia, the divergence might even be larger. If a mossy fiber forms 20 to 30 rosettes in a single folium, the divergence inside the folium should be to 400—600 granule neurons.

On the basis of the same reasoning, a convergence of roughly 4 to 5 mossy afferents upon the average granule neuron could be assumed. On account of the large overlap in the distribution fields of mossy fibers belonging to different afferent systems, even this small numerical level of convergence may be functionally important; and it will later be seen that, at least with some granule neurones, summation of the synaptic excitatory actions of two or more mossy fibers is necessary for generating an impulse discharge (Section C).

Although, as will be seen in sub-sections B 3 and 4, many individual profiles of Golgi axons can be seen in a single glomerulus, they probably all belong to the same axon ramification. This can be gathered from Golgi pictures illustrated by CAJAL (1911) and more recently by Fox et al. (1967), as well as from Fig. 71 B. That all glomeruli are supplied by Golgi axons is obvious from Golgi pictures like in Fig. 15 A with complete staining of the Golgi neuron neuropil. On the other hand the reasoning developed in Chapter I (Fig. 16) would indicate that there is little if any convergence of Golgi axons on the glomerulus.

It is quite impossible to give even a crude estimate of the fraction of glomeruli invaded by Golgi dendrites (Fig. 72), but they are certainly sufficient in number to enable the Golgi cells to get a fair sampling of the functional state of the mossy fibers of the respective territory. This is especially so if account is taken of the profuse branchings of the mossy afferents inside the folium to give around 20—30 presynaptic expansions.

2. Ultrastructure of the Glomerulus

The glomeruli are ovoid or polyhedric bodies with a longer diameter of about 20 μ, wrapped by a single thin glial lamella (Fig. 17), which is not everywhere conspicuous because of the many dendritic and axonal branches entering and leaving the glomerulus. The mossy fiber rosette occupies the central position in the glomerulus (Figs. 68, 69, 70); and, if cut longitudinally through the axis, it can be recognized as a large, slightly curving or sigmoid presynaptic profile having a central core with numerous neurofilaments (Fig. 70) and clusters of mitochondria. If cut transversally (Fig. 69) the bulbous side branches of the axial part become most apparent. This fits nicely with the shape of mossy endings as known from light microscopy of classical impregnation pictures (Fig. 68). The mossy fiber rosette is not necessarily an ending, the fiber may leave the glomerulus at its opposite pole and have further rosettes.

As seen from Figs. 17, 67, 69 and 70 the rosette is covered by numerous postsynaptic profiles of spheroid or ovoid shape, having diameters between 0.5 and 1 μ on the average. These profiles were already correctly recognized by GRAY (1961) as belonging to the granule dendrites. They are deeply impressed into the surface of the mossy fiber rosette, having membrane thickenings at the contacts with the rosette opposite to accumulations of synaptic vesicles (Figs. 67, 71 and 74). However, there are also symmetrical desmosomoid contacts between the dendritic terminals (Figs. 67, 74) that are termed by GRAY (1961) dendritic attachment plaques. It was recognized first by KIRSCHE et al. (1965) and independently by SZENTÁGOTHAI (1965 b) that the postsynaptic sites are not simply the dendrites, which can be

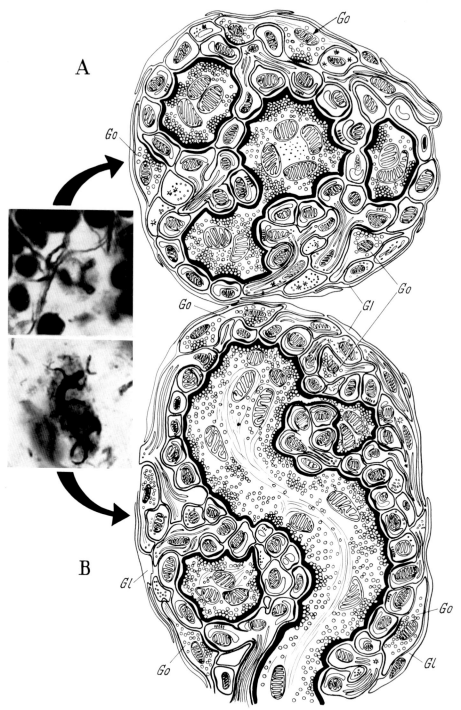

Fig. 68. Photographs and diagrams to show how the glomerulus presents itself in the transverse (A) and in the longitudinal section (B), both in the light microscope (left) and in the EM pictures (right). The diagrams showing the EM structure are abstracted from low power views of many glomeruli (like those in Figs. 69 and 70), both in the cat and the human cerebellar cortex. The mossy fiber rosette is drawn in thick outlines. The smaller terminal Golgi axons (Go) can be recognized in abundance in the outer part of the glomerulus. Gl shows glial sheath. Photograph at upper left from Gros-Bielschowsky and at lower left from Cajal stain, both in the adult cat

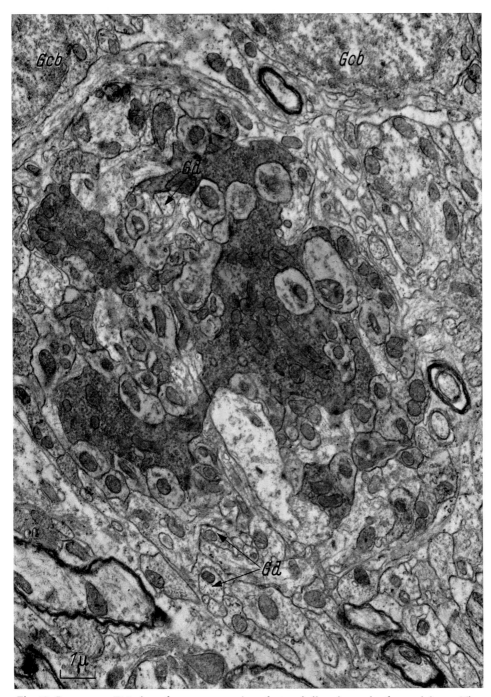

Fig. 69. Low power EM view of transverse section of a cerebellar glomerulus from adult cat. The several elements are shown in different colours: mossy rosette in blue; dendritic protrusions (postsynaptic units) of granule neurons in red; Golgi axons in yellow. Elements that cannot be recognized clearly or non terminal parts of granule dendrites are left uncoloured, the preterminal parts of granule dendrites (Gd) can be recognized on the basis of their strong tubular apparatus. Two granule cell bodies (Gcb) can be seen at top

well recognized on the basis of their strong tubular apparatus (Figs. 17, 69 and 70), but terminal bulbs or protrusions of the dendrite having a very characteristic struc-

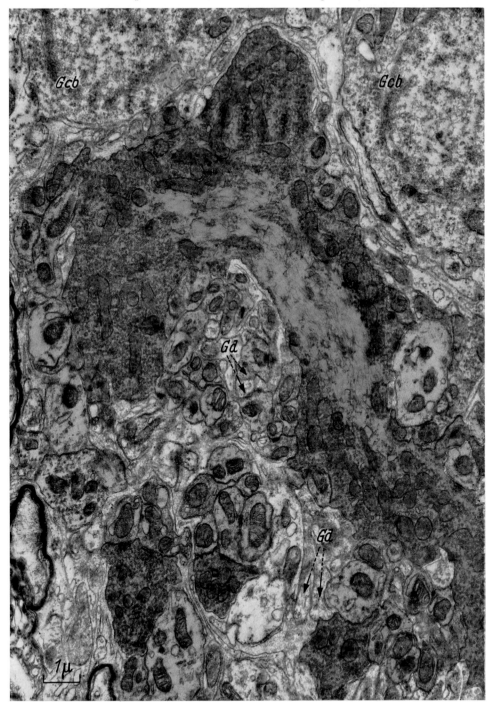

Fig. 70. Low power EM view of longitudinal section of a cerebellar glomerulus from adult cat. Otherwise as in Fig. 69. Granule cell bodies at top

ture. With respect to the importance of these postsynaptic units a separate sub-section 4 will be devoted to their detailed description. A crude estimate of the number of these postsynaptic units — shown in red colour in Figs. 69 and 70 — can be gained by multiplying the number of units found in transverse sections of glomeruli with that of full size units that would have room along the longitudinal axis of average glomeruli. When a certain percentage is deducted on account of the fact that the glomerulus is not a cylinder but an ovoid, one arrives at the very approximate guess of around 300—400 postsynaptic units of granule dendrites per glomerulus. Since, according to the calculations made in sub-section 1, about 20 granule dendrites invade the average glomerulus, one should expect that each dendrite ought to have about 15—20 postsynaptic units — i.e. sites. Estimates made from the magnificent high power photographs of Golgi pictures recently published by Fox *et al.* (1967) and counts made with oil immersion from our own material give approximately this number of bulges on the average claw shaped granule dendrite arborization.

As seen in Figs. 69, 70 and 71 there are additional axonal profiles, mostly be-longing to rather thin beaded fibers (Fig. 71) that seem not to be in connexion with the mossy rosette. They appear also to be lighter than the mossy rosettes, particularly in the monkey (Fox *et al.* 1967). The termination of Golgi axons has been described already by CAJAL (1911) and attempts to recognize them under the EM were started by SZENTÁGOTHAI (1962a) employing the combination of light and EM pictures. However, the Golgi axons can be recognized much better by experi-mental degeneration techniques, an account of which will be given briefly in the next sub-section 3.

The participation of Golgi neuron dendrites was very cursorily mentioned by CAJAL (1911), but in the later literature this connexion has been neglected com-pletely. Quite recently HÁMORI and SZENTÁGOTHAI (1966b) have been able to trace descending dendrites of typical Golgi neurons to glomeruli both under the light microscope (Fig. 14) and under the electron microscope (Fig. 72), using as criterion for their identification the strange finger-shaped processes of the descend-ing Golgi dendrites described in Chapter I (Fig. 17). The Golgi dendrites engage in broad synaptic contacts with the mossy expansion (Fig. 72), which are of specific structure and differ characteristically (Fig. 72) from the contacts with dendritic protrusions of granule neurones. The finger-like processes of the descending Golgi dendrites can be found also at the contact regions, where they are regularly placed between the regions having synaptic membrane thickenings and protrude into deep invaginations of the mossy rosette (Fig. 72). On the basis of this structural cri-terion the characteristic postsynaptic profile shown by Fox *et al.* (1967) in their Fig. 20 could be interpreted more probably as being a Golgi dendrite. The direct Golgi dendrite mossy fiber contacts so far identified are with rather proximal parts of the dendrites. Since the dendrites, or some of their branches at least, con-tinue to descend into the granular layer, their apical parts may have further synapses with mossy rosettes, for example as in Fig. 14, but many of these synapses may escape recognition under the EM. Golgi axons do not form synapses either with Golgi cell dendrites or with the mossy fiber rosettes (HÁMORI and SZENTÁGOTHAI, 1966b).

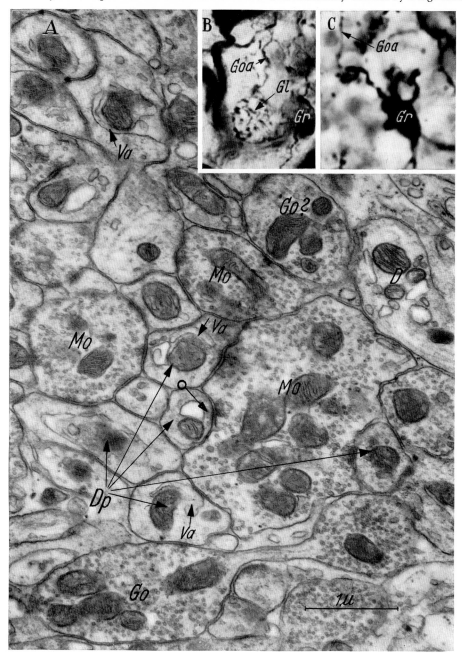

Fig. 71 A—C. Golgi axon endings (*Go*) can be recognized in cortical part of a glomerulus under the EM (A) on the basis both of their beaded character (below), and of their small caliber recognizable in the Golgi pictures (*Goa* in B and C), as compared to the large caliber of the mossy rosette (*Mo*). Since this is a tangential section of the glomerulus, only smaller side branches of the rosette (*Mo*) come into the picture. Dendritic protrusions (*Dp*) of the granule dendrites show characteristic single mitochondrium in their centre with vacuole (*Va*) wrapped around. Ringed arrow points to postsynaptic rows of granules, B and C, Golgi picture of granule cells (*Gr*) and Golgi axons (*Goa*) showing particularly in B that the delicate beaded axon system of the glomerulus (*Gl*) arises from single preterminal Golgi axon (*Goa*). All pictures from adult cat

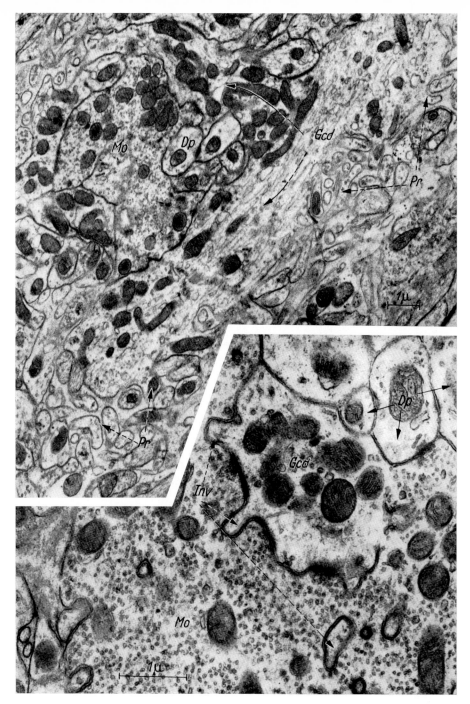

Fig. 72. A Golgi cell dendrite (*Gcd*) which is recognizable from its characteristic finger-like processes (*Pr*) along its entire right (lower) margin takes mossy terminal (*Mo*) into its fork. An extended contact line between the two elements has numerous synaptic attachment plaques. Some spheroid protrusions (*Dp*) obviously belong to granule cell dendrites. Lower inset shows that a large mossy ending (*Mo*), containing numerous synaptic vesicles, has synaptic contacts with Golgi cell dendrite (*Gcd*) whose short processes protrude into deep invaginations (*Inv*) of the mossy ending. At top right there are some characteristic dendritic protrusions (*Dp*) of granule cells, having synaptic contacts both with the mossy fiber and the dendro-dendritic attachment plaques described by GRAY (1961). (HÁMORI and SZENTÁGOTHAI, 1966 b)

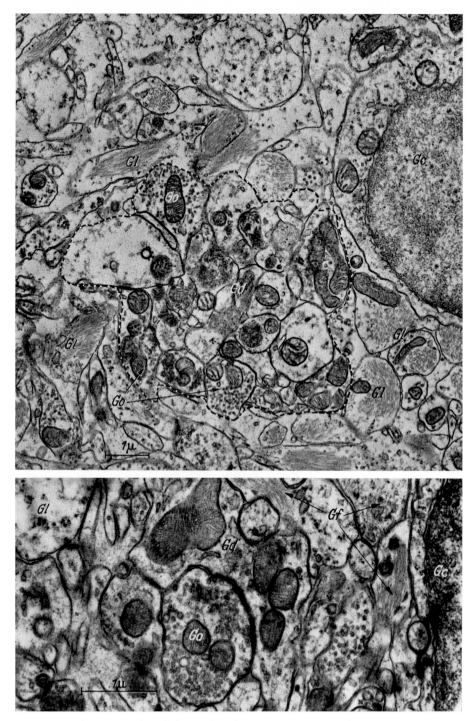

Fig. 73. Cerebellar glomerulus of chronically (for 2 months) isolated folium. The approximate outlines of the shrunken glomerulus are indicated by dashed line. A granule cell with nucleus (*Gc*) is at right. The center of the glomerulus is occupied by the dendrites of granule cells (*Gd*), which have taken the place of the mossy terminal that had disappeared completely. They are surrounded

3. Identification in the Glomeruli of Golgi Axonal Elements by Degeneration Analysis

After transection of afferent pathways that terminate in mossy fibers — for example the spinocerebellar tract — the mossy fibers show clear signs of degeneration that can well be recognized under the EM. However, the study of fresh degeneration is less favourable for the study of local axonal elements than the procedure of investigating "persisting elements" in experimental interferences with longer survival periods. That the large central axonal profiles of the glomeruli are the mossy fiber rosettes is obvious from their structure and needs no experimental proof. Using chronically isolated cerebellar folia HÁMORI (1964) showed convincingly that the beaded terminal axons in the outer zones of the glomeruli are indeed — as suspected — the Golgi axons. Using similar techniques MEAD and VAN DER LOOS (1964) have made an attempt to identify the mossy terminals as sites of cholinesterase activity, Golgi axon endings having monoamino-oxidase activity; however, the situation remains still uncertain and specific cholinesterase appears to be present also in the membrane of Golgi terminals. By using the technique of chronically isolated folia or of the chronically deafferented cerebellum Fox et al. (1967) and HÁMORI and SZENTÁGOTHAI (1966b) have confirmed that the Golgi terminals are the small beaded axons, and that these make synaptic contacts either with granule cell dendrites, somewhat "downstream" from their contacts with the mossy fiber rosettes, but nevertheless inside the glomeruli, or with the outer side of the dendritic protrusions opposite to their contacts with the mossy expansion. The Golgi axon terminals and their synapses persist in chronically isolated folia (Fig. 73) much better than the dendritic protrusions of the granule neurons, which, if deprived of their synaptic contacts with the mossy fiber, undergo severe atrophy. Thus the remnants of the glomeruli in the chronically isolated folium consist of a few dendritic profiles occupying the central position in the glomerulus and synapsing with slightly hypertrophic Golgi axon endings on their outer surfaces (Fig. 73).

4. The Postsynaptic Structural Units

As mentioned already in sub-section 2, the granule dendrites have postsynaptic sites of very peculiar structure, which are spheroid protrusions both at the end and sides of the claw-shaped terminal branches of the dendrites. Many details of these postsynaptic units can be seen in Figs. 67 and 71, and some others are assembled in Fig. 74. Each protrusion characteristically contains a single mitochondrion and an endoplasmic vacuole — or sometimes a group of vacuoles — wrapped around the mitochondrion. Quite often one can recognize a row of postsynaptic dense

by the surviving Golgi axon (Go) endings. The outer regions of the neurophil are filled with hypertrophic glial profiles (Gl), containing characteristic bundles of glial filaments and glycogen particles. Lower inset shows the same at higher magnification with a Golgi axon ending (Go) in synaptic contact with a granule cell dendrite (Gd). Granule cell body (Gc) is seen to the right. Glial profile (Gl) to the left contains only glycogen particles, while other profiles more to the right contain glial filament bundles (Gf). (HÁMORI and SZENTÁGOTHAI, 1966b)

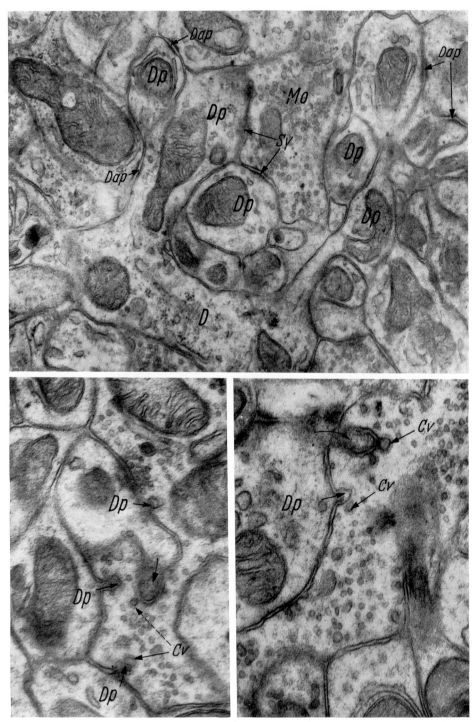

Fig. 74. Above: Arborization of granule cell dendrites (*D*) and their terminal bulbs or dendrite protrusions (*Dp*) that establish synaptic contacts (*Sy*) with tangentially cut part of mossy rosette (*Mo*). Desmosomoid attachment plaques (*Dap*) of symmetric structure between dendritic ends are frequent. — Below: Microspines of the dendritic protrusions (*Dp*) (arrows) are embedded into invaginations of axonal profiles. At the invaginations the formation of vesicular structures can be seen that resemble the bodies described by Gray (1961) as complex vesicles (*Cv*)

granules situated beneath the thickened part of the subsynaptic membrane, much like those described in sympathetic ganglia by TAXI (1962). Desmosomoid attachment plaques between dendritic protrusions (Figs. 67 and 74) with symmetric thickenings of both membranes are frequent. A very peculiar feature regularly encountered in some material, while almost completely lacking in others from the

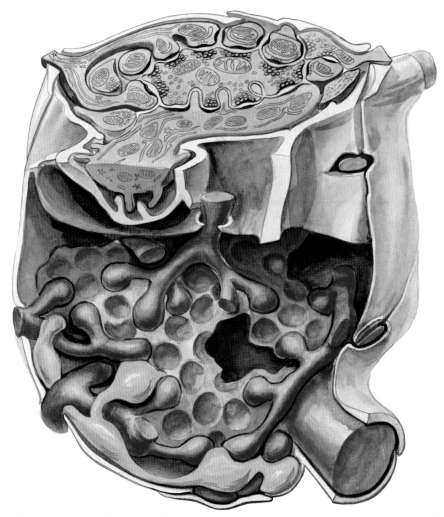

Fig. 75. Stereodiagram illustrating the structure of the cerebellar glomerulus. Mossy rosette blue, granule dendrites red, Golgi axon yellow, Golgi dendrite green, glial capsule grey

same species, are microspines of the dendrite protrusions invaginating the mossy rosettes (Fig. 74). They never occur at sites of specified contacts, i.e. membrane thickenings, but always at some distance. So called "complex vesicles" are often found in immediate neighbourhood of the invaginations in the rosettes. One wonders whether their absence in some and presence in other material does not indicate that this structure is the morphological substrate of slow functional change or exchange in materials between the synapsing elements. The occurrence of complex vesicles in immediate neighbourhood of the invaginations might indicate also that it is a mechanism of vesicle formation. But all these assumptions are hypothetical and the strange observation needs further elucidation.

5. Summary of Glomerulus Structure

The cerebellar glomerulus is thus a highly complex, but structurally standard synaptic system. There is no evidence whatsoever of mossy rosettes having synaptic contacts with any other elements excepting granule dendrite protrusions and Golgi cell dendrites. Both kinds of contacts may occur in the same glomerulus. While the mossy rosette occupies the center of the glomerulus, the Golgi axon terminals contact the granule dendrites from the outside, opposite to their contacts with the mossy rosette and often centrad, i.e. "downstream" if the direction of impulse is considered. The unit character of the glomerulus is emphasized by its good insulation from the environment by a thin glial layer. Fig. 75 attempts to give a stereoscopic, somewhat diagrammatic view of the glomerulus summarizing all information presented in this Section B.

C. Potentials that a Mossy Fiber Volley generates in the Granular Layer

Various procedures have been employed in the attempt to investigate the responses produced in the cerebellar cortex by a mossy fiber input. For example, as indicated in Fig. 81 A, B, stimuli have been applied through electrodes in the following locations: on the dorsal or ventral spino-cerebellar tracts in the cervical cord; on the nerves of the forelimb; in the external cuneate nucleus or the lateral reticular nucleus. But routinely there is a stimulating electrode in the region of the fastigial nucleus (the juxta-fastigial or J.F. electrode in Fig. 76); and stimuli so applied usually excite Purkinje cell axons and/or climbing fibers as well as mossy fibers (Figs. 47 C, D; 79 A; 90).

As illustrated in Fig. 76, the technique of transfolial (T.F.) stimulation has frequently been employed in order to give pure mossy fiber inputs.

There is an extremely wide dispersal of the branches of a single mossy fiber, some going at least as far as the adjacent folium (Fig. 19). Hence, by a kind of axon-reflex in the branching mossy fibers (Fig. 76), it is possible by T.F. stimulation to subject the cerebellar cortex to the action of a mossy fiber volley uncontaminated by the other inputs, which could be via climbing fibers and Purkinje cell axons (ECCLES, LLINÁS and SASAKI, 1966c; ECCLES, SASAKI and STRATA, 1967a), as so often occurs with J.F. stimulation. Alternate stimulation through J.F. and T.F. electrodes provides the information required for identifying the components of the J.F. responses that are due to the mossy fiber input. More recently SASAKI and STRATA (1967) have accomplished a systematic analysis of the pure mossy fiber inputs produced by stimulation of the lateral reticular nucleus, the external cuneate nucleus, and the spinocerebellar tracts (Fig. 81 A, B). The only complication was that, with stimuli applied over the DSCT, there was superimposed on the mossy fiber response a much later (about 10 msec) response attributable to climbing fibers (Chapter VIII).

1. Presynaptic and Postsynaptic Potentials

A weak T.F. stimulus generates in the granular layer a potential wave form (Fig. 77 A), which is similar to that recorded extracellularly in simple monosynaptic systems, such as the monosynaptic activation of motoneurones or interneurones in the spinal cord (ECCLES, 1957, pages 36—38). There is an initial diphasic (positive-negative, $P_1 N_1$) spike potential generated by the mossy fiber impulses after a

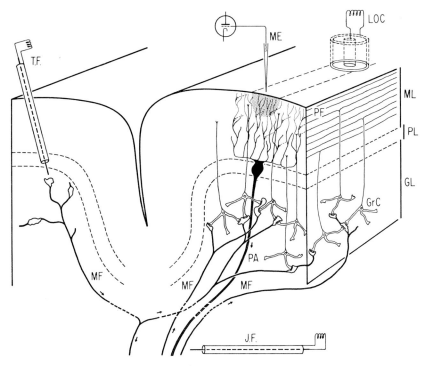

Fig. 76. *Perspective drawing of two cerebellar folia* to show the anatomical relays from mossy fibers (*MF*) through granule cells (*GrC*) and their axons, the parallel fibers (*PF*), to Purkinje cells and the experimental arrangements for juxtafastigial (J.F.), transfolial (T.F.) and local (LOC) stimulations. *ML:* molecular layer. *PL:* Purkinje cell layer. *GL:* granular layer. A recording micro-electrode (*ME*) is drawn in position for penetrating the cerebellar cortex through the parallel fiber beam elicited by the LOC stimulation. The J.F. electrode stimulates mossy fibers in the depth of the white matter, and the T.F. concentric electrode, with the tip placed in the granular layer of adjacent folium, activates mossy fibers there. Both of these mossy fiber volleys converge onto the recording locus, as shown by arrows. (ECCLES, SASAKI and STRATA, 1967 a)

fairly long trasfolial path, and a later slow negative wave, the EPSP. In Fig. 77 B the negative phase of the initial presynaptic spike has a latency of 0.5 msec, which indicates fairly rapid conduction in the transfolial mossy fiber pathway from the adjacent folium. The synaptic delays in A and B may be measured from the onset of N_1 (first arrow) to the onset of the EPSP, the respective values of 0.3 and 0.4 msec being typical durations for the synaptic delays of central synapses.

As would be expected for a directly excited nerve response, the presynaptic component follows a frequency of 500/sec in Fig. 77 C. At this frequency the

EPSP component rapidly fails, so leaving as the principal repetitive response the succession of triphasic presynaptic spike potentials, the initial $P_1 N_1$ being followed by a terminal positivity. Similarly in D and E, where the J. F. stimulus excited only mossy fibers, so producing an initial $P_1 N_1$ wave and a later EPSP, only the pre-synaptic $P_1 N_1$ potentials are well maintained during the repetitive stimulations at 330 and 500/sec.

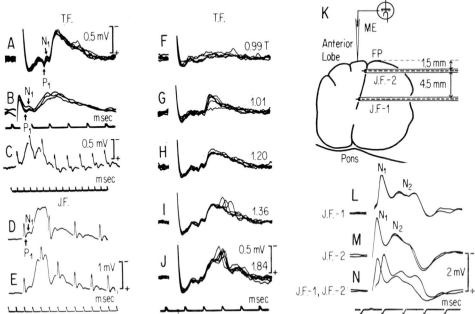

Fig. 77 A—N. *Field potentials produced by impulses in mossy fibers and by excitatory synaptic currents in granule cells.* In A, T. F. stimulation was given to a folium next but one to the recording site. F to J were recorded with the same arrangements, as A and B but under less favourable conditions several minutes later. The strength of the T. F. stimulus was increased from F to J as indicated relative to the threshold strength. Depth of the recording microelectrode was at $500\,\mu$ from the surface of the cerebellar cortex. Similar potential sequences at $500\,\mu$ depth in another cerebellar cortex are illustrated in B. As seen in C only the $P_1 N_1$ potential followed the repetitive T. F. stimulation at a frequency of 500/sec. In D and E J. F. stimulation excited only mossy fibers, and with repetitive stimulation only the $P_1 N_1$ response survived at 500/sec (E). L—N: N_1 and N_2 field potentials recorded with a microelectrode (*ME*) at a fixed position in the granular layer and elicited by two different J. F. electrodes which have been placed at a depth of 6.0 mm (J.F.-1) and 1.5 mm (J.F.-2) from the surface of the cerebellar cortex, as illustrated schematically in K, *FP* being the fissura prima. L shows the potential sequence set up by the J.F.-1 stimulation and M that by J.F.-2, the depth of the microelectrode being at $450\,\mu$. N is a superimposed record of responses to J.F.-1 and J.F.-2 stimulations. (Eccles, Sasaki and Strata, 1967 a)

The series of finely graded T. F. stimulations (Fig. 77 F to J) show that the EPSP exhibits quite a large all-or-nothing component (G), which must be the response evoked by a single mossy fiber. With a considerable increase in the T. F. stimulation, there seem to be further small increases in the EPSP. Under such conditions small spike potentials are often superimposed on the EPSP wave (Fig. 77 I, J), and further evidence will be presented later in support of their identification as impulse discharges in single granule neurones.

Evidence has been given in Chapters V and VI that with J.F. stimulation the dominant component of the diphasic $P_1 N_1$ response undoubtedly is the antidromic spike in Purkinje cell axons, somata and dendrites. For example the Purkinje cell IPSP produced by a parallel fiber volley produces a large depression of the N_1 spike component (Figs. 50, 51, 52, 61). Nevertheless, the experiment illustrated in Fig. 77 K—N shows that the mossy fiber spike potential is superimposed upon the antidromic Purkinje spike.

In the experimental arrangement (Fig. 77 K) one stimulating electrode is as usual in the juxta-fastigial region, and the other is at a depth of 1.5 mm from the surface of the cerebellar cortex and is 4.5 mm closer to the recording site. Fig. 77 L and M show respectively the N_1 and N_2 potentials with the usual locus for J. F. stimulation and with a 4.5 mm shorter conduction distance. The initial part of N_2 is the EPSP of granule cells, and later there are superimposed spike potentials of Golgi and granule cells as in Figs. 41 and 77 J. The recording electrode is in a fixed position and records are taken in alternating sequence with stimulus strengths chosen so as to match the respective N_1 and N_2 waves as closely as possible. In L the summits of both the N_1 and the N_2 waves had 0.26 msec longer latency than in M, the difference being well displayed in the superimposed traces of N. It can be concluded that in this experiment the conduction velocities of the mossy fiber impulses responsible for evoking the N_2 wave by synaptic action are approximately the same as for the Purkinje axon impulses that directly produce the bulk of N_1. The calculated velocity of about 17 m/sec for both Purkinje axons and mossy fibers is in good agreement with their equivalent diameter and their medullated character. Mossy fibers are medullated throughout their length, even into the granular layer (GRAY, 1961; Fox et al., 1967).

The $P_1 N_1$ potential produced by a pure mossy fiber input is seen with responses evoked in the granular layer by stimulation of the LRN (Figs. 81 C; 82 J, L) and of the VSCT (Fig. 81 E). As expected these $P_1 N_1$ potentials are not depressed by a conditioning LOC stimulus (Figs. 81 D, F; 82 K, M; SASAKI and STRATA, 1967). The conduction velocities for these mossy fiber volleys are usually in the range of 30 to 40 m/sec, which, as would be expected, is considerably faster than the velocity indicated in Fig. 77 K—N for the profusely branching terminals of the mossy fibers.

2. Spike Potentials from Cells in the Granular Layer

As described and illustrated in Chapter I (Figs. 7, 15, 16), neurohistological investigations disclose the existence in the granular layer of two quite distinct types of nerve cell: the enormous population of the very small granule cells; and the much more rare, but much larger, Golgi cells, of which there are several subvarieties. On the basis of these histological findings it is possible to design experimental tests that distinguish sharply between the spike potentials generated by these two cellular components. In Chapter IV there are accounts of spike potentials recorded in the granular layer at a depth of about 500 μ that may with assurance be identified as due to Golgi cells.

For example, in Fig. 39 N—Q there are high frequency repetitive responses generated by the synaptic excitatory action of a parallel fiber volley, and Fig. 40 A—J illustrates the facilitatory action of one parallel fiber volley on the responses evoked by a subsequent volley. These Golgi cells conform with the most common histological variety in that their dendrites are preponderantly in the molecular layer where they receive excitatory synapses from parallel fibers (cf. Figs. 15, 16). These cells are excited by juxta-fastigial stimulation, but with such a long latency (cf. Fig. 39 M and Table 1) that the pathway can be presumed to be by mossy fibers to granule cells to parallel fibers to excitatory synapses on the Golgi cell dendrites in the molecular layer, and not by the synapses that mossy fibers make directly with Golgi cell dendrites in the granular layer (Fig. 72). In Fig. 41 A—H are responses of a cell that is identified as a Golgi cell because of its depth (450 μ) and its excitation by a parallel fiber volley (A—C) though much less powerfully than the Golgi cells of Figs. 39 O—Q and 40 A—J. But in addition a mossy fiber volley set up by J. F. stimulation monosynaptically evokes a spike discharge (Fig. 41 D—G). It may be presumed that the dendrites of this Golgi cell are distributed less to the molecular and more to the granular layer. And corresponding to the deep Golgi cells with dendrites confined to the granular layer, there is the cell at 480 μ depth (Fig. 41 I—L) with a strong monosynaptic excitation by mossy fibers and no spike response to a parallel fiber volley. The conditioning action of a parallel fiber volley sharply distinguishes these deep Golgi cells from granule cells, the former being not inhibited (Fig. 41 B, L), whereas, as we shall now see, granule cells invariably are (Figs. 78, 83 A—F).

In Fig. 78 A stimulation of the superficial radial nerve evokes after a latency of 7.5 msec a brief burst discharge of a cell in the granular layer, the pathway probably being via the cuneo-cerebellar tract with its mossy fiber terminations (GRANT, 1962; HOLMQVIST, OSCARSSON and ROSÉN, 1963). This response is completely inhibited by a conditioning LOC stimulus in B, there being progressive recovery at longer testing intervals in C and D. There is a similar burst response to another cell (Fig. 78 E) in response to the mossy fiber volleys set up by stimulation of the external cuneate nucleus (LCN), and it is completely inhibited by a preceding similar stimulus at brief intervals (F, G) and even at 25 msec (H) there is reduction of the second response to one spike. In Fig. 78 J, K and L a preceding LOC stimulus of progressively increasing strength also results in an inhibition of the discharge (I) evoked by a LCN stimulus. The identification of this cell as a granule cell is supported by the finding that a LOC stimulus evokes a single discharge (M—O), presumably by antidromic invasion from the parallel fiber that is its axon.

The spike potentials of granule cells are to be recognized by the following criteria, on the basis of which the spikes of Figs. 77 I, J and 78 are identified as being produced by granule cells: they must be recorded in the granular layer, that is 400 to 700 μ deep to the surface of the folium; they do not fire antidromically to a J. F. stimulus, as do Purkinje cells (Fig. 42), nor orthodromically in response to a parallel fiber volley as do most Golgi cells (Figs. 38—40), which also lie in the granular layer (Chapter IV); they are not activated synaptically by a parallel

fiber volley, but they may be invaded antidromically (Fig. 78 L—O). It is important to remember that strong LOC stimulation can directly set up impulses in
mossy fibers, just as occurs with T.F. stimulation, which then synaptically evoke
the discharges of granule cells. However such responses are easily distinguished
from the Golgi cell discharges evoked by a LOC stimulus, because a preceding LOC
stimulus results in an increased Golgi cell discharge (Fig. 40 A—C, I, J) and in
inhibition of granule cell discharges (Fig. 78). In general the granule cell spikes

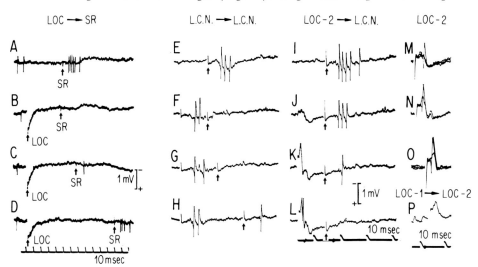

Fig. 78 A—P. *Responses of single granule cells.* In A a single granule cell was fired repetitively by
a single stimulus to the superficial radial nerve (*SR*). In B to D this response was inhibited by a
conditioning LOC stimulus which preceded the *SR* stimulus at increasing intervals. Stimulus artifacts
are marked with arrows. E. Repetitive firing of a granule cell evoked by a stimulus to the external
cuneate nucleus (*L.C.N.*), with inhibition in F—H by a preceding similar *L.C.N.* stimulus. In
J—L the response to a *L.C.N.* stimulus (control in I) is progressively more inhibited as the strength
of the conditioning LOC-2 stimulus in increased. M—P: Presumed antidromic invasion of a granule
cell by LOC-2 stimulation is seen as a unitary spike superimposed on the field potential and is
inhibited by LOC-1 in P. All records E—P have same time and potential scales; stimuli marked
with arrows. (ECCLES, LLINÁS and SASAKI, 1966 c)

have the very small size that would be expected for such small cells, and the spike
potentials of a single cell are difficult to isolate clearly from the background of
spike potentials generated by the densely packed adjacent granule cells.

The only neuronal element that could be concerned in the inhibitory action on
the mossy fiber-granule cell synapses in the glomeruli of the granular layer is the
Golgi cell, because it alone has synaptic endings on the dendrites of granule cells
(Figs. 71, 73, 75). Parallel fiber volleys powerfully excite Golgi cells by the synapses on their dendritic spines (Chapter IV), and it is postulated that the Golgi cell
axonal terminals in the glomeruli cause the inhibition of granule cells demonstrated in Figs. 78 and 83 A—F. Furthermore, the inhibition produced by mossy
fiber stimulation (Fig. 78 E—H) is similarly explained, for the excited mossy
fibers in turn activate granule cells and the parallel fibers stemming therefrom, and
in addition mossy fiber impulses *directly* excite Golgi cells (Figs. 41, 72).

On the other hand, the axonal terminals of Golgi cells do not form synapses on the dendrites of Golgi cells (HÁMORI and SZENTÁGOTHAI, 1966b), a finding which is in agreement with the failure of parallel fiber volleys to inhibit the mossy fiber — Golgi cell synapses (Fig. 41 F, L; 82 E—H). In contrast, a conditioning J. F. stimulus depresses the production of a Golgi cell spike by a later testing J. F. stimulus (Fig. 41 H and J). Two alternative explanations can be offered: the inhibitory action of Purkinje cell axon collaterals on Golgi cells (Fig. 105 A—H; ECCLES, LLINÁS and SASAKI, 1966a), for which there is anatomical evidence (Figs. 18, 102 E); the diminished effectiveness of synapses for some time after their activation, which to a large extent appears to be due to diminished transmitter output (cf. ECCLES, 1964, pp. 83—93).

D. Depth Profiles in the Cerebellar Cortex

The further study of mossy fiber action requires an investigation of the potentials produced at all depths of the cortex and the effect of graded levels of Golgi cell inhibition on these potentials. Usually the large potentials produced by J. F. stimulation have been used for this purpose, but suffer from the disadvantage that there may be superimposed potentials produced by climbing fiber impulses. It is therefore important to have confirmatory evidence with pure mossy fiber inputs such as are produced with T. F. stimulation (Figs. 80 E, F; 82 C, D) or with lateral reticular nucleus (LRN) or ventral spinocerebellar tract (VSCT) stimulation (Figs. 81 C, D, E, F; 82 J—M). The investigations on chronically deafferented cerebella reveal that, with antidromic impulses in Purkinje cell axons, the initial large negative spike response is followed only by a slow positive wave of low amplitude and about 15 msec duration (Figs. 43, 44, 45, 50). No complex complicating wave forms are therefore introduced if the J. F. stimulus excites Purkinje axons.

In Fig. 79 A there is a depth spectrum of the field potentials generated by a J. F. stimulus. Since the complex wave forms produced by a mossy fiber volley have a standard configuration, it is convenient to label the negative waves N_1 to N_4 and the positive P_1 to P_3. At depths of 350 to 550 µ the initial diphasic spike (positive-negative, $P_1 N_1$) leads on immediately to a brief negative wave (N_2), with traces of a double summit, that is abruptly terminated by a sharp positive wave (P_2), and subsequently there is a brief negative wave (N_4) and a terminal slow positive wave (P_3). The response at a depth of 250 µ appears to be transitional to the quite different wave form at depths of 200 to 100 µ. Over this range of depths the $P_1 N_1$ wave sharply decrements, as already fully described in Chapter V, and a negative wave (N_3) appears, its onset being synchronous with the onset of the P_2 wave in the granular layer. Since T. F. (Fig. 80 E), LRN (Fig. 81 C) and VCST (Fig. 81 E) stimulations evoke the same complex of wave forms under comparable conditions of recording, the whole complex from N_2 to P_3 must be evoked by the mossy fiber volley. The inhibitory action resulting from a parallel fiber volley has given very important information in the attempt to discover the mode of production of this complex wave form.

The traces of Fig. 79 B and C correspond to those of A, except that they are inhibited as a consequence of a LOC stimulus some 17.2 msec earlier, which is weak in B and stronger in C. The stronger LOC stimulus (C) reduces, but does not suppress, the N_2 wave at depths from 350 to 550 µ, but the P_2 wave is greatly reduced and N_4 and P_3 are suppressed. At depths of 100 to 200 µ, the spike-like components of N_3 are completely suppressed in C, there remaining only a slow negative wave that exactly conforms to the wave that would be expected for the synaptic excitatory potentials on Purkinje cell dendrites, the EPSP of Fig. 63 E. The weaker LOC stimulation in Fig. 79 B produces only a partial suppression of the spike components of the N_3 potential, which at depths of 150 and 200 µ can be seen superimposed on the background slow negative wave.

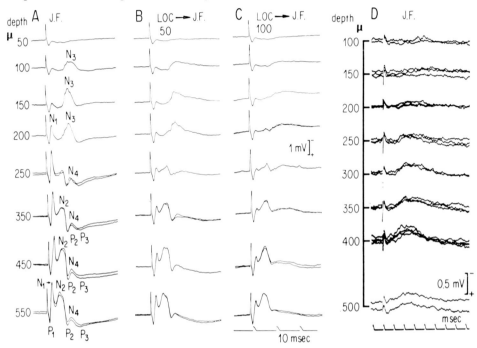

Fig. 79 A—D. *Depth profiles of potentials generated in cerebellar cortex by juxta-fastigial stimulation.* A—C show the potential wave forms evoked by a J.F. stimulus that excited both mossy fibers and Purkinje cell axons, and that are recorded by a microelectrode at the indicated depths below the surface. The labelling of the waves N_1 to N_4 and P_1 to P_3 is described in the text. B and C show the same depth profile of responses evoked by the same J.F. stimulus, but with conditioning by a weak and strong LOC stimulus (50 and 100 strength) 17.2 msec earlier. D shows responses evoked in another experiment at the indicated depths by a very weak J.F. stimulus that apparently excited only mossy fibers. (ECCLES, SASAKI and STRATA, 1967 a)

Fig. 80 A shows in another experiment a similar series of potentials that a J.F. stimulus evokes at all depths in the cerebellar cortex, but the N_1 wave is smaller and N_4 is larger. Just as in Fig. 79 B, conditioning by a parallel fiber volley converts the large N_3 wave at depths of 100 to 250 µ into a small slow potential wave on which are superimposed occasional small spikes (Fig. 80 B). Again, at depths of 300 to 400 µ in Fig. 80 B, conditioning by a parallel fiber volley greatly reduces the P_2 and N_4 waves of Fig. 80 A. In Fig. 80 C a weaker J.F. stimulus is seen to set up a similar series of potential waves at corresponding depths except that the N_4

wave is greatly reduced. The conditioning parallel fiber volley exerts a more effective inhibitory action (Fig. 80 D), the small surviving N_1 being followed at all

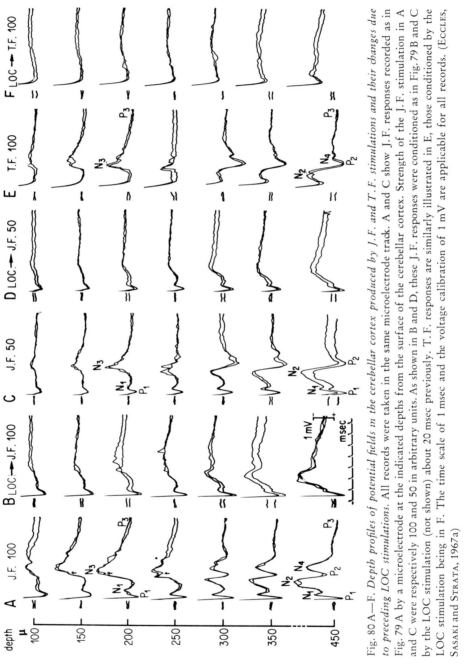

Fig. 80 A—F. Depth profiles of potential fields in the cerebellar cortex produced by J.F. and T.F. stimulations and their changes due to preceding LOC stimulations. All records were taken in the same microelectrode track. A and C show J.F. responses recorded as in Fig. 79 A by a microelectrode at the indicated depths from the surface of the cerebellar cortex. Strength of the J.F. stimulation in A and C were respectively 100 and 50 in arbitrary units. As shown in B and D, these J.F. responses were conditioned as in Fig. 79 B and C by the LOC stimulation (not shown) about 20 msec previously. T.F. responses are similarly illustrated in E, those conditioned by the LOC stimulation being in F. The time scale of 1 msec and the voltage calibration of 1 mV are applicable for all records. (ECCLES, SASAKI and STRATA, 1967a)

depths by a smooth slow negative potential wave. This wave is largest at 450 μ depth. More superficially it progressively declines in size and its summit is a little more delayed.

138

With T. F. stimulation in this same experiment (Fig. 80 E) the N_2 wave at depths of 300 to 400 μ resembles the weaker J. F.-evoked N_2 wave in C, and there is a similar sequence of a P_2 wave and a small N_4 wave. At 250 to 100 μ the N_3 waves are also comparable. Finally, in Fig. 80 F conditioning by a parallel fiber volley reduces the T. F.-evoked response to a slow negative potential resembling that in D, the only difference being a small surviving spike-like component of the N_2 wave at 400 μ depth.

Since the T. F.-evoked responses of Fig. 80 E and F are so similar to the J. F.-evoked responses of C and D, it is justifiable to assume as above that under the conditions of this experiment the J. F. stimulus, like the T. F. stimulus, is exciting mossy fibers, and that it is not exciting any of the climbing fibers passing to the region of the cerebellar cortex under investigation. The identification of climbing fiber responses will be described in Chapter VIII.

Further evidence for the purity of the mossy fiber responses of Figs. 79 A—C and 80 A—D is provided by the similarity of the depth profiles of LRN- and VSCT-evoked responses in Fig. 81 C and E and of the effects of conditioning by a LOC stimulus in D and F (SASAKI and STRATA, 1967).

E. The Mode of Production of the N_2 Potential

With the weak T. F. stimulation of Fig. 77 A, the N_2 wave has the typical configuration of an extracellularly recorded EPSP with a rise to a rounded summit in about 1 msec, from which there is a gradual decline over several milliseconds. In Fig. 79 D a weak J. F. stimulation also produces a small N_2 wave having the typical EPSP configuration, and this slow negative wave rapidly decrements in size with more superficial recording.

An N_2 wave with this EPSP configuration is much more readily obtained by employing a parallel fiber volley to inhibit the T. F.- or J. F.-evoked responses. For example, in Fig. 80 D the N_2 response is inhibited so that it has the EPSP configuration, being very similar to Fig. 79 D. It has already been noted that this potential is progressively diminished with more superficial recording, but retains this configuration of a slow negative wave. With T.F. and VSCT stimulation, inhibitory conditioning also converts the N_2 wave virtually into slow negative potentials (Figs. 80 F and 81 F).

Except when there is just threshold stimulation or the inhibition of weak responses, a mossy fiber input sets up an N_2 wave of a spike-like character which usually has a double summit (Figs. 77 L—N; 79 A; 80 A, C, E; 81 C, E; 82 E, J, L). Comparison of the inhibited records of Figs. 80, 81 and 82 with the corresponding uninhibited records suggests that the generation of impulses by Golgi cells and granule cells is likely to be concerned in the production of these spike-like N_2 responses.

When a fine microelectrode is very carefully manipulated in the granular layer, it is sometimes possible to record spike potentials from single granule cells and to maintain recording conditions stable during a systematic investigation. For example in Fig. 83 A unitary spike potentials are superimposed on the N_2 wave, there often being no more than a single spike in each trace. The spikes are seen to fluctuate

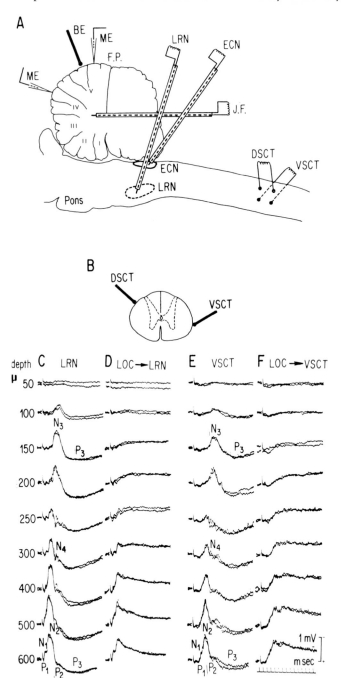

Fig. 81 A—F. A and B. Diagrams illustrating the experimental set up to stimulate juxta-fastigial region (*J. F.*), lateral reticular neclcus (*LRN*), external cuneate (*ECN*), dorsal spino-cerebellar tract (*DSCT*) and ventral spino-cerebellar tract (*VSCT*). Responses evoked by these stimulations were recorded with a microelectrode (*ME*) at various depths from the surface of the cerebellar cortex and also with a silver ball electrode (*BE*) from the surface of the cortex. C—F. Field potentials of the cerebellar cortex in lobulus IV produced by *LRN* (C) and *VSCT* (E) stimulations, and conditioned by a preceding LOC stimulation (by about 20 msec) in D and F. All records were obtained in the same microelectrode track at the indicated depths below the cortical surface. (Sasaki and Strata, 1967)

in latency, but to cluster at a time just later than the first summit of the N_2 wave and even during the earlier part of P_2 (Fig. 83 C, E). The time course of the N_2 wave is more easily appreciated in the inhibited responses of Fig. 83 D, F. This timing in relation to the N_2 wave is also shown in Fig. 77 I, J for a spike potential that likewise is assumed to be due to a granule cell.

In contrast to this relatively late position of the granule cell spikes, the Golgi cell spikes of Fig. 41 D, I, K, L are located very early on the N_2 wave, even with

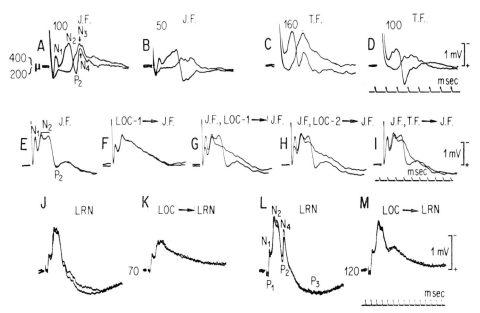

Fig. 82 A—M. *Field potentials evoked by mossy fiber volleys and their conditioning by preceding LOC or T. F. stimulation.* On each frame of A to D are superimposed traces recorded in the same microelectrode track at 200 μ and 400 μ depths with J.F. or T.F. stimulation of the indicated strengths in a linear scale. E shows a J.F. response recorded at 400 μ depth in another experiment and in F it was conditioned by a preceding LOC-1 stimulation. G is a superimposed record of similar conditioned and unconditioned responses. In H and I are superimposed traces as in G, conditioning being by a different LOC stimulation (LOC-2) in H and by a T.F. stimulation in I. Same time and voltage scales for A to D, and for E to I. (ECCLES, SASAKI and STRATA, 1967 a). J and L are potentials evoked by weak (70) and strong (120) stimulation of the lateral reticular nucleus and recorded in the granular layer at a depth of 450 μ. The inhibitory action of a preceding LOC stimulus is seen in K and M. (SASAKI and STRATA, 1967)

a just threshold stimulation (ECCLES, SASAKI and STRATA, 1967 a). It, therefore, is proposed that the double summit often exhibited by the N_2 wave (cf. Figs. 77 L—N; 79 A, B; 80; 82 E—M) arises because of the latency differential between the initiation of spike discharges in Golgi cells and granule cells respectively. It is certainly unexpected that there is this delayed initiation of spike discharges evoked monosynaptically in granule cells. However it has been demonstrated that summation of the excitatory actions of two or more mossy fiber impulses is required to initiate impulse discharges in granule cells (cf. Fig. 77 G—J), particularly when under the influence of Golgi cell inhibition (cf. Figs. 80 B, D;

141

81 D, F), whereas the large synaptic contact of a single mossy fiber expansion with a Golgi cell dendrite (Fig. 72) seems to be adequate to set up a dendritic spike potential (Fig. 41). Thus the delay of the granule cell spike is attributable to the delays involved in electrotonic transmission of the EPSP to the soma or axon hillock in order that summation to the firing level can occur.

The series of Fig. 82 E—I provides a good illustration of the composite nature of the double-peaked N_2 wave (E) that is evoked by a mossy fiber volley. In F a conditioning parallel fiber volley depresses the N_1 spike and also the second spike but not the first spike of N_2, this effect being well seen in the superimposed traces of G. Another parallel fiber volley has a similar action in H. In the superimposed traces of I, with conditioning by a previous J. F. stimulus, there is no depression of N_1, and only a slight depression and delay of the first component of N_2, but the second component is again much more depressed. The striking differential effect on the two components of the N_2 wave in F, G and H conforms precisely with the observations on the spike responses of single Golgi and granule cells in Figs. 41, 78 and 83 A—F.

In conclusion it can be stated that a mossy fiber volley causes the production of the N_2 wave in the granular layer by its excitatory synaptic action on both granule and Golgi cell dendrites in the glomerulus as described and illustrated by HÁMORI and SZENTÁGOTHAI (1966 a; 1966 b; and Section B of this Chapter). The N_2 wave is compounded of the EPSPs and spike potentials of both of these cell types.

F. The Mode of Production of the P_2 and N_3 Potentials

In the depth series of J. F. responses in Fig. 80 A the onset of the P_2 wave following N_2 in the granular layer is synchronous with the onset of the N_3 wave in the molecular layer. With all mossy fiber inputs there is this exact temporal correspondence when both P_2 and N_3 waves are well developed (cf. Figs. 79 A, 80 A, 81 C, E); and it is well illustrated by the superimposed traces in Fig. 82 A—D, where there is also a good correlation between the sizes of these respective waves if allowance be made for the antagonistic N_4 in A and C. In Figs. 79 B and 80 B conditioning by a parallel fiber volley reduces the size of P_2, and correspondingly there is a reduction of N_3; and in Figs. 79 C, 80 D, 81 D and F, when there is great reduction or abolition of P_2, there is only a very small slow N_3 wave in the molecular layer.

Evidently these positive (P_2) and negative (N_3) waves represent the field potentials generated by sources in the granular layer and sinks in the molecular layer. The great bulk of the core-conductor elements linking these two layers is provided by two neural constituents: the granule cells with their axons running perpendicularly into the molecular layer before bifurcating to form the parallel fibers; and the Purkinje cells that have their great branching dendritic trees in the molecular layer and their axons with their collaterals in the granular layer. There is good evidence that both of these structures are concerned in producing the observed field potential in the two layers — the granular P_2 wave and the molecular N_3 wave.

Since most granule cell spike discharges occur just at the end of the N_2 wave and at the onset of P_2 (Fig. 83 A), during the P_2 wave the granule cell somata and dendrites would be passive sources for the sinks generated by the propagation of these impulses along their axons — up to the molecular layer and then along the parallel fibers. The predicted diphasic (negative-positive) spike potentials are observed at an intermediate level deep in the molecular layer, for example at 250 μ in Figs. 79 A, B, C and 80 C, E. At these locations the initial negative component has a longer latency than the N_2 wave, as would be expected if it were due to impulses propagating up granule cell axons after their discharge at the second spike of the N_2 wave.

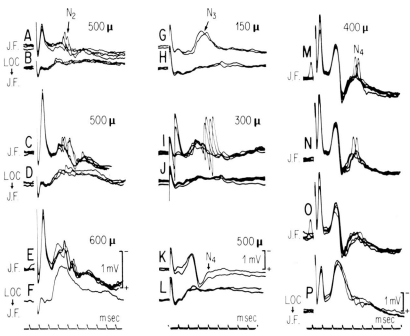

Fig. 83 A—P. *Neuronal spike potentials in relation to the potential waves set up by juxta-fastigial stimulation.* A, C and E show spike potentials (superimposed traces) evoked in several granule cells by J. F. stimulation, the inhibitory effects of a conditioning LOC stimulation (about 20 msec earlier) being shown in B, D and F respectively. E, F are responses of other granule cells 100 μ deeper. G, I and K show superimposed responses evoked at the indicated depths and in another experiment, the inhibitory effect of a conditioning LOC stimulation (about 20 msec earlier) being shown in H, J and L respectively. The superimposed traces of M to O show unitary spikes of a Purkinje cell sometimes superimposed on the N_4 wave produced by J. F. stimulation, P showing inhibitory effect of a conditioning LOC stimulation. (ECCLES, SASAKI und STRATA, 1967 a)

As the impulses discharged by the granule cells travel along the parallel fibers in the molecular layer, they will excite at the crossing-over synapses as described in Chapters IV and V, so setting up EPSPs in the Purkinje cell dendrites (cf. Figs. 47, 48 D—F, 84 A, F) as well as in the other dendrites of the molecular layer belonging to basket cells, outer stellate cells and Golgi cells (cf. Figs. 38 J and 39, L, M). Since both Purkinje cells and Golgi cells have somata deep to the molecular layer and profuse axonal branching in the granular layer, EPSPs generated on their dendrites would give rise very effectively to field potentials with active sinks in the molecular layer and passive sources in the granular layer. Presumably, such field potentials would contribute to the $P_2 N_3$ wave complex. When the responses to a mossy fiber input are inhibited by a conditioning parallel fiber volley, the N_3 potential has the typical configuration of an EPSP with a fairly rapid rise to a rounded summit and a much slower decline (Figs. 79 B at 100 μ; and 79 C at 200 to 100 μ; 80 B at 250 to 100 μ; 81 D at 200 to 100 μ). However, in the absence of such inhibition, it is evident that spike production in the molecular layer also contributes to the N_3 wave.

In Fig. 83 I at 300 μ depth there is a large unitary spike potential in 4 of the 5 superimposed traces of J. F. responses, the latencies ranging from 3.3 to 3.95 msec. This unitary response must arise from a Purkinje cell because in I there are three similar diphasic (positive-negative) spike potentials at the antidromic response latency — about 0.5 msec (cf. ECCLES, LLINÁS and SASAKI, 1966 e). At 150 μ depth there is a typical N_3 response (G), the negative potential at 300 μ (I) being transitional in latency between the N_2 wave at 500 μ (K) and the N_3 wave at 150 μ depth (G). However, the spike potentials at 300 μ occur, as expected, at the time of the latter part of the N_3 wave in G.

It is evident from these illustrations that the depth in the molecular layer at which large N_3 waves are recorded is too superficial for the recording of large Purkinje cell spike potentials. A comparable situation has been reported by ANDERSEN and LØMO (1966) for hippocampal pyramidal cells. The depth at which the impulses in the SCHAFFER collaterals evoke the largest extracellular EPSPs is unfavourable for recording the spike potentials generated by these EPSPs. However, as in Fig. 83 I large spike potentials are recorded from the dendrites nearer to the cell somata.

Thus it can be concluded that the principal components of the N_3 wave are produced, firstly, by the impulses in the granule cell axons, particularly in their longitudinal course as parallel fibers, and secondly, by the EPSPs generated by these impulses. The spike potentials generated in Purkinje cells also contribute to the N_3 wave at deeper levels of the molecular layer.

G. The Mode of Production of N_4 Potential

Since a mossy fiber input generates the discharge of impulses in Purkinje cells (Figs. 47 C, D, F and 83 I), and since these impulses would propagate down to the granular layer, it is important to see how well their latency fits them to be the generators of the N_4 wave. An invariable finding is that a large mossy fiber input is required to evoke an N_4 wave (cf. Fig. 80 A and C; Fig. 82 A and B, C and D, J and L) and it is very vulnerable to inhibition (cf. Fig. 79 A and C; Fig. 80 A and B; Fig. 82 L and M).

It was reported above that the Purkinje cell spikes in Fig. 83 at 300 μ depth correspond approximately in time to the small N_4 wave observed at 500 μ depth. In Fig. 83 M, N, with recording at 400 μ depth, unitary spike potentials of a Purkinje cell are superimposed on the N_4 wave. This Purkinje cell was firing spontaneously, and in two traces a spontaneous discharge so closely precedes the J. F. stimulus that the antidromic discharge is blocked in that trace (M, O), there being 3 to 5 superimposed traces in each record; hence the unitary spike may be identified as a Purkinje cell response. In Fig. 83 P, conditioning by a parallel fiber volley not only abolishes all unitary spike potentials, but it also virtually eliminates the N_4 wave. Similarly the N_4 wave in Fig. 79 A is inhibited by the conditioning LOC stimulation in a manner exactly paralleling the N_3 wave; the partial N_3 inhibition in B matches the partial N_4 inhibition, while in C both are totally inhibited. The latency of N_4 is also similar to the latency of the latter part of the N_3 wave. This correspondence of size and latency is well shown in Fig. 80 A, B and in the superimposed traces of Fig. 82 A and C.

If, as all these observations suggest, the N_4 wave is generated by the impulses discharged from Purkinje cells, impulse collision and refractoriness should cause a reduction in the antidromic spike potential (the N_1 wave) that is set up in Purkinje cells by a J. F. stimulus during and after the N_4 wave, and this is observed when the N_4 wave is large, but not when it is small or absent (ECCLES, SASAKI and STRATA, 1967 a).

H. The Mode of Production of the P_3 Wave

Following the N_3 and N_4 potentials in Figs. 79 A, 80 A, E, 81 C, E there is a slow positive wave (P_3) that is large at depths of 250 to 550 µ. Its time course and depth profile suggest that it is homologous to the positive wave produced by a parallel fiber volley set up by LOC stimulation (Figs. 58, 59), and hence that it is a consequence of the following sequence of actions: mossy fiber impulses exciting discharge of impulses from granule cells and so along parallel fibers — synaptic excitation of basket and outer stellate cells — inhibitory synaptic action on P-cell somata and dendrites with the consequent generation of the positive field potential. Fig. 79 C corroborates this explanation because inhibition of the granule cell discharge is accompanied by an apparent suppression of P_3, and with the lesser degree of granule cell inhibition in B there is a correspondingly lesser depression of P_3. An additional mode of production of P_3 is the Golgi cell postsynaptic inhibitory action on the granule cells. As a consequence there would be active sources in the granular layer to passive sinks on the axons of the granular cells (the parallel fibers in the molecular layer). The IPSPs responsible for the Purkinje cell component of the P_3 wave will now be studied by intracellular recording from P-cells.

I. Potentials Recorded Intracellularly from Purkinje Cells

1. EPSPs

Since EPSPs are recorded from Purkinje cells in response to parallel fiber volleys, it would be expected that T. F. or J. F. stimulation would also evoke EPSPs by the propagation of impulses along the pathway: mossy fibers to granule cells to parallel fibers.

Fig. 84 A and F are intracellular records of the EPSPs so evoked in response to J. F. and T. F. stimulation respectively, but the Purkinje cell is not activated to fire a discharge on account of partial deterioration (ECCLES, LLINÁS and SASAKI, 1966c). In Fig. 84 B—E the response to J. F. stimulation is conditioned by single stimuli of increasing strength through the LOC electrode 52 msec previously. As the conditioning strength is increased, the amplitude of the J. F.-evoked EPSP is very effectively decreased.

In Fig. 84 F—J, an EPSP evoked by T. F. stimulation is similarly depressed by a conditioning LOC stimulus. Evidently the J.F. stimulation is confined to mossy fibers, there being no sign of responses attributable to impulses in Purkinje cell axons or in climbing fibers. It will be noticed that the LOC stimulation evokes

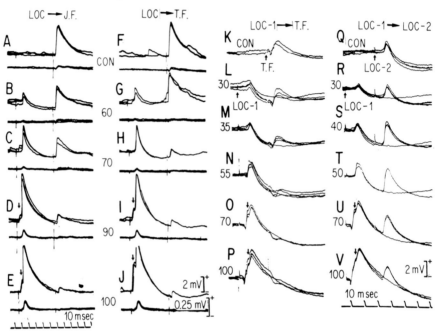

Fig. 84 A—V. *Intracellular EPSPs evoked in a Purkinje cell by various stimulations as indicated: J.F., T.F. and LOC.* A and F are control EPSPs produced by J.F. and T.F. stimulations respectively and B to E and G—J show depressions produced by a conditioning LOC stimulus of progressively increasing strength as indicated by the numbers 60 to 100. In records D, E and I, J direct mossy fiber activation by the LOC stimulus produces an EPSP (see arrows) preceding that directly evoked by parallel fiber activation. Series K—P resembles F—J, but in another experiment where the IPSP was large and not virtually neutralized by Cl⁻ injection out of the microelectrode as in A—J. Q to V is for same cell as in K—P, but with the response to a LOC stimulus (control in Q) conditioned by a previous LOC stimulus through another surface concentric electrode. Again the strengths of the conditioning LOC stimulations are indicated in an arbitrary linear scale. (ECCLES, LLINÁS and SASAKI, 1966 c)

only a small IPSP and not the large IPSP that usually follows activation of the parallel fibers. This reduction may be attributed to the spontaneous leakage of Cl⁻ ions into the impaled cell (COOMBS, ECCLES and FATT, 1955 a; ANDERSEN, ECCLES and VOORHOEVE, 1964; ECCLES, LLINÁS and SASAKI, 1966 f), and has the desirable consequence that the amplitude and duration of the EPSPs evoked by parallel fiber impulses can be determined with very little distortion by the simultaneously occurring IPSP.

Another example of this depression of the Purkinje cell EPSPs is illustrated in the intracellular records of Fig. 84 K—P. It will be noted in Fig. 84 K that the

T. F.-evoked EPSP reverses in about 10 msec to an IPSP (cf. subsection 2 below). The EPSPs produced by T. F. stimulation are progressively more depressed as the conditioning LOC stimulation is increased in strength (note the strengths in arbitrary units for records L—P). On the other hand, the EPSPs evoked in the same Purkinje cell by direct parallel fiber stimulation (LOC-2 stimulus) appear to be increased by the conditioning LOC-1 stimulations (Fig. 84 Q—V). The depression of the EPSPs generated by the T. F. stimulation is thus not occurring in the actions of parallel fiber impulses on the Purkinje cells, but must take place at the cerebellar glomeruli by the Golgi cell inhibitory action.

2. IPSPs

A mossy fiber input also produces IPSPs of Purkinje cells corresponding to the extracellularly recorded P_3 wave in Figs. 79 A; 81 C, E; 82 J, L; 83 E and M—O. As suggested in Section H of this Chapter the pathway would be: granule cells to parallel fibers to stellate or basket cells and so to inhibitory synapses on Purkinje cells. Fig. 85 D shows at high and low amplification both the intracellular and extracellular potentials generated by the parallel fiber volley evoked by a LOC stimulus. Subtraction of the latter from the former reveals that the induced membrane potential change is solely a hyperpolarisation (IPSP) having a latency of 3.8 msec and a voltage of —22 mV, thus resembling Fig. 48 G—K. A weak J. F. stimulus (Fig. 85 A) also evokes an IPSP of similar time course but smaller size. Stronger J. F. stimulation (B, C) excites the climbing fiber supplying this Purkinje cell (cf. Fig. 93); and, following the depolarization so induced, there is the prolonged hyperpolarization characteristic of the IPSP. Subtraction of the corresponding extracellular potential in C gives a value of —15 mV for the IPSP.

The full time courses of the IPSPs produced by J. F. and LOC stimulation can be compared in the respective series of Fig. 85 F—I and J—N, which are recorded at a slower sweep speed. Both of these series show responses at high and low amplifications to graded stimulations at the indicated strengths scaled in arbitrary units. The J. F. stimulation in H and I evokes an initial climbing fiber response, just as in B and C. However, subsequently to this response, the IPSP has virtually the same time course as when it is uncomplicated in this way, either with weaker J. F. stimulation (F, G), or with LOC-evoked IPSPs of comparable size (L—N). A total duration in excess of 120 msec for the IPSP is indicated by these records, which is in very good agreement with the duration of the inhibitory action on the antidromic invasion of Purkinje cells (Chapter V, Figs. 52, 53).

The finding that a mossy fiber input evokes an IPSP equivalent to that evoked by LOC stimulation (Figs. 85 and 86) is in accord with the explanation given in Section H of this Chapter for the slow late positive wave (P_3) that is observed extracellularly. Under various test situations the P_3 wave exhibits a behaviour similar to that of the slow positive wave produced by LOC stimulation.

Throughout the series of Fig. 85 E to N, small spike-like potentials appear at a fairly regular frequency of almost 100/sec. Similar potentials were observed by GRANIT and PHILLIPS (1956), the rhythmic wavelets or prepotentials. Possibly these potentials are generated by a rhythmic firing locus on some injured area of the cell, for example a small dendrite damaged by the microelectrode. However this may be, the response in Fig. 85 is valuable in signalling the duration of the IPSP, because it is completely suppressed throughout almost the whole duration of the IPSP; and, when it reappears at the terminal stage of the IPSP, it initially

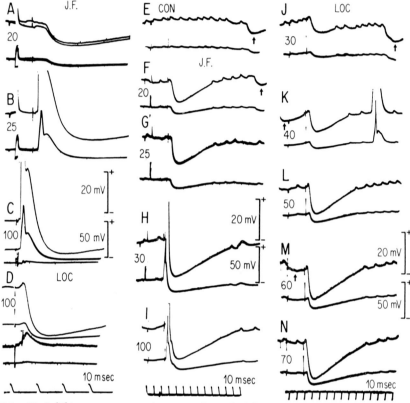

Fig. 85 A—N. *Inhibitory post-synaptic potentials evoked by LOC and J.F. stimulations.* Intracellular recording with a 10 MΩ potassium citrate microelectrode at 800 μ depth and with −50 mV resting potential. All intracellular records are shown at the same high and low amplification. E is control record of base line. In A—C, J.F. stimulation at the indicated strengths in arbitrary units. Immediately under the J.F. (100) response is the corresponding just extracellular trace at low amplification. In F—I there also was J.F. stimulation at the indicated strengths in arbitrary units, but at slower sweep speed (see time scale). In D there was LOC stimulation at strength 100, there being corresponding just extracellular traces immediately below and at the high and low amplification. J—N are LOC-evoked responses at the indicated strengths and same sweep speed as E—I. (ECCLES, LLINÁS and SASAKI, 1966 f)

fires at a low frequency and only resumes its initial frequency after the termination of the IPSP. It is thus a sensitive indicator of low levels of inhibitory action.

The IPSP generated by a mossy fiber input is depressed by a LOC stimulation in the same way as the EPSP in Fig. 84 A—P. For example the IPSP evoked in a Purkinje cell by J.F. stimulation (Fig. 86 A) is greatly depressed by preceding LOC stimulations of increasing strength (B—F). In another Purkinje cell (Fig. 86 G, H) the IPSP produced by LOC stimulation of the parallel fibers (G, upper record) is not much depressed by a conditioning volley through the same electrode (G, lower record), but in H this conditioning volley causes a much larger depression of a J. F.-evoked IPSP. Evidently, just as with the J. F.-evoked EPSP (Fig. 84 A—P), the parallel fiber volley has a powerful depressant action because it excites Golgi cells that inhibit the mossy fiber-granule cell relay.

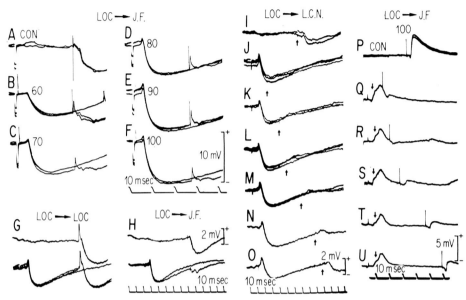

Fig. 86 A—U. *Golgi cell inhibition of IPSPs evoked in Purkinje cells by J. F. and L. C. N. (external cuneate nucleus) stimulation.* Record A is a control IPSP evoked in a Purkinje cell by a J. F. stimulation. In B—F, a preceding LOC stimulation of increasing strengths produced a graded depression of the J. F.-evoked IPSP, so that in E and F there was an almost complete suppression of the J. F.-evoked IPSP. The stimulus strengths are marked on the records in relative values. Upper record in G illustrates an IPSP evoked by a LOC stimulation in another Purkinje cell, and the lower record shows that a preceding LOC stimulation produced little change in this IPSP. On the contrary, as seen in H, an IPSP evoked in the same cell by J. F. stimulation was markedly depressed when conditioned by a LOC stimulation. Record I shows an IPSP evoked in a Purkinje cell by stimulating the L. C. N. In J—O, time course of the depression of this IPSP by a preceding LOC stimulation is seen at increasing time intervals. The arrows indicate the L. C. N. stimulus artefact. P—U. Time course of the Golgi inhibition that a conditioning LOC stimulus produces in the J. F.-evoked EPSP recorded in a Purkinje cell. P is the control EPSP produced by J. F. stimulation. As seen in Q to U, the depression of the EPSP by the LOC stimulus was greater at the shorter intervals. (ECCLES, LLINÁS and SASAKI, 1966 e)

J. The Time Course of Golgi Inhibition of the Mossy Fiber-Granule Cell Relay (Eccles, Sasaki and Strata, 1967 b)

Golgi cell inhibition of granule cell discharges has a duration in excess of 100 msec (Fig. 78 A—D), and there are corresponding durations for the presumed Golgi cell inhibition of the J. F.-evoked responses in the granular and molecular layer. When attempting to plot the time course of the inhibition of the mossy fiber-granule cell relay, several test responses can be used in addition to the discharges of granule cells. The most convenient are the N_3 and P_2 waves that are generated by the granule cell discharges as described in Section F of this Chapter. For example in Fig. 87 A the N_3 wave evoked by a J.F. stimulus and recorded at a depth of 150 μ (see the inset records) is used in determining the time course of the inhibition that is set up by a parallel fiber volley acting through Golgi cells and their inhibition of the mossy fiber-granule cell relay. The plotted points show that the inhibition appears with a testing interval as brief as 2—3 msec, the maximum being attained at about 14 msec, from which there is a slow, approximately expotential, decline. In Fig. 87 B the Golgi cell inhibition evoked by J.F. stimulation exhibits an even faster onset to a maximum with testing intervals as brief as 5 msec, after which there is a decline similar to that in A.

This rise of the Golgi cell inhibition to a maximum and the decay therefrom is much faster than the basket cell inhibition that is plotted in Figs. 52 G and 53 B, where there is a flat maximum with test intervals as long as 30 to 50 msec. By utilizing the P_2 wave to test for inhibition of the mossy fiber-granule cell relay it is possible to compare the time courses of the Golgi cell and basket cell inhibitions of the same test response. In Fig. 87 C and D the inset records show the way in which the P_2 and N_1 waves are measured, the former testing the Golgi cell and the latter the basket cell inhibition (cf. Fig. 52 G). The P_2 test gives a time course for Golgi cell inhibition (C) comparable with that given by the N_3 test in Fig. 87 A, while the basket cell inhibition (D) has the slower rise and much delayed decline already seen in Figs. 52 G and 53 B.

Fig. 86 I to O and P to U illustrate two other methods of testing for the time course of the Golgi cell inhibition evoked by a parallel fiber volley. In I to O the testing response is the IPSP evoked by a mossy fiber input (L.C.N. stimulation), and in O there is almost complete recovery by 90 msec. In P to V the testing response is the EPSP evoked by J.F. stimulation. The maximum inhibition occurs at the brief test intervals, Q and R, and there is considerable recovery at the longest test interval (U) of about 60 msec. These methods of testing thus give time courses comparable with those of Fig. 87 A and C.

It is a remarkable finding that there is such a large temporal discrepancy between the two kinds of inhibitory action set in train by a parallel fiber volley (Figs. 52, 53 and 87). The slow onset of the basket cell inhibition may be attributed to the special structure of the Purkinje cell baskets. This unique synaptic mechanism has the very extensive endings of the basket cell collaterals wrapping around the axonal pole of the Purkinje cell soma and the adjacent pre-axon, the whole complex being ensheathed in a glial lamella (Fig. 56; HÁMORI and SZENTÁGOTHAI, 1965; Fox et al., 1967). Furthermore, there are aggregates of vesicles in the presynaptic terminals at some distance from the presumed receptor sites on the Purkinje cell soma and pre-axon. Possibly the slow onset and long duration of the basket cell inhibition can be attributed to these anatomical features that cause both a gradual build up of transmitter action and its long continuance.

It has been suggested (PALAY, 1964; HÁMORI and SZENTÁGOTHAI, 1965; Fox et al., 1967) that this glial encapsulation of the basket terminals might have the same action as in the axon cap of the Mauthner cell (FURUKAWA and FURSHPAN, 1963), but there has been no evidence for this fast electrical inhibition. It is now postulated that the encapsulation serves to prevent the rapid dissipation of the inhibitory transmitter, which thus continues to act synaptically for 50 msec or more after release, so effecting the slow build up to the maximum of basket cell inhibitory action. In this way functional meaning may be given to the strange "bearded" structure of the basket terminals (Figs. 55, 56; HÁMORI and SZENTÁGOTHAI, 1965)

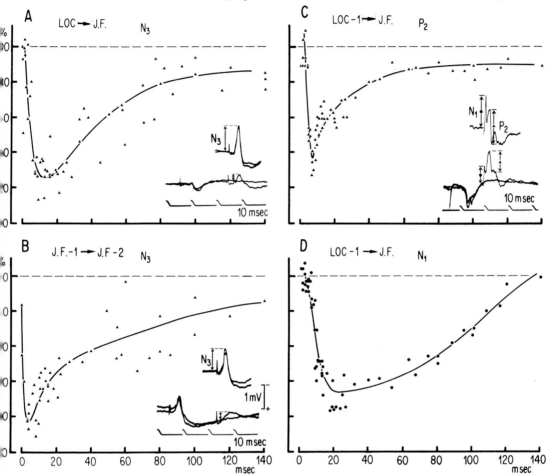

Fig. 87 A—D. *Time courses of Golgi cell and of basket cell inhibition.* In A and B the inhibitions were tested by a N_3 wave produced by J. F. stimulation and recorded at 150 μ depth (see specimen records). The Golgi cell inhibition was produced in A by a LOC stimulus on-beam for the recording site, and in B by a J. F. stimulation through a different electrode from that used for testing. C and D were recorded at 400 μ depth, the inhibitions being produced by a LOC stimulus on beam. As shown in the specimen records, Golgi cell inhibition was tested by the P_2 response to a J. F. stimulus (C), and the basket cell inhibition by the N_1 reponse to the same stimulus (D). (ECCLES, SASAKI and STRATA, 1967 b)

with the concentrations of vesicles remote from the actual synaptic sites. It is suggested that transmitter may even be liberated remote from its site of action and that it diffuses there within the encapsulated space. A related concept of an "effective synaptic space" surrounded by a diffusional barrier has been proposed by EMMELIN and MCINTOSH (1956) for the sympathetic ganglion cell.

K. The Transverse Profile of the Golgi Cell Inhibition

It was shown in Chapter VI that a narrow beam of excited parallel fibers evokes an inhibition of Purkinje cells that extends for as far as 1000 μ on either side of the beam (cf. Figs. 61, 62, 65). There is a remarkable correspondence between this wide

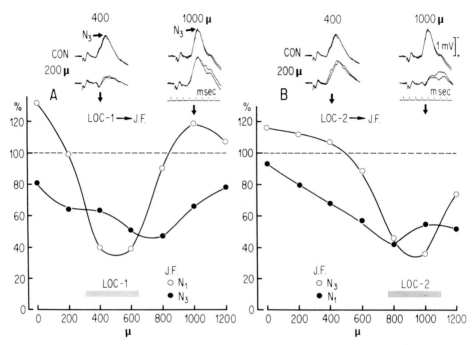

Fig. 88 A and B. *Comparison of the transverse profiles of the basket cell and Golgi cell inhibitions set up by parallel fiber volleys.* The plotting in A and B resembled that in Fig. 62 A except that the effects produced by the LOC-1 and LOC-2 beams have been plotted separately in A and B, though actually recorded in the same microelectrode tracks at 200 μ spacing in the transverse plane indicated in the abscissae. As shown in the specimen records at 400 μ and 1000 μ positions in A and B, the N_3 waves evoked by J. F. stimulation and recorded at 200 μ depth were employed in sampling the inhibitory action of the LOC-1 and LOC-2 volleys respectively, whose transverse distributions are indicated by the shaded rectangles. The conditioned N_3 waves are plotted (open circles) as percentages of the mean controls to give the transverse profiles of the Golgi cell inhibition. The N_1 waves recorded at 400 μ depth in the same microelectrode tracks are similarly measured and plotted (filled circles) to give the transverse profiles of the basket cell inhibition. (ECCLES, SASAKI and STRATA, 1967 b)

transverse spread of inhibition and the axonal distributions of the basket and stellate cells (Figs. 8, 11, 54) that form those synapses on Purkinje cells (Figs. 55, 56, 57) that are assumed to be responsible for this inhibition. On the other hand the axon of a Golgi cell has a distribution no wider than its dendritic expansion (Figs. 13, 16); hence the distribution of Golgi cell inhibition to the mossy fiber-granule cell relay would be expected to be much more limited.

The topography of the inhibitory action on Purkinje cells has been determined by using as a test response the antidromic spike potential extracellularly recorded from Purkinje cells (Figs. 61, 62). The N_3 wave produced by J. F. or T. F. stimulation is chosen as providing the simplest and most reliable test for mapping the extent of the Golgi cell inhibition that is induced by a narrow beam of excited parallel fibers. In Fig. 88 A and B a parallel fiber volley induces a Golgi cell inhibition of the N_3 wave (open circles, and specimen records in insets) that extends for no more than 200 μ on either side of the beam (shaded rectangles) of excited parallel fibers. In contrast the Purkinje cell inhibitions induced by the same parallel fiber volleys (filled circles) typically have a very extensive distribution, comparable with that plotted in Fig. 62. This restricted distribution of Golgi cell inhibition of the N_3 wave is observed in all experiments. Of course, if the LOC stimulus excites mossy fibers as well as parallel fibers, a much wider distribution of Golgi cell inhibition would be expected. There will be further discussion of the topography of inhibitory action in Chapter XII.

L. Conclusions

The findings of the physiological investigations on the mode of action of mossy fibers in the cerebellar cortex (ECCLES, LLINÁS and SASAKI, 1966 c; ECCLES, SASAKI and STRATA, 1967 b) are in remarkable accord with the structures revealed by the Golgi technique and the electron microscope (Figs. 67—75; HÁMORI and SZENTÁ-GOTHAI, 1966 b; Fox et al., 1967). The responses of every component of the complex synaptic apparatus, the glomerulus, can now be recognized in the electrophysiological investigations. On account of the minute size of all components only extracellular recording has been possible. There has been some investigation of unitary responses, but the greater part of the investigation has been concerned in the analysis of the electric field potentials under carefully controlled conditions.

Fig. 89 A—F summarizes diagrammatically the field potential analyses of the J.F.-evoked mossy fiber responses in the cerebellar cortex (cf. ECCLES, SASAKI and STRATA, 1967 a; SASAKI and STRATA, 1967). A and B show typical field potentials generated by a J.F. stimulation and recorded with a microelectrode at 200 μ and 500 μ depths respectively. The field potentials are changed to C and D by a conditioning local (LOC) stimulation applied about 20 msec previously. The field potentials in A and B can be analysed into the activities of the elementary neuronal components in the molecular and the granular layer as illustrated in E and F. The $P_1 N_1$ potential is caused largely by antidromic impulses in Purkinje cell axons, somata and dendrites (N_{1P} in E and F) and partly by impulses in mossy fibers (N_{1m} in F). The mossy fiber impulses produce EPSP currents in Golgi cells and in granule cells that are recorded in the granular layers as the N_2 wave (N_{2E} in F), the spike potentials in the Golgi cells adding the early negative peak of the N_2 wave (N_{2G} in F, cf. Fig. 41) and those in the granule cells the second negative peak (N_{2g} in F, cf. Figs. 82 E—H, 83 A—F). The impulses discharged along the axons of granule cells up to the molecular layer contribute to the P_2 potential in the granular layer and the N_3 wave in the molecular layer (N_{3g} in E). The larger later component of the N_3 wave has been attributed to the EPSP currents (N_{3E} in E), the local responses and the spikes (N_{3P} in E) that the parallel fiber volley generates in the Purkinje cells and in the interneurones (ECCLES, SASAKI and STRATA, 1966). The impulses thus evoked in the dendrites of Purkinje cells propagate down to the

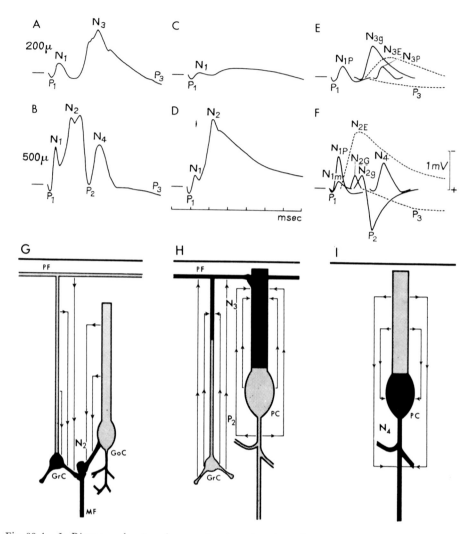

Fig. 89 A—I. *Diagrams showing the postulated modes of production by a mossy fiber volley of the potential waves in the cerebellar cortex.* A—F. Diagrammatic illustrations of the field potentials generated by a J.F. stimulation, and their postulated constituents. A to D are traced from oscilloscope pictures at 200 (A, C) and 500 (B, D) μ depths, C and D showing the depression of the J.F.-evoked responses by a conditioning LOC stimulation. E and F show the constituent potentials that are postulated to compose the A and B potentials. Further explanation in text (SASAKI and STRATA, 1967). In G to I: *PC*, Purkinje cell; *GrC*, granule cell; *MF*, mossy fiber; *GoC*, Golgi cell; *PF*, parallel fiber. By convention the excited elements are shown dark. The areas occupied by impulses are very dark, and synaptically excited areas are dark grey, progressively lightening with electrotonic spread. Extracellular lines of current flow are shown flowing into the depolarized areas (active sinks) from passive sources. G. An impulse in the mossy fiber is shown exciting in a glomerulus the dendrites of both granule and Golgi cells and so generating the field potentials of the N_2 wave. H. An impulse discharged from the granule cell up its axon to the parallel fiber is shown synaptically exciting a Purkinje cell dendrite and so generating directly and by its synaptic action the P_2 and N_3 field potentials. I. An impulse is shown propagating through the Purkinje cell soma and down its axon and axon collaterals and so generating the N_4 field potential. (ECCLES, SASAKI and STRATA, 1967 a)

somata and axons in the ganglionic and granular layers, producing the N_4 wave there (F). The inhibitory action of Golgi cells upon granule cells and that of superficial stellate and basket cells upon Purkinje cells have accounted for the late slow P_3 wave. A preceding LOC stimulation produces the inhibitory action of Golgi cells upon granule cell activities and so suppresses the N_3 potentials in the molecular layer and the P_2 potentials in the granule layer, as seen in Fig. 89 C and D.

Fig. 89 G—I illustrates in diagrammatic form the explanations for the electrical potential waves that a mossy fiber sets up in the cerebellar cortex. The initial diphasic spike, $P_1 N_1$, is the standard wave form generated by impulses propagating up to nerve terminals, in this case the mossy fiber impulses, and needs no special diagrammatic illustration. Usually with J.F. stimulation there is also the much larger diphasic spike potential produced by impulses propagating antidromically up the Purkinje axons to invade the Purkinje cells (Fig. 89 F).

In Fig. 89 G a mossy fiber is shown synaptically exciting dendrites of both a granule and a Golgi cell, the excited areas of depolarization being darkly shaded. The lines of extracellular current flow account for the negativity of the granular layer relative to the molecular layer, which is the observed N_2 wave. The slow EPSP type of N_2 wave (Figs. 77, 79 D, 80 D) is attributable to the inadequacy of the synaptic depolarization of the granule cell dendrites, summation of the synaptic depolarizations on two or more dendrites being required for impulse generation. Otherwise the N_2 wave has the configuration of a spike potential with a clear double composition indicated in Fig. 89 B and F. An explanation has been suggested in Section E above for this clear separation between the latencies of spike generation in Golgi cells and granule cells.

Fig. 89 H illustrates the two mechanisms that have been proposed for the generation of the linked waves, molecular layer negativity (N_3) and granular layer positivity (P_2). Again the shading indicates the depolarized areas of the membranes. As impulses propagate from the granule cells up the parallel fibers, the granule cells will be passive sources (P_2) to the active sinks in the molecular layer (N_3). This initial phase leads on to the postulated later phase of N_3 and P_2 that is also treated diagrammatically in Fig. 89 H. There are an immense number of excitatory synapses of parallel fibers on each Purkinje cell (over 100,000); hence the parallel fiber impulses very effectively depolarize Purkinje cells, as shown by the shading, there being produced in this way active sinks in the molecular layer to passive sources in the ganglionic and granular layers. When the mossy fiber input is weak, or when the Purkinje cells are inhibited by basket and stellate cell activity, only EPSPs are produced in the Purkinje cells (Figs. 79 C at 100 to 200 μ depth and 80 B at 100 and 150 μ); but otherwise spike potentials are generated, which may be seen as components of the N_3 wave (Figs. 80 A, C, E; 81 C, E; 83 I).

The postulated mode of production of the N_4 wave is illustrated in the much simpler diagram of Fig. 89 I. The impulses discharged from the Purkinje cells along their axons and axon collaterals will give rise to active sinks in the granular layer to passive sources in the molecular layer. When the N_4 wave is large there may even be a simultaneous positive wave superficially in the molecular layer (ECCLES, SASAKI and STRATA, 1967 a).

Chapter VIII

The Climbing Fiber Input and its Excitation of Purkinje Cells

A. The Synaptic Distribution of a Climbing Fiber

The simple synaptic contacts made by a climbing fiber have been adequately described in Chapter II B and illustrated in Figs. 21, 23 and 24. Each climbing fiber has a primary synaptic relation to a single Purkinje cell. This synaptic contact is of very unusual extent, by reason of the long parallel relation between the branches of the climbing fiber and of the smooth dendrites of the Purkinje cell. The contact is not truly parallel or continuous, but is interrupted, so that there are probably hundreds if not thousands of separate contacts between any climbing fiber and its Purkinje cell. Even if one or the other of the short side branches terminating in a small knob were to touch a neighbouring Purkinje cell, as surmised by SCHEIBEL and SCHEIBEL (1954), this small contact would be insignificant functionally. Furthermore, as one can see on longitudinal or even better on oblique sections of folia with all Purkinje cells stained, there is no interlacing between the dendrites of neighboring Purkinje cells in the longitudinal direction of the folium. Between each of these dendritic arborizations there is a small space that is occupied by the dendritic arborizations of basket and stellate neurones (Fig. 110). Most of the side branches of the climbing fibers are so short that they can only make synaptic contacts on the same Purkinje cell. There are, however, also longer side branches of the climbing fiber that give synapses to basket and outer stellate cells, as described in Chapter II, Section B, and the existence of these axo-somatic synapses of climbing fiber collaterals has been confirmed by degeneration and EM analysis on Golgi neurones and basket cells (Fig. 36; HÁMORI and SZENTÁGOTHAI, 1966a) — and their existence on stellate cells is highly probable.

B. Experimental Methods

The enormous extent of the apparently one-to-one synaptic contacts made by each climbing fiber onto its Purkinje cell (Figs. 21 and 90 A) provides perhaps the most remarkable synaptic mechanism in the nervous system — a monosynaptic pathway which would be expected to have an enormously high safety factor as well as an all-or-nothing functional action. By utilizing the discovery of SZENTÁGOTHAI and RAJKOVITS (1959) that these climbing fibers come very largely, if not entirely, from the nerve cells of the inferior olive (Chapter II B), it has been possible to investigate the action of this synapse virtually uncomplicated by other cerebellar responses (ECCLES, LLINÁS and SASAKI, 1964, 1966d). As shown in Fig. 90, a stimulating electrode has been implanted in the accessory inferior olive (I.O.) and also one in the white matter deep to the cerebellar cortex in the juxta-fastigial region

(J. F.). A third electrode (LOC) has been placed upon the surface of the cerebellar folium under investigation, one millimeter or so away from the actual site of insertion of the recording microelectrode.

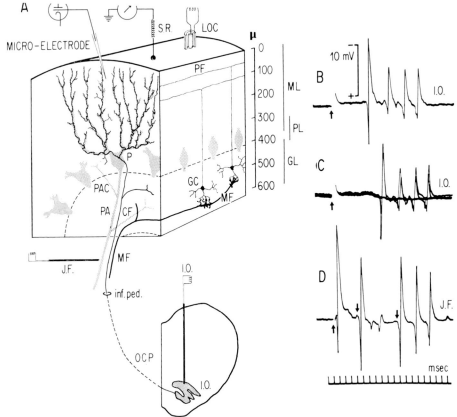

Fig. 90 A—D. *The recording of climbing fiber responses of Purkinje cells.* A. The experimental arrangements resemble in general those of Figs. 33 and 37, but there is in addition a concentric stimulating electrode (I. O.) in the dorsal accessory component of the inferior olive, that excites climbing fibers running by the olivo-cerebellar pathway (*OCP*) through the inferior peduncle and ending in the remarkable climbing ramification on the dendrites of Purkinje cells. B and C show extracellular responses of a Purkinje cell to a climbing fiber impulse set up by the I. O. stimulus at the arrow. In C the stimulus was just threshold for the climbing fiber, the stimuli being subliminal in two of the four superimposed sweeps. In D, following the antidromic invasion of the cell by J.F. stimulation (up-going arrow), there are two sets of responses (down-going arrows); the first was produced by direct stimulation of the climbing fiber, the second by reflex activation via the inferior olive (cf. Figs. 92, 93, 94). (ECCLES, LLINÁS and SASAKI, 1966 d)

C. Extracellular Recording of Spike Potentials

In Fig. 90 B the inferior olive (I. O.) stimulus evokes a complex series of spike potentials at a depth of 250 µ in the cortex of the cerebellar vermis. By careful adjustment of stimulus strength this whole complex is displayed in Fig. 90 C as a unitary response that is superimposed on a low background potential. There is an initial large diphasic spike potential (positive-negative) and a succession of spike potentials of the same polarity but of various smaller sizes. For example, in

Fig. 90 C there are four superimposed traces with the stimulus just straddling threshold, the stimulus being below threshold in two and in two above. The two latter give four successive superimposed spikes.

Since the Purkinje cells represent the only efferent system of the cerebellar cortex, a stimulus applied to the juxta-fastigial region (J. F. in Fig. 90 A) would be expected to excite the axons of Purkinje cells and of no other cells in the cerebellar cortex; and in Fig. 90 D there is at the first arrow an antidromic spike potential having a configuration closely resembling the initial spike evoked from the inferior olive at first downward arrow; hence it can be concluded that this spike is evoked in the same Purkinje cell. Each subsequent spike potential in Fig. 90 B, C, D has the same configuration as the antidromic spike in D, the smaller size being attributable to background depolarization of the Purkinje cell and to relative refractoriness at that high frequency of response. Therefore, these spikes also are produced by the same Purkinje cell. The all-or-nothing property of the spike complex in Fig. 90 C establishes that a single neural element coming from the inferior olive has a powerful excitatory influence on this Purkinje cell, the synaptic depolarization being so prolonged that it generates four impulses, and so large that the spike mechanism is greatly depressed. From the histological pictures of the climbing fiber synapse (Chapter II B; Figs. 21, 23) it would be expected to have such a powerful action. Other examples of unitary responses of Purkinje cells to climbing fiber impulses are shown at CF in Fig. 91 E, F after the initial antidromic spike.

D. Intracellular Recording from Purkinje Cells

The intracellularly recorded responses to an inferior olive stimulus are in good agreement with the extracellular response. For example, the first spike in Fig. 91 B indicates antidromic invasion from a juxta-fastigial stimulation and so provides Purkinje cell identification; and, in response to an inferior olive stimulation (Fig. 91 A), there is an initial spike with a latency of 5.8 msec and a later large slow potential on which are superimposed several small spikes. The whole spike complex evoked by inferior olive stimulation usually has a duration of 5—8 msec (cf. Fig. 92 A, B).

E. The Projection from the Inferior Olive to Purkinje Cells

The pathway from the inferior olive to the cortex of the cerebellum traverses the contralateral restiform body (BRODAL, 1954) and those climbing fibers going to the vermis should pass close to the fastigial nucleus. This expectation is confirmed by the finding (Fig. 91 B, C) that juxta-fastigial (J. F.) stimulation frequently evokes responses in Purkinje cells which are identical with those that are produced by stimulation of climbing fibers (CF) by means of the electrode in the inferior olive (Fig. 91 A; as also in Fig. 90 B and D and Fig. 92 A and E). Similarly GRANIT and PHILLIPS (1956) found that juxta-fastigial stimulation often evoked large and prolonged depolarizations of Purkinje cells, and these 'D potentials' are now identifiable as climbing fiber responses.

In the extracellular records of Fig. 91 D—F, graded J. F. stimulation evokes when weak the antidromic spike response of a Purkinje cell (D). In E the stimulus is just straddling threshold for a complex response which occurs after the initial spike potential (ANT) in the cell that is antidromically invaded, and which consists of a series of two or three small spikes (CF), the whole complex resembling that evoked a little later in that same cell by inferior olive stimulation.

Figure 91 G gives another example of juxta-fastigial stimulation evoking first an antidromic spike potential and then a later spike superimposed on a prolonged

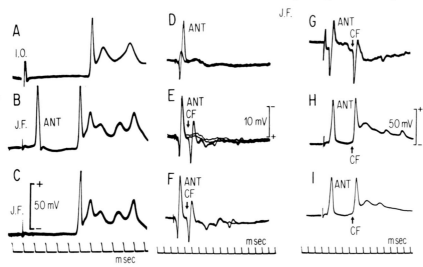

Fig. 91 A—I. *Responses evoked in Purkinje cells by climbing fiber impulses.* A—C. Intracellular records from Purkinje cells activated from the inferior olive and by juxta-fastigial stimulation. B and C responses were evoked by J.F. stimulation; in B the cell was antidromically activated, while in C the stimulus strength was subthreshold for antidromic invasion. In both there was a later spike followed by a prolonged complex depolarization that was virtually identical with that evoked by I. O. stimulation in the same cell (A), the only difference being its longer latency. In D, E and F extracellular spikes were evoked by J. F. stimulation at different strengths. In D the stimulus strength was straddling threshold for the antidromic activation (ANT) of the cell. In E a small increase to the stimulus strength produced a second response in an all-or-nothing manner (CF). In F a further increase in the stimulus strength evoked both responses on every occasion. In G are the extracellularly recorded responses from another Purkinje cell that also were evoked by J. F. stimulation and that closely resemble F. In H and I are intracellular records of the same cell showing, after the antidromic invasion, a second spike (arrow) followed by a long lasting depolarization (about 9 msec). The late potentials evoked by the J. F. stimulation in E to I are produced as indicated (CF) by the activation of a single climbing fiber. The potential scales of E and H are for D—G and H, I respectively. (Eccles, Llinás and Sasaki, 1966 d)

positive potential. Subsequently the microelectrode impaled this same Purkinje cell, and juxta-fastigial stimulation then evokes (Fig. 91 H, I) an initial antidromic spike potential and about 3.6 msec later a similar spike potential followed by a large depolarization on which small spikes are superimposed. These responses closely resemble those illustrated in Fig. 91 A—C from a different experiment. The illustrations of intracellular CF responses are seen to conform to a standard pattern, which is regularly observed when the Purkinje cell is in good condition.

In interpreting Fig. 91 it has so far been assumed that both the juxta-fastigial and the inferior olive stimulation set up a single discharge in the climbing fiber belonging to the Purkinje cell impaled by the microelectrode. However, with many Purkinje cells this assumption is not valid.

For example in Fig. 92 A—D, as the Purkinje cell deteriorates so that the spike potentials completely fail in D, it is seen that the single I. O. stimulus sets up four discharges in the climbing fiber at a frequency of about 500/sec. This repetitive discharge must also be occurring in A, B and C and be responsible for much of the later waves of these traces. However the concurrent series with J. F. stimulation

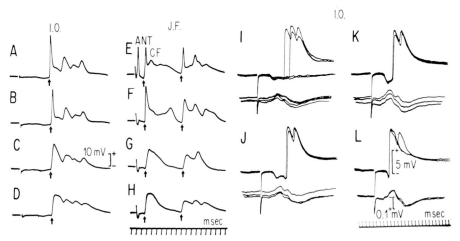

Fig. 92 A—L. *Intracellular records evoked by climbing fiber stimulation.* Records A to H show a Purkinje cell in the process of deterioration; potentials A to D and E to H were evoked respectively by I.O. and by J.F. stimulation, the records being arranged in the serial order of the state of deterioration. In records E to H the second arrow marks the "reflex" activation of the climbing fiber by J.F. stimulation. Same potential and time scales for A—H. I—L. Intracellular records from a Purkinje cell showing different latencies for the synaptic potential evoked by I.O. stimulation. Lower records are the simultaneous potentials recorded at the surface of the cerebellar cortex with their own potential scale. The stimulus strength was increased from I to L. Note in I and L the all-or-nothing nature either of this whole synaptic potential or of its later component. (ECCLES, LLINÁS and SASAKI, 1966 d)

(Fig. 92 E—H) shows that a single CF impulse can produce a prolonged depolarization with superimposed partial spikes as in the J.F.-evoked responses of Fig. 91. In Fig. 92 E the J. F. stimulus evokes an initial antidromic spike that is followed by a typical CF response with a latency of 1.75 msec (first arrow) and at the second arrow there is a second CF response with a latency of 9.3 msec, which is considerably longer than the latency for the I. O. stimulus (6.2 msec in A—D). With deterioration of the Purkinje cell there is first a failure of the antidromic spike potential but not of the spikes evoked by CF impulses (F). Finally in H there is failure even of the partial spikes, revealing that the first CF response is a simple EPSP, whereas the second is generated by three discharges at about 500/sec, much as in D. The response at the second arrow will be considered below. For the present it is sufficient to note that, when J. F. stimulation evokes a CF response with short latency, as in Fig. 91 B, C, H, I, it is always due to a single impulse (cf. Figs. 91, 92, 93).

Fig. 92 I—L presents further evidence on the repetitive discharge that a single inferior olive stimulation may evoke in the climbing fiber innervating the Purkinje cell under observation. In Fig. 92 I a just-threshold stimulation evokes either an EPSP with a triple summit having a latency of 7.3 msec and successive peaks at about 2 msec intervals, or a double-peak EPSP having a latency of 9.0 msec. With further increase in the stimulus strength (J) the latency is identical with the shorter value in I; and, with still further strengthening, there is further reduction in latency, to 6.0 msec in K and to 4.4 msec in L. At the same time it will be noted that there is virtually no change in the latency of the potential (lower traces) simultaneously recorded from the surface of the folium within 1 mm from the recording microelectrode. It seems that the weaker stimuli to the inferior olive are exciting presynaptic pathways to the cell of origin of the climbing fiber, and that only with the strongest stimuli (L) is this cell or its axon directly excited.

The differential latency for the two modes of stimulation (inferior olive and J. F.) usually lay between 1.0 and 3.6 msec, the actual conduction distance between the two sites of stimulation (cf. Fig. 90 A) being about 20 mm; hence conduction velocities would range between 5 and 20 m/sec. These values are in good agreement with the observed fiber diameters of 1—5 µ (SZENTÁGOTHAI-SCHIMERT, 1941).

Wide ranges of stimulation strength through either the inferior olive or J. F. electrodes almost invariably fail to disclose the convergence of two climbing fibers on to a single Purkinje cell; but two out of more than 100 cells exhibited a clear superposition of two unitary responses, i. e. there was a double climbing fiber innervation of these two Purkinje cells (ECCLES, LLINÁS and SASAKI, 1966 d, Fig. 9).

Fig. 93 shows at fast (A—B) and slow (C—E) speeds the double unitary responses (arrows indicating both first and second responses) often evoked in a Purkinje cell by a J. F. stimulation, there being an interval of 6.0—6.5 msec between the two responses both with extracellular (A) and intracellular (B—E) recording. Presumably the depressed size of the second unitary response is attributable to its superposition on the residual depolarization following the first response. The double character of the synaptically evoked response in Fig. 93 is seen particularly clearly when deterioration prevents the generation of spike potentials by the neurone (D, E).

Further examples of such delayed responses to J. F. stimulation are illustrated in Fig. 93 F—I. In F, J. F. stimulation evokes a climbing fiber response consisting of an initial spike trailing on to a smooth declining depolarization of several milliseconds duration. In G—I there is either a single delayed EPSP (second arrow in G) or a sequence of EPSPs (H, I), which in I generates a second spike. These sequences of EPSPs closely resemble those evoked by inferior olivary stimulation (Fig. 92 D, I—L). The unitary character of this complex response is exhibited in the superimposed responses of Fig. 93 I.

In Fig. 94 A—D from another experiment the delayed response usually has this sequence of EPSPs, which are shown in the superimposed records to appear at regularly spaced intervals, just as in Fig. 92 D, H, I—L. In Fig. 94 A and C stimulation through one J. F. electrode evokes an initial simple EPSP, as in Fig. 92 H, and in addition the later response of 1, 2 or 3 EPSPs, as in Fig. 92 E—H.

In Fig. 94 B and D, stimulation by the other J. F. electrode evokes only the later complex response. Apparently this electrode is relatively further from the climbing fiber supplying the impaled Purkinje cell, which consequently is not directly excited.

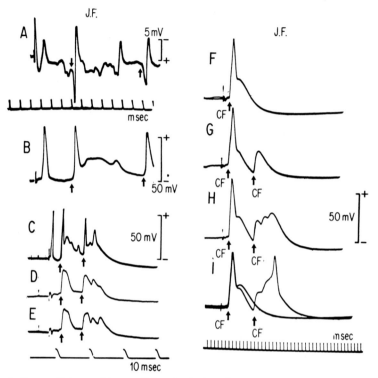

Fig. 93 A—I. *Extracellular and intracellular Purkinje cell potentials evoked by reflex activation of a climbing fiber by J. F. stimulation.* All records from A to E are from the same cell. In A extracellular Purkinje spikes show an initial antidromic activation, then the direct CF response at the first arrow and the reflex CF response at the second arrow. After impalement of the cell (B) there is the same sequence of the antidromic spike, then the direct and reflex CF responses at the arrows. C gives the same responses at slower sweep speed. Records D and E were taken after the spike generation had deteriorated and show the direct and reflex CF responses at the same latencies as in C. In F to I the intracellular potential produced in another Purkinje cell by direct CF activation was superimposed on the large IPSP produced by the simultaneous activation of inhibitory interneurones via the pathway — mossy fibers to granule cells to parallel fibers thence to basket and stellate cells. In records G, H and I the reflex activation of the CF at the second arrows produced single and multiple synaptic potentials which summated and were able to generate a second spike in I. (ECCLES, LLINÁS and SASAKI, 1966 d)

F. Interpretation of Climbing Fiber Responses

The delayed responses to J. F. stimulation resemble the responses evoked by inferior olive stimulation, as for example in Fig. 92 E—H and A—D, and their longer latency gives time for transmission from the J. F. stimulating electrode to the inferior olive; hence it can be postulated that they are reflex responses from the inferior olive — the J. F. stimulus excites antidromic impulses in climbing fibers, and on reaching the inferior olive the impulses act via recurrent axon collaterals

(Fig. 94 E) to evoke the discharge of impulses from the inferior olive cells. The situation will thus be identical with that obtaining when, with inferior olive stimulation, there is also activation of the recurrent collaterals.

Direct investigation of the responses of the inferior olive with intracellular and extracellular recording (ITO, OCHI and OBATA, 1967) reveals that antidromic activation by cerebellar stimulation induces two or more repetitive responses of

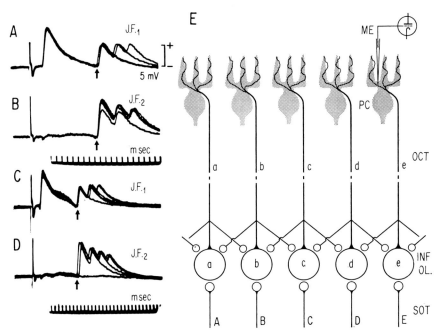

Fig. 94 A—D. *The repetitive reflex responses of inferior olivary cells.* In A with a J.F. stimulation there is an initial direct CF-evoked EPSP that is intracellularly recorded from a Purkinje cell, and at the arrow are the reflex EPSPs. In B, J.F. stimulation through another electrode evokes only the reflex CF EPSPs. C and D are similar to A and B respectively, but are recorded at a slower sweep speed. All records are formed by the superposition of 4 or 5 traces, the all-or-nothing character of the reflex response being shown in D. (ECCLES, LLINÁS and SASAKI, 1966 d). E gives a diagrammatic illustration of the recurrent axon collaterals in the inferior olive that are postulated as causing the reflex responses. The intracellular recording by the microelectrode, ME, is shown from the Purkinje cell innervated by the climbing fiber, *e,* of the olivocerebellar tract, *OCT*. Further description in text

cells at 1.2 msec intervals. They therefore have also postulated that the axons of inferior olive cells have collaterals that excite other olive cells.

The postulated manner of operation of the axon collaterals in the inferior olive can be described in relation to a greatly simplified model (Fig. 94 E). There are three initial assumptions in the operation of this simplified model: that each afferent fiber to the olive has an excitatory synapse on one olivary cell; that each olivary cell sends recurrent collaterals to two adjacent cells; that one excitatory synapse is adequate to evoke the discharge of an impulse from an I. O. cell. It is further assumed that the Purkinje cell under observation by ME is supplied by the cell and fiber e. We may now suppose that in Fig. 92 I the weakest stimulus evokes discharges in a and b fibers either directly or by excitation of the presynaptic fibers A and B. A discharge in fiber e and a CF-evoked response of the Purkinje cell will then be observed only after the serial relays through recurrent collaterals: b to c to d to e; and a to b to c to d to e. Consequently there will be the observed double response in Fig. 92 I with latency of 9.0 msec. With the response in I at the briefer latency (7.3 msec) and also in J with the response to stronger stimulation, fiber c will be excited as well, hence the shortening of the latency by the synaptic delay of the b to c transmission. The still shorter latency in K can be attributed to the stimulus exciting d fiber, and finally, in L, fiber e is directly excited and the I. O. response has a minimal latency.

As already suggested, the repetitive discharges are due to the serial activation of the recurrent axonal relays in response to a more remote initial stimulation. For example, if a, b, c, d, and e are directly excited by the strong initial I. O. stimulus, then, after the initial discharge in fiber e, the inferior olive cell e would be bombarded by the axon collateral of d and so be induced to fire a second impulse. However, if this likewise happens to cell d in response to axon collaterals from cell c, there will be a further bomdardment of cell e at one synaptic delay still later, i. e. a third discharge could be induced in e; and so even for a fourth. It might therefore be suggested that an indefinite series of discharges might be produced. However, there seems never to be more than four discharges in a series (Fig. 94 D), so the additional assumption is required that these high frequency responses build up an increased threshold of the I. O. cells either by cumulative refractoriness or by the action of inhibitory pathways, which certainly are very effective in the inferior olive (ARMSTRONG, ECCLES, HARVEY and MATTHEWS, 1967). The action of inhibition is also suggested in Fig. 92 I—L, where the strongest stimulation (L) is the one with least tendency to repetitive firing, though the opportunity for recurrent collateral activation would be largest.

Fig. 94 E also allows the development of a satisfactory explanation for the reflex responses that J. F. stimulation often evokes from the inferior olive. Stimulation of the climbing fibers by the J. F. electrode will result in the antidromic propagation down fibers such as a, b, c, d and e to the inferior olive with the axon-collateral activation of the I. O. cells as investigated by ITO, OCHI and OBATA (1967). It will be appreciated that the developing situation will then be identical with that already described for an I. O. stimulus. Reference to Fig. 92 shows how closely the repetitive responses to reflex activation of the inferior olive from J. F. stimulation (H) resemble those obtained by direct I. O. stimulation (D). The reflex responses to the first J. F. stimulations in Fig. 96 K—O are likewise seen to give repetitive discharges of the I. O. cell comparable with those directly evoked by the I. O. stimulation in F—J.

In all these figures the intervals between the successive discharges are longer (about 2 msec) than those observed by ITO, OCHI and OBATA (1967) for the unitary cell discharges in the inferior olive (1.2 msec). Presumably the longer times observed for the successive responses of Purkinje cells are due to slower conduction for impulses travelling in the relatively refractory period, an effect which could be cumulative for a brief series.

Fig. 97 A—C illustrates the remarkable ability of a climbing fiber to drive a Purkinje cell to a high frequency of discharge. In the brief repetitive series of A at 70/sec, each J.F. stimulus produces a response not much depressed relative to the initial responses in A and in Fig. 95 K, L. In each case the initial response is the antidromic spike (a) and a later CF complex (cf) of three or four spikes. In the faster stimulation in B (108/sec) the CF complex with three spikes (cf) still is well maintained for the six stimuli, but no stimulus after the first evokes the

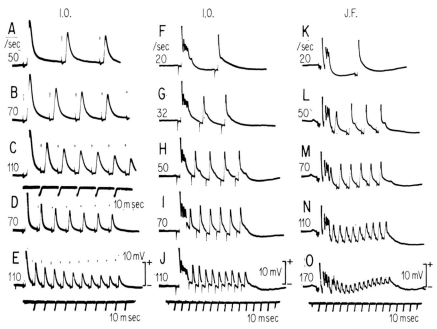

Fig. 96 A—O. *Intracellular records of the CF EPSP produced in Purkinje cells by repetitive I. O. and J. F. stimulation.* Series A—E and F—J show responses of two different Purkinje cells to I.O. stimulation, while K—O gives the responses of the same cell as in F—J, but for J.F. stimulation. The stimulation frequency is noted at the left of each record as number of stimuli per second, and the time and voltage scales are given for each series. (Eccles, Llinás, Sasaki and Voorhoeve, 1966)

initial antidromic spike (a). Presumably the propagation down the Purkinje cell axon of the last spike discharge of each CF response prevents by refractoriness the next antidromic spike.

With the still more severe tetanus of Fig. 97 C (16 stimuli at 180/sec) there is a rapid failure of large spikes, and irregular small spike potentials continue during the remainder of the tetanus. However, after the tetanus there is a remarkable after-discharge of large spike potentials commencing at the high frequency of about 350/sec and declining to 180/sec just before failing. The increase in spike size with slowing of frequency may be entirely attributable to refractoriness. Comparable responses of Purkinje cells were observed by Granit and Phillips (1956) following tetanization by an electrode in the fastigial region, and likewise these may be attributed to the repetitive stimulation of climbing fibers.

Fig. 97 D, E shows the similar responses evoked in another Purkinje cell of that same experiment by quite brief tetani, which respectively are seven at 330/sec and twelve at 240/sec. In both there is the same deep depression of spikes during the tetanus and for about 10 msec thereafter, but subsequently there is a recovery of the spike size. The spikes of the after-discharge have a characteristic frequency

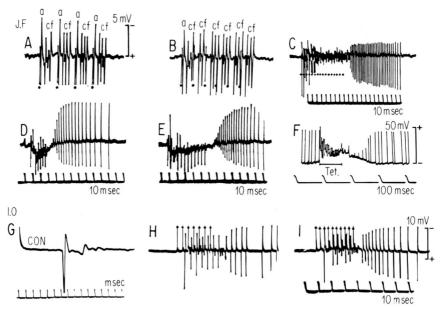

Fig. 97 A—I. *Extracellular and intracellular spike activity evoked in Purkinje cells by repetitive CF activation in response to tetanic J.F. or I.O. stimulation. A—C are responses of same Purkinje cell as in Fig. 95 J—L, the J.F. stimulation being repeated at 70/sec and 108/sec for A and B respectively. In A every J.F. response consisted of the two components a and cf. Record B shows that antidromic invasion failed after the first J.F. stimulation. In record C a tetanus at 180/sec produced a failure of the large spike potentials after six stimulations, and shortly after the tetanus there was a prolonged after-discharge. Records D and E illustrate similar responses evoked in another Purkinje cell. In F, an intracellular record from a Purkinje cell shows the prolonged depolarization and spike inactivation produced by summation of the repetitively produced CF EPSPs by a tetanic J.F. stimulation for the duration of the horizontal line. The depolarization outlasts by 100 msec the duration of the stimulus. The same potential scale obtains for records A—E. There are separate scales for F. Record G shows a typical CF response of a Purkinje cell following I.O. stimulation. In H and I brief repetitive I.O. stimulation was followed by an after-discharge. In A—C and H, I the stimuli are marked by dots.* (ECCLES, LLINÁS, SASAKI and VOORHOEVE, 1966)

pattern, which declines progressively from an initial high rate to as low as 100/sec (D) before failing. The frequency is higher after the 12 stimuli (E) than after 7 (D).

Finally, in Fig. 97 F intracellular recording from another Purkinje cell in this same experiment shows the large maintained depolarization during the tetanus (19 stimuli at 230/sec), and the slow decline for almost 100 msec thereafter, though there is no associated generation of spike discharge as in C, but merely a recovery of the spontaneous discharge frequency. This build-up of residual depolarization is

170

also noted in the more severe tetani of Fig. 96 I, J, M, N, O, but is less well developed, presumably because this Purkinje cell is so badly deteriorated.

It is assumed that in Fig. 97 repetitive activation of climbing fibers is responsible for all the subsequent after-discharge of the Purkinje cell, because at lower frequencies the CF response is dominant (Figs. 95 K, L; 97 A, B). Fig. 97 G—I shows that this characteristic type of response is produced by a brief tetanic stimulation of the inferior olive, and hence undoubtedly is due to climbing fiber activation. The characteristic CF-evoked response in G has a latency of 6.1 msec. A tetanus of seven stimuli at 220/sec produces a well-developed after-discharge (H), and, with a further increase to ten stimuli at 325/sec (I), the after-discharge almost matches those of Fig. 97 C, D, E. There is similarly a brief interval (7—12 msec) after the last stimulus just before the after-discharge commences, and the size of the spikes shows the same characteristic increase during the after-discharge.

3. Comment

With repetitive activation there has invariably been a diminution in potency of climbing fiber synapses. With double stimulation (Fig. 95 A—I) this diminution of the second response has the slow time course which characterizes many synapses (cf. Curtis and Eccles, 1960; Hubbard, 1963) and which has been attributed (Eccles, 1964) to the slow recovery from the depletion of the immediately available transmitter, although receptor desensitization may also contribute. With repetitive stimulation, the faster the frequency, the more rapid and severe is the decrease in the EPSP of the successive responses (Fig. 96). As is usually observed with synapses, virtual stabilization of the EPSP size occurs after about ten responses. In these respects the climbing fiber synapses exhibit no unusual features. However, the potency of the climbing fiber synapse is such that, even with the considerable depression occurring at frequencies as high as 100/sec, each impulse continues to evoke multiple discharges (Fig. 97 B).

The failure of Purkinje cell spikes during still higher frequencies of climbing fiber activation (Fig. 97 C—F, H, I) is due not to a deficiency in the EPSP produced by the successive impulses, but to the too intense depolarization produced by summation of the successive EPSPs (Fig. 97 F); as a consequence the spike-generating mechanism is suppressed, as was originally described by Granit and Phillips (1956).

After cessation of the stimulation this depolarization declines with a relatively slow time course (Fig. 97 F). Evidently there is a continuing action of the accumulated transmitter for at least 100 msec after a brief tetanus. As the depolarization gradually declines, spike generation of the soma and dendrites again becomes more and more effective, as indicated by the increasing size of the extracellular spike potentials in Fig. 97 C—E, H, I. During these after-discharges there is the expected correlation of increasing size of Purkinje cell spike potentials and slowing of frequency. With more severe tetani after-discharges persist for several seconds, which has already been reported by Granit and Phillips (1956). Evidently there can be a large accumulation of the excitatory transmitter at climbing fiber synapses, and its dissipation can be extremely slow.

H. Inhibition of the CF-Evoked Responses of Purkinje Cells

1. Extracellular Recording

The potency of the synaptic excitation produced by a single climbing fiber impulse is displayed by its resistance to a powerful inhibition of Purkinje cells. In the extracellular record of Fig. 98 A a CF impulse evokes the discharge of four impulses from a Purkinje cell. In B to D a preceding parallel fiber volley evokes

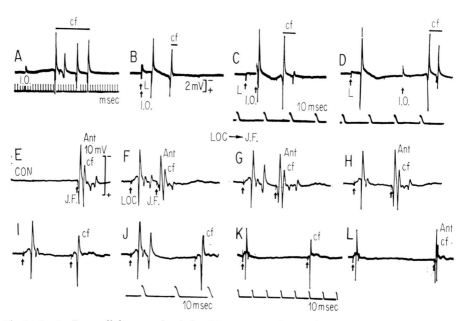

Fig. 98 A—L. *Extracellular records of the CF responses of a single Purkinje cell evoked by I.O. or J.F. stimulation, and conditioned by a LOC stimulation.* A gives control of I.O.-evoked response and in B—D this response is conditioned by a LOC stimulus at arrow labelled L at progressively longer testing intervals. Note that the LOC stimulus alone evoked a spike potential and a later positive wave (cf. Fig. 47 G). In E—L the CF response was evoked by J.F. stimulation as shown. In the control, E, the J.F. stimulus evoked an initial antidromic spike (*Ant*) followed by the CF response (*cf*) of the Purkinje cell. Note that in F—L the conditioning LOC stimulus evoked spike responses of the Purkinje cell, presumably due to parallel fiber stimulation. Note inhibition of the antidromic spike in I to K and also the depression of the late spikes of the *cf* response. (Eccles, Llinás, Sasaki and Voorhoeve, 1966)

a single impulse discharge (cf. Fig. 47 A, B, E, G, H) followed by a slow positive wave, during which, as we have seen in Chapters V and VI, the Purkinje cell is powerfully inhibited by the action of both basket cells and stellate cells. Under such conditions there is suppression of the antidromic invasion of the Purkinje cell (Fig. 98 I—K) and also of spike discharges generated by a subsequent parallel fiber volley (Fig. 47 G). However, in Fig. 98 B—D, at the optimal interval for inhibition (B), the CF impulse evokes a single discharge of the Purkinje cell and at longer intervals in C and D this inhibition can be seen to decline, though even at the longest test interval (D) the inhibition is still strong enough to reduce the CF-evoked response from 4 to 2 impulses.

In Fig. 98 E—L the climbing fiber response is evoked by juxta-fastigial (J. F.) stimulation, and so there is the complication arising from the excitation of the axon of that Purkinje cell with the consequent production of an early antidromic spike (Ant) potential (control in E) that precedes the CF response. At test intervals of 14—37 msec after the conditioning LOC stimulus (I, J, K), the Purkinje cell is so deeply inhibited that the antidromic invasion is suppressed; yet the initial spike (cf) produced by the climbing fiber impulse survives undiminished. However, as in Fig. 98 B—D, the subsequent partial spike complex is depressed, and there is still not full recovery at a test interval of 55 msec (L), by which time the antidromic invasion is restored.

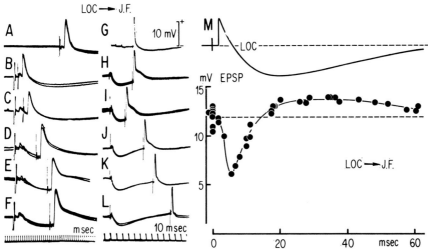

Fig. 99 A—M. *Intracellular records of a Purkinje cell showing the time course of the interaction between the IPSP evoked by parallel fiber stimulation (LOC) and the CF EPSP evoked by J. F. stimulation.* Record A shows the control EPSP evoked by J. F. stimulation. In B—F, the EPSP was superimposed at different intervals after the initiation of the IPSP. H—L give another series from the same cell taken at slower sweep speed, G being the control EPSP. M is a plot of the time course of the interaction between the CF EPSP and the LOC IPSP. The records were taken from another series from the same Purkinje cell as that illustrated in A—L. The amplitude of the EPSP in millivolts (ordinate) is plotted against the interval in milliseconds between the LOC stimulation and the J. F. stimulation. The drawing in the upper part of the figure shows the time course and amplitude of the synaptic potentials evoked in that Purkinje cell by the LOC stimulation, with the same time and voltage scale as for the plotting underneath. The initial parallel fiber EPSP is followed by the prolonged IPSP produced by the inhibitory interneurones (ECCLES, LLINÁS, SASAKI and VOORHOEVE, 1966)

2. Intracellular Recording

In the intracellular records of a Purkinje cell (Fig. 99) the control CF response (an EPSP) to juxta-fastigial (J. F.) stimulation (A) is superimposed on the IPSP produced by action of basket and outer stellate cells that are excited by the pathway, mossy fibers to granule cells to parallel fibers (Chapter VII, Figs. 85, 86). With conditioning by the IPSP produced by the LOC stimulus, there is an increase in height of the CF-evoked EPSP (in D—F), and it declines to a prolonged depolarization, at least relative to the course of the conditioning IPSP. At the shortest conditioning intervals (B, C), there is a depression of the CF-evoked EPSPs and an occlusion of the IPSPs of the conditioning and testing responses. The effect of the background IPSP on the CF-evoked EPSP is well illustrated in the potentials recorded from this same cell at a slower sweep speed (G—L).

When the CF-evoked depolarizing potential is measured at its height above the control background formed by the conditioning response and plotted as in the lower curve of Fig. 99 M, it is reduced in size (Fig. 99 B, C) when superimposed on the initial phase of increasing IPSP; on the other hand it is potentiated when it is later, during the maximum hyperpolarization and the recovery therefrom. These changes may be readily explained on the basis of the ionic conductance theories of excitatory and inhibitory postsynaptic potentials (cf. ECCLES, 1964). The decrease at testing intervals from 3 to 12 msec is doubtless due to the shunting effect of the high membrane conductance during the incrementing phase of the IPSP, which is given by the downward deflection in the upper trace of Fig. 99 M. At longer intervals this raised conductance will decline progressively, and the size of the CF-evoked EPSP becomes more influenced by the increased membrane potential, as has already been described (ECCLES, LLINÁS and SASAKI, 1966 d, Fig. 14).

3. Comment

There are thus two opposed actions of the inhibitory synapses. In Fig. 99 M this incrementing action is seen to preponderate beyond 15 msec. The shunting inhibitory conductance would meanwhile have declined; nevertheless the membrane hyperpolarization continues to increase until the later slow decline sets in.

In Fig. 99 D—F and H—J, the CF-evoked EPSP exhibits a remarkable slowing in decline when it occurs during the IPSP. The most probable explanation of this slowing is that the intense ionic currents produced by the activated CF synapses very effectively discharge the hyperpolarization of the IPSP, which subsequently can be rebuilt only by the action of any inhibitory transmitter still lingering in the inhibitory synaptic areas. As would be expected on this explanation, the rebuilding in Fig. 99 is much more effective early in the IPSP than later, and there is little or no trace of it very late in the IPSP (Fig. 99 K, L).

The excitatory power of a single climbing fiber synapse is demonstrated by its generation of an impulse discharge from a Purkinje cell even when it is subjected to the most intense inhibition from basket and stellate cells (Fig. 98 B, I, J). With Purkinje cells under good conditions of extracellular recording there seems never to be an inhibitory suppression of the first discharge to a CF impulse; but the later discharges can be very effectively inhibited.

I. Extracellular Field Potentials

In the molecular layer the field potential produced by a volley of CF impulses (Fig. 100 A) resembles the N_3 potential produced by a volley of mossy fiber impulses (Figs. 79, 80, 81).

The depth profile in Fig. 100 A shows typically a maximum of the initial negative wave at a depth of 100 to 200 µ and at depths below 200 µ there is an increment of a later and slower positive wave. This potential profile can be satisfactorily explained by the excitatory action of the climbing fiber synapses on the Purkinje cell dendrites. This explanation assumes that, in general accord with the usual histological descriptions (cf. Fig. 21), the climbing fiber (CF) synapses on the Purkinje dendrites are most numerous at a depth of 100 to 200 μ, with the consequence that both the EPSPs and the spike potentials generated thereby produce a maximum negative field potential at this depth.

In Fig. 100 the potential profile of A is not greatly altered in B when elicited during the powerful postsynaptic inhibition of the Purkinje cells that is produced by a stimulus through the local surface electrode (LOC). Later an explanation will be given for the findings that the inhibitory action increases the initial negative

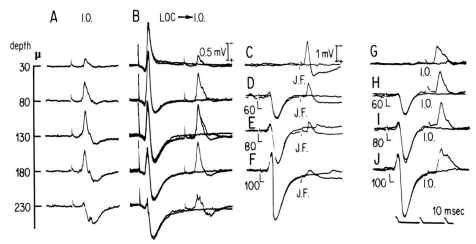

Fig. 100 A—J. *Field potentials produced in the cerebellar cortex by a single climbing fiber (CF) volley during conditioning by a LOC, stimulus.* In A, an inferior olive (I.O.) stimulation evoked a typical potential field recorded at the different depths below the surface of the cerebellar cortex. When the I.O. stimulation was preceded by a conditioning local (LOC) stimulation in B, an increase of the negative component was observed. (ECCLES, LLINÁS, SASAKI and VOORHOEVE, 1966). C—J are responses evoked in another experiment at 150 μ depth, there being conditioning by a preceding LOC stimulus of the N_3 response to a J. F. volley in C to F, and of the CF response to I.O. stimulation in G to J, the respective controls being given in C and G. The strengths of the LOC stimulus (L) are shown in an arbitrary linear scale for D to F and H to J. (ECCLES, 1965)

potential at all depths, and that there is a reduction of the later positive wave, particularly at levels deeper than 150 μ.

The contrast between the negative potentials evoked in the molecular layer by mossy and climbing fibers is displayed in Fig. 100 C—J. C gives the N_3 potential wave recorded at a depth of 150 μ in response to J. F. stimulation (cf. Chapter VII), and in D—F this wave is diminished by a parallel fiber volley evoked by LOC stimulation; the greater the parallel fiber response, the more profound the inhibition. This inhibitory depression contrasts with G—J, where similar parallel fiber stimulation does not diminish the I.O.-evoked climbing fiber response below the control value in G. This difference would be expected if the inhibition in D—F is due to Golgi cell action on the mossy fiber-granule cell synapse (Chapter VII); whereas the climbing fiber stimulation of the Purkinje cells is monosynaptically produced, there being no interneuronal synaptic relay on which inhibitory action can be exerted. Furthermore, there is accord between Fig. 100 J, and the finding in Fig. 98 B, I that even the most powerful postsynaptic inhibitory action on Purkinje cells fails to suppress the initial spike discharge evoked by a climbing fiber impulse.

There have been several previous reports on conditioning of evoked responses of the cerebellar cortex (Dow, 1939; Jansen, 1957; Jansen and Fangel, 1961). Unfortunately the recorded electrical responses were not subjected to analytical procedures which would allow their identification as due to the mossy fiber or climbing fiber inputs into the cerebellum, or to combinations of both these inputs. Usually there was a severe depression of the testing response at intervals as long as 100 to 200 msec, but some responses evoked by stimulation of the inferior olive (Jansen, 1957) or of the cerebral cortex (Jansen and Fangel, 1961) showed relatively little depression even at test intervals of 10 to 20 msec. Jansen and Fangel noted that it was the long latency component of the complex spike potential that was resistant to depression and suggested that it was probably the climbing fiber response of Purkinje cells, whereas the earlier components so susceptible to depression were due to the responses that the mossy fiber input evokes in granule cells.

J. Discussion

Initially, two explanations can be offered for the effect of inhibition in increasing and prolonging the negative field potentials (cf. Fig. 100 J) produced by CF stimulation. There are, first, the increased and prolonged EPSPs that are observed during the hyperpolarization of the IPSP (Fig. 99); secondly, during the inhibition there is depression of the later spike complex produced by climbing fibers (Fig. 98 B—D, I—L). The more superficial dendritic regions of the Purkinje cells (200 µ to surface) are but little invaded by impulses (Figs. 43, 50, 51; Eccles, Llinás and Sasaki, 1966 e) and so act as sources to the deeper sinks produced by the impulses (Fig. 46); hence the diminution of these sinks by inhibition would diminish the sources and so increase the later stages of the negative field potential, particularly at superficial levels.

Under normal physiological conditions it can be assumed that the background excitation of Purkinje cells by the parallel fiber synapses is controlled by the input through mossy fibers to granule cells to their axons, the parallel fibers. The negative feedback on this excitatory input by the pathway, parallel fibers to Golgi cells to the inhibitory synapses on granule cells (Chapter VII) would produce a "disfacilitation" of the Purkinje cells, much as has been demonstrated for the cerebellar inhibitory influence on motoneurones (Terzuolo, 1959; Llinás, 1964) and on neurones of the red nucleus (Tsukahara, Toyama, Kosaka and Udo, 1964). Thus experimentally applied parallel fiber stimulation in Fig. 100 B and H—J by exciting Golgi cells removes the background excitatory effect that is produced on Purkinje cells by the mossy fiber → granule cell → parallel fiber pathway; and so it exerts a hyperpolarizing influence on Purkinje cells. Such a hyperpolarization would be accompanied by an increase of the over-all resistance of the post-synaptic membrane (LLINÁS, 1964), and thus provides a third explanation of the increased size of the CF-evoked EPSP when superimposed on the hyperpolarization produced a parallel fiber volley.

In the normal functioning of the cerebellum it must be of great significance that single climbing fibers have such an intense excitatory action that, even when at a relatively high frequency, each impulse may evoke several discharges from a Purkinje cell as in Fig. 97 B. Furthermore, our experiments (ECCLES, SASAKI and STRATA, unpublished observations) indicate that a powerful inhibition can succeed only in reducing this frequency of Purkinje cell discharge to one for each climbing fiber impulse, not to blocking all discharge. Inhibitory action may also be of importance in preventing a high frequency of climbing fiber impulses from effecting an inactivation response of the Purkinje cell as in Fig. 97 C—F, H, I. Thus it can be postulated that climbing fiber impulses have a dominating control on the Purkinje cell discharges and that multiple discharges normally evoked by each impulse can be reduced to a varying degree by inhibition, but not blocked. Therefore, for any given testing input by CF impulses, the frequency of the evoked Purkinje cell discharge signals the level of the background excitatory and inhibitory synaptic action on the cell from instant to instant, the excitation being by the parallel fiber synapses, the inhibition by the basket and stellate cell synapses. This operative feature will be further considered in Chapters XII and XV.

Chapter IX

The Axon Collaterals of Purkinje Cells

A. The Distribution and Mode of Termination

The recurrent collaterals of Purkinje axons take their origin from the proximal as well as more remote parts of the axon. Thus, they can reach closely neighboring regions of the cortex within the same folium as well as in adjacent and even in rather remote folia. According to the classical description of CAJAL (1911) the recurrent collaterals are myelinated and ascend in oblique direction through the deeper strata of the granular layer. Upon reaching the upper stratum of this layer they bend into a tangential direction, and by branching profusely they give rise to a dense plexus situated beneath the layer of the Purkinje cell bodies. This plexus is referred to generally as the "infraganglionic plexus". Branches arising either directly from the Purkinje cell axons or from the infraganglionic plexus, ascend to the level above the Purkinje cell bodies, where another tangential plexus of myelinated fibers is established: the so-called "supraganglionic" plexus. The course of the fibers in the infraganglionic plexus is predominantly parallel to the transversal plane of the folium, but the supraganglionic plexus in the molecular layer is longitudinally oriented (Fig. 101). Under the EM the fibers, especially of the upper plexus, can be recognized easily from their myelin sheaths (FOX, SIEGESMUND and DUTTA, 1964), there being no other myelinated fibers in the molecular layer except the rare Cajal-Smirnov fibers.

Using the degeneration technique, FREZIK (1963) could show that, while there are very few if any recurrent Purkinje collaterals of the vermis reaching beyond the immediate vicinity of their origin in the longitudinal direction of the folium, in the transverse plane of the folia quite considerable distances can be bridged by these connexions. For example, in the sagittal plane of the vermis, recurrent Purkinje axon collaterals could be traced from lobe VII B of LARSELL as far as lobe V A. Essentially similar results were obtained by EAGER (1963 b, 1965) who found that the majority of association systems is of relatively short interfolial character with some predominance of connexions in the sagittal plane. Long association pathways have been traced from anterior paravermal regions to caudal folia of the homolateral crus II and from crus II a crossed pathway to the contralateral crus II and paramedian lobule. It is a remarkable observation of EAGER (1965) that instead of being distributed throughout the folium, degeneration was confined to a surface area corresponding roughly in position to the area of damaged cortex giving rise to the pathway. A similar *quasi* point-to-point relationship between cortical areas and those to which they send association fibers could be observed also in our own material.

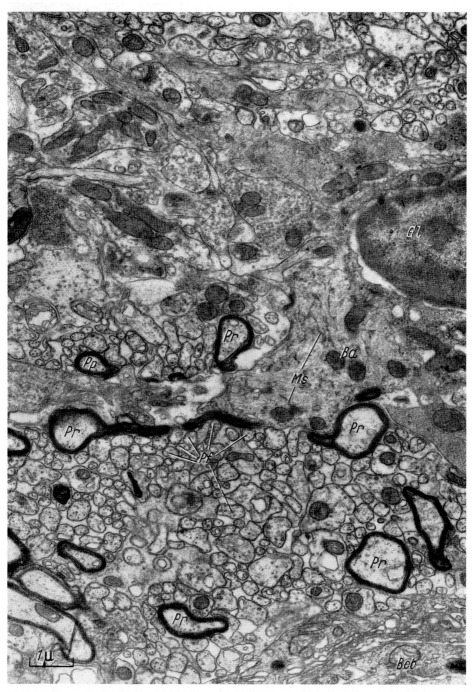

Fig. 101. Supraganglionic plexus of recurrent Purkinje axon collaterals (*Pr*) in the molecular layer. These fibers are myelinated and their course is longitudinal, i. e. parallel to the parallel fibers (*Pf*). Basket cell body (*Bcb*) is seen below. Basket axon (*Ba*) can be recognized on the basis of its filamentous structure and membrane systems (*Ms*). *Gl* = glia cell

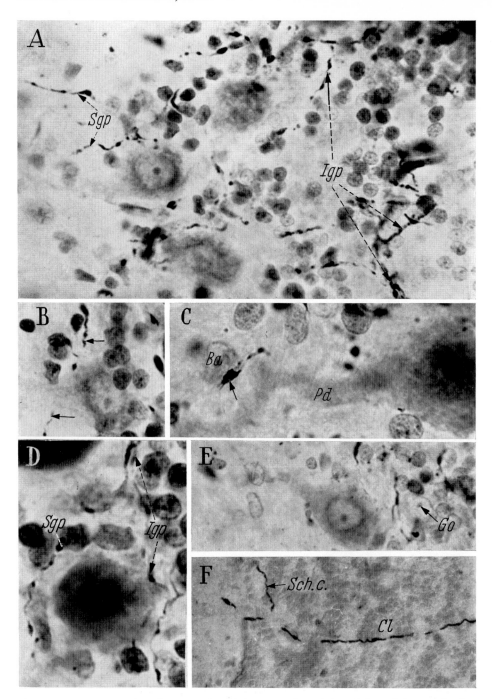

Fig. 102 A—E. Degeneration of recurrent Purkinje axon collaterals in a folium of the vermis of an adult cat five days after the removal of three adjacent folia. Nauta procedure. A. Degenerated axon fragments in the infraganglionic plexus (*Igp*) and the supraganglionic plexus (*Sgp*) can be recognized. The latter fragment rows due to their seemingly ascending course might be mistaken as climbing fibers. Howevers, this is a delusion in consequence of slightly oblique sectioning plane (as seen from the irregular positions of Purkinje cell bodies), and the longitudinal course of the

FREZIK (1963) described the mode of termination of intercortical association fibers as being unequivocally due to degeneration of the infraganglionic and of the supraganglionic plexus. Moreover, he compared the characteristic distributions of degeneration fragments in the course of the degeneration of pathways terminating exclusively either by mossy fibers (see Fig. 20), or by climbing fibers (Fig. 22), with the degeneration pattern found at the sites of termination of association fibers. From this he drew the conclusion that the supra- and infraganglionic plexuses of CAJAL are indeed the preterminal parts of association pathways, which thus must be mainly recurrent Purkinje axon collaterals.

It is most surprising that EAGER (1965) on the basis of very similar findings arrived at the conclusion that intercortical association fibers might terminate as climbing fibers. With respect to the importance of this question a reinvestigation of FREZIK's (1963) material and a comparison with the figures of EAGER (1965) was undertaken. Although some figures of EAGER raise doubts with respect to the fixation or to the possible postoperative vascular damage of the molecular layer[1], it is clear from the two investigations that both the supraganglionic and the infraganglionic plexuses were degenerated. As also to be seen from Fig. 102, partly reproduced from FREZIK (1963), the degeneration of association systems corresponds exactly to the classical description of the course of recurrent Purkinje axon collaterals and has no resemblance whatever to the distribution of fragments that is described by SZENTÁGOTHAI and RAJKOVITS (1959) as occurring after olivary lesions. Whereas the fragments of climbing fibers are always closely associated to the main dendrites of the Purkinje cells (Fig. 22), the association fibers are not. Of course, in cases of such massive degeneration as shown by EAGER (1965), degeneration fragments may by chance look as running parallel with larger Purkinje dendrites. But on close inspection under high power it becomes clear that the degeneration fragments of association fibers in the supraganglionic plexus are only crossing the Purkinje dendrites. A source of error is introduced by the fact, unknown from light microscopy, but appearing clearly under the EM (Fig. 101), that the supraganglionic plexus is oriented predominantly in the longitudinal axis of the folium. In transverse sections of about 20—30 μ thickness this may very well generate the false impression that the rows of fragments are ascending in the molecular layer. The relatively good staining in the Nauta procedure of association

[1] Degeneration appears to be too massive in many pictures.

recurrent collateral branches (see Fig. 101) in the supraganglionic plexus. — B. Row of degeneration fragments (arrows) can be seen to cross principal dendrite of Purkinje cell. — C. Row of fragments (oriented transversally to sectioning plane, i.e. parallel to folium axis) approaches basket cell body (Ba), recognizable from nucleus. Degeneration fragments have no relation to Purkinje dendrite (Pd). — D. Details of degeneration in infraganglionic (Igp) and supraganglionic plexus (Sgp) — E. Fragments of infraganglionic plexus get into close relation with Golgi cell (Go) recognizable from pale nucleus. — F. Degeneration in the granule layer of climbing fiber (Cl) after olivary lesion (from SZENTÁGOTHAI and RAJKOVITS, 1959), shown for comparison. Note undivided radial course of fragment row, giving a single side branch immediately below the Purkinje cell layer, the Scheibel (1954) collateral (Sch.c), and the main branch beginning to ascend through the ganglionic layer. It is lost generally from sight due to loss of myelin sheath and defective staining of unmyelinated fiber fragments in the molecular layer (see also Fig. 22) fibers is most probably connected with their being myelinated, as was correctly surmised by EAGER (1965); but this again is a strong argument against the termination of association systems as climbing fibers, which are well known to lose their myelin sheath at the Purkinje cell level. This can be seen also under the EM, and at the level of the large Purkinje dendrites they are certainly unmyelinated (HÁMORI and SZENTÁGOTHAI, 1966 a).

The termination and the synaptic relations of the recurrent Purkinje axon collaterals are still not fully defined. In neurofibrillar preparations, CAJAL (1911) saw numerous boutons terminaux in contact with the primary and secondary dendrites of Purkinje cells, and suggested that they corresponded most probably to the terminals of Purkinje collaterals. This assumption is in good agreement with the level at which the supraganglionic plexus is located. But there are two other kinds of cells to which terminal branches of the Purkinje axon collaterals could easily have access: the basket and the Golgi cells. In CAJAL's time the numerous endings covering the cell bodies of these neurons were not known, and in addition CAJAL may have been biased by his general idea that axon collaterals terminate on the same kind of cell as that from which they originate. Of course, this idea has now been shown to be erroneous in many places: e. g. the initial motor axon collaterals, and the collaterals of thalamic neurons.

As mentioned in Chapter IV, the terminal knobs on both Golgi cells (Fig. 18) and basket cells (Fig. 36) are at least of two different kinds: the neurofibrillar kind is the ending of climbing fibers, while the vesicular is shown to be of local origin by the degeneration experiments of HÁMORI and SZENTÁGOTHAI (1966 a). In the case of the Golgi cells there are no other axon terminals from which terminal side branches could reach the Golgi cells easily. Indirect reasoning would support the assumption that the vesicular terminal knobs are recurrent Purkinje axon endings, and quite convincing evidence for this has presented itself recently in EM studies (Fig. 103).

The strange tubular system discovered by ANDRES (1965) was mentioned already in Chapter I, and has been shown by HÁMORI (unpublished) to be specific for Purkinje axons and their endings (Fig. 5); hence it can be used for identification of the synaptic terminals of Purkinje axons. So far, this characteristic tubular system has been found in terminals situated in the immediate neighborhood of basket cells, but not in the numerous vesicular (i. e. non-climbing fiber) synapses on the large Purkinje dendrites, and in synaptic terminals on Golgi cell somata; however, as mentioned in Chapter I such negative observations are equivocal. The question, therefore, of the termination of Purkinje axon terminals needs further elucidation with the aid of degeneration studies combined with observation under the EM. Although no final judgement is possible as yet, it appears from experiments under progress, that very few if any recurrent Purkinje axon collaterals contact Purkinje dendrites, whereas their synaptic contacts with basket and Golgi cells can be demonstrated by secondary degeneration (Figs. 102, 103). Fox et al. (1967) give a beautiful illustration of synapses made by a Purkinje axon collateral on a large smooth dendrite in the molecular layer, which conceivably could be a Purkinje dendrite. They also give Golgi pictures of presumed synapses of Purkinje axon collaterals on somata of Purkinje cells and Golgi cells.

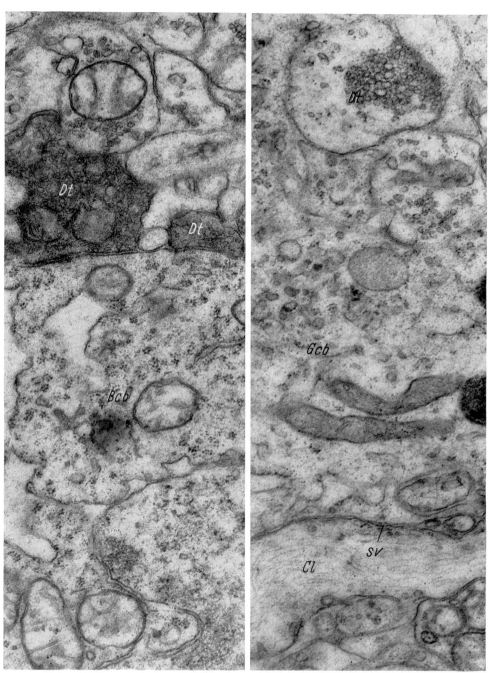

Fig. 103. Degeneration of recurrent Purkinje axon terminals (*Dt*) (left) on basket cell body (*Bcb*) and (right) on Golgi cell body (*Gcb*). Adult cat cerebellar folium of the vermis after destruction of three neighboring folia of the same lobe five days earlier. Boutons in contact with basket cell body show the high density that is most characteristic for the five day stage degeneration. The Golgi cell body (left) is cut tangentially with vesicular boutons (compare Fig. 18) impressed into its surface. Degeneration (*Dt*) appears in one of the boutons as agglutination of synaptic vesicles in one part of the terminal. Below an intact neurofilamentous climbing fiber collateral (*Cl*) is seen attached to cell surface having only few synaptic vesicles (*Sv*) at site of contact

B. Physiological Evidence for Synaptic Actions of Purkinje Axon Collaterals

1. On Purkinje Cells

As described in Section A, histological investigations have in general failed to discover synapses on Purkinje dendrites and somata that can with assurance be attributed to Purkinje axon collaterals. It can be concluded that, if present, these synapses are infrequent, and hence relatively ineffective.

Since Purkinje cells have been shown to have a direct inhibitory action on the cells of Deiters nucleus (Chapter XIII; ITO and YOSHIDA, 1964, 1966; ITO, OBATA and OCHI, 1966) and of the intracerebellar nuclei (ITO, YOSHIDA and OBATA, 1964; ITO, YOSHIDA, OBATA, KAWAI and UDO, 1967), a similar synaptic inhibitory action would be expected for the axon collaterals of Purkinje cells. The chronically deafferented cerebellum gives opportunity for testing this inference. Since, presumably, the inhibitory action is weak, it is important to test for it by the sensitive index that is provided by the spontaneous rhythmic discharge of a Purkinje cell in chronically deafferented cerebella (ECCLES, LLINÁS and SASAKI, 1966 e).

Fig. 104 A gives a consecutive series of records in which single J.F. stimuli are applied during such a rhythmic discharge. In each of these four records the stimulus evokes an antidromic response marked by the arrows, and this is followed by a silence of 52 to 146 msec, which is much longer than the longest cycle (35 msec) of the rhythm before the stimulation. However, this silence is much briefer than the silence produced by the inhibitory action of a single parallel fiber volley, the range being 325 to 380 msec for this rhythmic response, one example (325 msec silence) being illustrated in Fig. 104 A (cf. Fig. 106). In the deafferented cerebellum the mode of generation of the spontaneous rhythm is unknown; nevertheless the typical inhibitory action of the parallel fiber volley establishes that it is a sensitive indicator of inhibitory action on Purkinje cells. Hence it can be concluded that the antidromic volley in the Purkinje axons exerts a considerable inhibitory action on this Purkinje cell. The variability in the duration of the silence may be attributed in part to variations in the rhythmic mechanism itself, as disclosed by the irregularities in the rhythm before the silent periods, and in part to variations in a weak inhibitory mechanism.

The most regular rhythmic discharge that we have observed is illustrated in Fig. 104 B, C from another chronically deafferented cerebellum. In B the J. F. stimulation is just at threshold for the axon of the Purkinje cell under observation, setting up a discharge in three examples and failing to do so in four others. In the former the interpolated antidromic impulse is followed by a pause in the rhythm which in each case is a little longer than compensatory, i. e. the sum of the intervals before and after the interpolated response is longer than two normal cycles, the mean value for 14 observations being 2.19. On the other hand, in the latter group of four, the rhythmic discharge appears to be unaffected; yet as shown by a small potential wave (marked by arrows) this stimulus excited other Purkinje axons. When the J. F. stimulus strength is increased so that antidromic impulses are set up in a larger number of Purkinje axons, the pauses are always more than compensatory, the mean value being 2.49 for the series of 18 that is partly illustrated in

Fig. 104 C, which is highly significant ($P \ll 0.01$). It can be concluded that in this experiment antidromic impulses in the Purkinje axons also exert a weak inhibitory action on Purkinje cells.

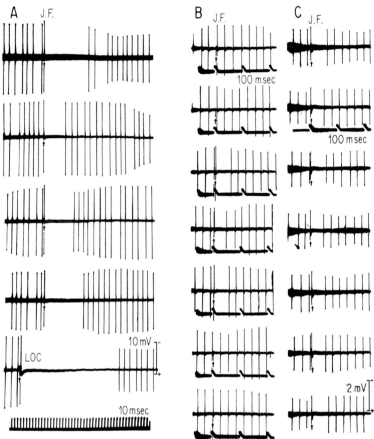

Fig. 104 A—C. *Inhibitory action on the spontaneously rhythmic discharges of Purkinje cells in the chronically deafferented cerebellum.* In the four upper records of A a single J. F. stimulus was applied at the arrows and evoked an antidromic response of the Purkinje cell followed by a silence of variable duration. In the lowest record a much longer silence was produced by a single parallel fiber volley. The variations in the spike heights are due to slight movements caused by respiration. B and C illustrate the weaker inhibition that a J. F. stimulus exerts on a rhythmic Purkinje cell in another chronically deafferented cerebellum. In B the stimulus was just at threshold and in this consecutive series of traces it excited the Purkinje cell antidromically only in the middle three. In C the J. F. stimulus was 2.5 times the threshold strength and on every occasion an antidromic spike was set up and followed by a fairly long silence (ECCLES, LLINÁS and SASAKI, 1966 e)

Altogether, thirteen rhythmically discharging Purkinje cells of the deafferented cerebellum have been tested for the inhibitory action of impulses in Purkinje cell axons, and inhibition has been demonstrated in 9, including the two illustrated in Fig. 104.

It is important to recognize that this inhibitory action is very weak relative to the inhibition generated by parallel fiber volleys, hence the double antidromic volley technique fails to demonstrate any inhibitory depression beyond that attributable to refractoriness (Fig. 44), though the antidromic spike potential wave is very effective in demonstrating the inhibition produced by a parallel fiber volley (Figs. 50, 51, 52, 53).

2. On Inhibitory Interneurones

In Section A it was seen that Purkinje axon collaterals make synapses on the somata and dendrites of basket and Golgi cells. If these synapses are inhibitory, an antidromic volley in Purkinje axons would be expected to diminish the response of Golgi or basket cells to a testing parallel fiber volley.

In Fig. 105 A—H this suggestion is tested by the response of a Golgi cell to a parallel fiber volley at various intervals after a conditioning J. F. stimulation. There is depression of the testing response, so that instead of the control response of 4 spikes (A) there is reduction to 2 spikes at 40 to 74 msec (F—H). At briefer intervals there is less depression, but there is never the facilitation observed with two parallel fiber stimulations (Fig. 40). Evidently, in addition to its initial excitatory action that evokes usually a single discharge from the Golgi cell (Fig. 39 M and Table 1), J. F. stimulation produces a prolonged inhibition.

The inhibitory effectiveness of J. F. stimulation can be assessed by testing it at a fixed interval by the responses evoked by parallel fiber stimulations of various strengths. In Fig. 105 I—P, at a testing interval of about 20 msec, the J. F. stimulation is very effective on the responses to relatively weak parallel fiber stimulation, reducing the number of spikes from 4 to 1 (I, M) and from 5 to 2 (J, N); but with stronger stimulation the depressions are less spectacular, from 6 spikes to 3 (K, O) and from 8 to 6 (L, P).

3. Discussion

The inhibitory action that may be postulated for impulses in the axon collaterals of Purkinje cells is so weak that it may have but little functional importance as a negative feed-back control of Purkinje cell activity; nevertheless it is highly significant because it corroborates the general principle (a development of DALE's Principle) that all the synapses made by the axonal branches of a neurone have the same function: in this case there is inhibitory action by the synaptic terminals of Purkinje cells in three sites: the intracerebellar nuclei (ITO, YOSHIDA and OBATA, 1964); Deiters nucleus (ITO and YOSHIDA, 1964, 1966); and at the synapses of the Purkinje axon collaterals onto Purkinje cells, basket cells and Golgi cells.

In experiments such as those of Fig. 105 the J. F. stimulus would be exciting mossy fibers and climbing fibers as well as Purkinje axons. However, mossy fibers would be expected to have purely an excitatory action on Golgi and basket cells by the granule cell-parallel fiber pathway, and collaterals of climbing fibers would also be expected to be excitatory; hence it seems likely that the inhibition of Fig. 105 is genuinely due to Purkinje axon collaterals. This inference has now been corroborated by investigations on the chronically deafferented preparations (LLINÁS, personal communication). In such preparations J. F. stimulation completely silenced repetitively discharging basket cells, being apparently more powerful than in Fig. 105. Possibly, because of the section of the Purkinje axons, there was a hypertrophic reaction of the Purkinje axon collaterals.

It is surprising that, despite its very effective excitation of parallel fibers, J. F. stimulation is much less effective than LOC stimulation in evoking discharges from Golgi, basket or stellate cells (Chapter IV; ECCLES, LLINÁS and SASAKI, 1966a). For example, in Figs. 38 J, 39 L and M, J. F. stimulation evokes only a single discharge in contrast to the multiple discharges evoked by parallel fiber volleys. Sometimes J. F. stimulation evokes a double discharge (Fig. 105 B—H), but triple discharges are rare (Table 1). It can now be suggested that this ineffectiveness of

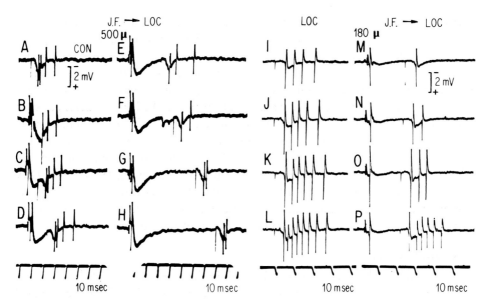

Fig. 105 A—P. *Inhibitory actions of juxta-fastigial stimulation on the responses that parallel fiber volleys evoke in presumed inhibitory interneurones.* In A—H the inhibitory action of the juxta-fastigial stimulus was tested over a wide range of stimulus intervals, 4 msec in B to 74 msec in H, the control response to the testing parallel fiber volley being shown in A (depth, 500 μ). In I—P the first column shows responses evoked by a parallel fiber stimulus of progressively increasing strength, while in the equivalent responses of the second column there was conditioning by a juxta-fastigial stimulus 20 msec earlier (depth 180 μ). (ECCLES, LLINÁS and SASAKI, 1966a)

the J. F. stimulation is attributable to the inhibitory action of the Purkinje cell axon collaterals, which considerably curtails the repetitive discharges of Golgi and stellate cells in Fig. 105.

These actions of Purkinje axon collaterals are examples of positive feed-back action upon Purkinje cells, arising as a consequence of disinhibition (cf. WILSON and BURGESS, 1962). The discharge of impulses by Purkinje cells inhibits both the basket and stellate cells that are inhibitory to Purkinje cells (ANDERSEN, ECCLES and VOORHOEVE, 1964; ECCLES, LLINÁS and SASAKI, 1966b, e, f).

Again the Purkinje cell discharge also inhibits Golgi cells that are inhibitory to granule cells, which in turn excite Purkinje cells (ECCLES, LLINÁS and SASAKI, 1966c; ECCLES, SASAKI and STRATA, 1967a). In all cases, the more the Purkinje cells discharge, the more the inhibitory cells are depressed and so the more the Purkinje cells are released from inhibition.

Chapter X

Spontaneous Activity in the Cerebellar Cortex

ADRIAN (1935) first described the existence of high frequency (about 200/sec) potential waves on the surface of the cerebellum. There has been much investigation of these waves and there is general agreement that they are generated by the physiological events in the cerebellar cortex (BROOKHART, MORUZZI and SNIDER, 1951), and rapidly disappear on deterioration of the cortex (DOW, 1938; MORUZZI, 1957). However, they persist after section of all the cerebellar peduncles (CREPAX and INFANTELLINA, 1955). Microelectrode investigation of the cerebellar cortex has as yet not disclosed the manner of production of the cerebellar waves, though it has shown that in the lightly anaesthetized cortex there is a background activity of most cellular components (Figs. 106, 107; BROOKHART et al., 1950, 1951; DOW and MORUZZI, 1958; GRANIT and PHILLIPS, 1956, 1957; ECCLES, LLINÁS and SASAKI, 1966a, 1966c, 1966e, 1966f). In this chapter an account will be given of investigations on the spontaneous background discharges of the various types of cells.

A. Granule Cells

A relatively high resistance microelectrode in the granular layer of the cerebellar cortex often records a fine background noise, but only occasionally is it possible to position the electrode so that this noise is resolved into the repetitive spike discharges of one or a very few granule cells, as in Fig. 107 A. In B, the spontaneous activity of all these cells is silenced for a period of 100 msec by a single LOC stimulation, and in D there is a similar inhibition (also 100 msec) following a J. F. stimulation. Presumably these inhibitions are produced by the Golgi cells (cf. Chapter VII, sections B and J) that are excited by LOC and J. F. stimulation (Chapter IV). In C stimulation of the inferior olive (I. O.) has a small inhibitory action, which presumably is due to the Golgi cells that are excited by the axon collaterals of climbing fibers (cf. Chapter II B and Table 1).

B. Purkinje Cells

The background discharge of Purkinje cells has been frequently described (BROOKHART et al., 1950, 1951; GRANIT and PHILLIPS, 1956, 1957). There are firstly the discharges of single impulses in a more or less regular rhythmic series, and secondly the spontaneous Purkinje cell responses that we now can recognize as being evoked by climbing fibers.

In Fig. 106 two Purkinje cells are firing spontaneously at a frequency of about 200/sec, which is higher than the usual discharge rate (BROOKHART et al., 1950, 1951; GRANIT and PHILLIPS, 1956, 1957; DOW and MORUZZI, 1958). A single LOC stimulus suppresses the discharges for about 100 msec for the small spikes and

120 msec for the large. At the frequency of 5/sec there is time for full recovery of the Purkinje cell discharges before suppression by the next stimulus, but at 10/sec only one Purkinje cell recovers between the successive stimuli. A stimulation frequency of 16/sec suffices to suppress all discharges, but recovery occurs at just over 100 msec after the last stimulus. Finally, at 100/sec stimulation, the complete suppression takes rather longer (150 msec) before firing is resumed at an initially lower frequency.

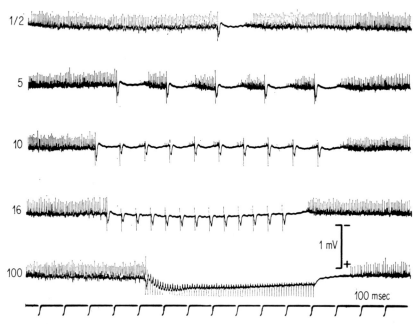

Fig. 106. *Inhibition of spontaneous discharges of Purkinje cells.* The spontaneous firing of two Purkinje cells giving the large and small spike responses were inhibited by LOC stimulation at the indicated frequencies. (ANDERSEN, ECCLES and VOORHOEVE, 1964)

It was originally suggested that this powerful inhibitory action is wholly due to the IPSPs that parallel fiber volleys evoke in Purkinje cells by the pathway through basket cells (ANDERSEN, ECCLES and VOORHOEVE, 1964). However, if the repetitive Purkinje cell discharge is excited by continuous background discharge of the granule cells (cf. Fig. 107 A) and so of parallel fibers, then Golgi cell inhibition of the granule cells (Fig. 107 B and D) would contribute very effectively to the periods of silence in Fig. 106. According to both explanations the silence would be expected to be of the observed duration — rather more than 100 msec.

In Fig. 104 A—C the background discharge of Purkinje cells occurs even in the chronically deafferented cerebellum. This common finding that the Purkinje cells are continuously discharging even in the chronically deafferented cerebellum (cf. CREPAX and INFANTELLINA, 1955) is surprising, and shows that a continuous excitatory barrage along the input lines is not necessary for maintenance of the Purkinje cell discharge. One possibility is that the chronically deafferented granule cells are spontaneously discharging on account of a denervation sensitivity (cf.

CANNON and ROSENBLUETH, 1949). Alternatively, the Purkinje cells themselves may be generating the discharge, and certainly in many cases this can be attributed to mechanical injury by the microelectrode, since the frequency can be raised or lowered by small movements of the microelectrode. In Fig. 104 B, C, the discharge is seen to be remarkably regular, but some Purkinje cells are grossly irregular. LOC stimulation regularly produces prolonged silence in this discharge, the silence being 325 msec in the lowest trace of Fig. 104 A.

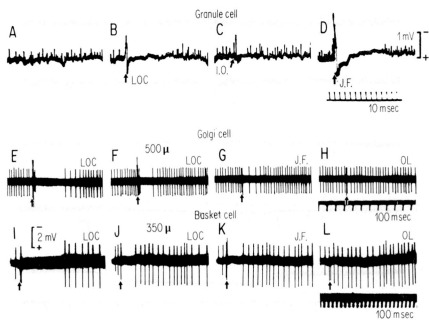

Fig. 107 A—L. *Inhibition of spontaneous discharges of granule cells and of inhibitory interneurones.* The spontaneous discharge of several granule cells in A is inhibited by LOC, I. O., and J. F. stimulation. Presumably the LOC stimulation was effective because of its excitation of mossy fibers. (ECCLES, LLINÁS and SASAKI, 1966 c). The inhibitory interneurone at 500 μ depth in E—H was silenced by a strong and weak parallel fiber volley in E and F, and by J.F. stimulation in G, while in H inferior olive stimulation caused at most a brief slowing of the discharge. The inhibitory interneurone at 350 μ depth in I—L also was silenced by a strong and weak parallel fiber volley in I and J, and by J.F. stimulation in K, while in L inferior olive stimulation caused no significant change. All stimuli indicated by arrows. (ECCLES, LLINÁS and SASAKI, 1966 a)

Many Purkinje cells exhibit spontaneous climbing fiber (CF) responses, as illustrated in Figs. 85 K and 108 P—S at arrows, and first reported by GRANIT and PHILLIPS (1956). These responses are identical with the CF responses evoked by inferior olive or juxta-fastigial stimulation, as may be seen by comparing the spontaneous response in the lower trace of Fig. 85 K with the J. F.-evoked responses in the lower traces of Fig. 85 H, I, after due allowance for the IPSP that curtails the latter part of the depolarization. As described in Chapters II B and VIII, the spontaneous CF responses can be presumed to arise on account of impulse discharges from the cells of the inferior olive. Usually these discharges are infrequent (1 to 2/sec) and exhibit no regular rhythm.

C. Inhibitory Interneurones

All inhibitory interneurones of the cerebellar cortex discharge spontaneously at a low and rather irregular frequency, which usually is between 7 and 30/sec (Fig. 107 E—L). This rhythmic discharge provides a suitable background for revealing any direct or indirect action that the various forms of stimulation have on the interneurones. Invariably the repetitive discharge generated by a parallel fiber volley (cf. Figs. 38, 39, 40) is followed by a silence of the background discharge for several hundred milliseconds, as in the presumed Golgi cell of Fig. 107 E, F. Juxta-fastigial stimulation also produces a silence (Fig. 107 G) but of briefer duration, usually 100 to 200 msec; and often, as in G, the inhibitory action may be more properly considered as a slowing of discharge rather than a silence. Fig. 107 H shows that inferior olive stimulation has almost no action.

Comparable inhibitory actions are exhibited in Fig. 107 I—L for a presumed basket cell at a depth of 350 μ. Weak and strong parallel fiber (I, J) and J.F. stimulations (K) result in silences for 1000, 310 and 370 msec respectively, and stimulation of the inferior olive (L) has little or no action.

It must not be assumed that the observed silent periods are due to inhibitory actions directly exerted on the inhibitory interneurones. A more probable explanation can be based on the postulate that these background discharges are due to a continued excitatory action on the interneurones by the pathway: mossy fibers to granule cells to parallel fibers; and that the various stimulations employed in Fig. 107 E—G and I—K inhibit the pathway by exciting Golgi cells that in turn inhibit the mossy fiber-granule cell transmission (Chapter VII; ECCLES, LLINÁS and SASAKI, 1966c; ECCLES, SASAKI and STRATA, 1967a, 1967b). The postulated excitation of presumed Golgi cells by parallel fiber and juxta-fastigial stimulation has been illustrated above (Figs. 39 M—Q, 40 A—J). However, an alternative pathway has also been demonstrated for the inhibitory action of J.F. stimulation on inhibitory interneurones, as is illustrated in Fig. 105, and it has been suggested in Chapter IX that this inhibition could be due to Purkinje axon collaterals. This axon collateral inhibition could contribute to the silence that J.F. stimulation produces in Fig. 107 G and K. Moreover the same axon collateral inhibition could be contributing to the silences in E, F, I and J because the LOC stimulation would be evoking discharges from Purkinje cells (Fig. 47).

D. The Inhibitory Synaptic Noise of Purkinje Cells

In Fig. 85 there are numerous examples of spontaneously occurring IPSPs that appear to be identical with small evoked IPSPs, as for example at arrows in E, F, J, K and M. In Fig. 48 I and J the arrows indicate the onset of small spontaneous hyperpolarizations that presumably also are IPSPs. GRANIT and PHILLIPS (1956, Fig. 7) illustrated two similar examples of spontaneous IPSPs, the small hyperpolarizations silencing the repetitively discharging Purkinje cell for about 100 msec.

Particularly favourable conditions are provided for recording the spontaneous IPSPs when they are inverted by a large increase in intracellular concentration of chloride ions as in Figs. 108 and 109. In Figs. 108 Q and 109 J, K, a J.F. stimulation suppresses the spontaneous IPSPs for about 200 msec, and suppression is also produced by the presumably pure mossy fiber input that is evoked by external cuneate nucleus stimulation (Fig. 108 R). This suppression shows that the spontaneous IPSPs are not quantal like the miniature endplate potentials, but presumably are attributable to the background discharges of basket cells that are illustrated in Fig. 107 I—L; hence these IPSPs may appropriately be termed in-

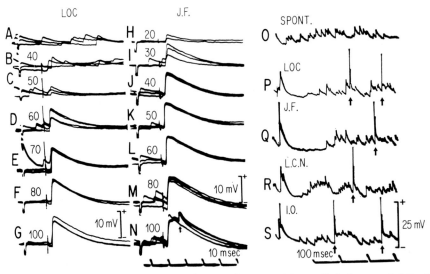

Fig. 108 A—S. *Inhibitory synaptic noise and inverted IPSPs of intracellularly recorded Purkinje cells.* A microelectrode of 10 MΩ filled with KCl recorded from the Purkinje cell at 300 μ depth, IPSPs being inverted by the chloride diffusion out of the electrode. A shows inhibitory synaptic noise in a series of three superimposed traces. In B—G LOC stimulation was progressively increased, as shown by the strengths on the arbitrary scale. In H—N there was similarly a progressively increasing J. F. stimulation with strengths as indicated. (ECCLES, LLINÁS and SASAKI, 1966 f). Record O illustrates the background inhibitory synaptic barrage inverted by Cl⁻ injection into another Purkinje cell. In P, this background bombardment was suppressed for about 140 msec by a LOC stimulation. A suppression was found also in records Q, R and S with J.F., L.C.N. and I.O. stimulation respectively. Note the spontaneous climbing fiber EPSP marked with arrows in records P, Q, R and S. (ECCLES, LLINÁS and SASAKI, 1966 c)

hibitory synaptic noise, being the counterpart of the excitatory synaptic noise first described by BROCK, COOMBS and ECCLES (1952). It is thus postulated that single impulses in the presynaptic terminals of a basket cell are responsible for producing these randomly occurring IPSPs of Purkinje cells in Figs. 48 and 85. The inhibitory synaptic noise has a magnitude in accord with this postulate. As many as 20 basket cells make synaptic contact with one Purkinje cell (Chapter VI, section A1), but some of these contacts are much more extensive than others; hence the expectation that the inhibitory noise would display the observed range of size when measured relative to the maximum evoked IPSPs in Figs. 85, 108 and 109.

An applied depolarizing current can reverse synaptically induced depolarizations whether these are EPSPs (COOMBS, ECCLES and FATT, 1955 b) or IPSPs reversed by chloride (COOMBS, ECCLES and FATT, 1955 a); but much less current is required for the latter. The action of applied depolarizing currents thus sharply distinguishes between the depolarizing IPSPs and EPSPs for the Purkinje cell giving the responses of Fig. 108 A—N.

In the three superimposed traces of Fig. 108 A, there are nine randomly occurring unitary IPSPs having a size range from 0.8 to 3.3 mV. In B—G LOC

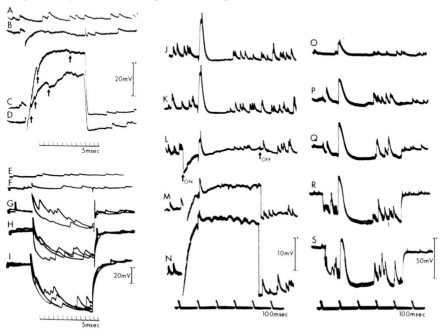

Fig. 109 A—S. *Effect of polarizing DC currents on inhibitory synaptic noise and inhibitory synaptic potentials.* A—D and J—S are responses of the same cell as in Fig. 108 A—N, A showing background inhibitory noise, B the effect of a weak depolarizing DC current, and C and D of a strong depolarizing current that reversed the noise (see arrows). J and K show effect of interposed J. F. stimulation on the inhibitory noise, the stimulus strength being similar to that of Fig. 108 N and similarly showing the small superimposed climbing fiber response. In L—N this J. F. response was superimposed on a depolarizing DC current of progressively increasing size. O gives effect of J. F. stimulation as in J and K but at lower amplification. In P—S this J. F. stimulation was superimposed upon a background hyperpolarizing DC current. E—I show response from another Purkinje cell also recorded with a KCl microelectrode, and with inverted IPSPs as shown in control trace E. In F a small applied hyperpolarizing DC current gave a small increase in the unitary components of the noise, while in G—I a large current caused a large amplification of the inhibitory synaptic noise. (Eccles, Llinás and Sasaki, 1966 f)

stimulation of progressively increasing strength evokes IPSPs of similar time course and as large as 10.3 mV, the smallest (B, C) having a size comparable with the inhibitory synaptic noise. LOC stimulation of strength 50 or more suppresses all inhibitory noise for the duration of the trace and the full duration of the LOC-evoked suppression is seen in Fig. 108 P. In Fig. 108 H to N this suppression also occurs even with the weakest J. F. stimulation (H). It is suggested that this suppression of the spontaneous basket cell discharge (cf. Fig. 107 I—K) is due to the LOC or J. F. excitation of Golgi cells (Figs. 39 M—Q, 40 A—J), which in turn inhibit the mossy fiber granule cell synapses on the background excitatory path to basket cells (Fig. 107 E—G). The IPSPs of the two traces in Fig. 108 H are within the size range for unitary responses, but alternatively the larger could be a double response. The superimposed traces of Fig. 108 D and I give a clear indication that the evoked IPSPs are compounded of varying numbers of unitary IPSPs.

In Fig. 109 F—I hyperpolarizing DC current pulses have the expected effect of greatly amplifying the inverted unitary IPSPs of the inhibitory noise (E), and as well reveal additional small components so that in G—I a ten-fold range in size is displayed. In Fig. 109 B the inhibitory noise of A is apparently abolished by a weak depolarizing current, which presumably displaces the membrane potential to the equilibrium potential for the inverted IPSP. The much larger depolarizing currents (C, D) even reverse the inhibitory noise to the hyperpolarizing potentials indicated by arrows.

The effects of polarizing DC currents on evoked IPSPs and on the unitary IPSPs of inhibitory noise are displayed in Fig. 109 J—S for the same Purkinje cell as Fig. 108. In Fig. 109 J, K the IPSP evoked by J. F. stimulation has a small superimposed EPSP produced by the climbing fiber, as is shown by the arrow at the faster sweep speed in Fig. 108 N. The suppression of inhibitory noise by J.F. stimulation in Fig. 109 J—S has been noted above. Possibly it is caused by two distinct excitatory actions of the J. F. stimulation, namely on Golgi cells and on Purkinje axons, as has been suggested above for the inhibition of spontaneous discharges of the inhibitory interneurones (Fig. 107 E—K): firstly, the Golgi cells excited by the mossy fibers directly or by the mossy fiber-granule cell relay to parallel fibers exert an inhibitory action on the mossy fiber-granule cell synapses (Chapter VII and Figs. 78—83), which are assumed to be continuously discharging excitatory impulses (Fig. 107 A—D) via parallel fibers to the inhibitory interneurones; and, secondly, impulses in the collaterals of the Purkinje axons exert a direct inhibitory action on inhibitory interneurones (Fig. 105).

In Fig. 109 L a weak depolarizing DC current reduces the sizes both of the evoked IPSP and of the inhibitory noise, and in M a larger current virtually neutralizes both these inhibitory responses. Finally, with a still larger current (N), there appears to be inversion of the inhibitory noise. Hyperpolarizing DC currents in Fig. 109 P—S have the opposite effect, increasing many fold both the evoked IPSP and the inhibitory noise. With the largest hyperpolarizing current (S) the evoked IPSP is as large as $+50$ mV and the unitary components of the noise are as large as $+25$ mV. It will be noted that, following the applied currents in Fig. 109 L—N and P—S, there is an immediate return of the inhibitory noise to the size that prevailed before the application of the current.

Chapter XI

Architectural Design of the Cerebellar Cortex

Before embarking on the attempt (Chapter XII) to explain both structurally and functionally the operational features of the cerebellar cortex, it may now be the appropriate occasion to try to get a more synthetic view of its minute architecture. Our approach in Chapters I and II was of necessity more analytic, the attempt there being made to describe separately each of the several neuronal elements and their connexions. Although some synthesis has already been given in the morphological Sections of Chapters III and VII on the two main synaptic arrangements, there is an attractive prospect in the attempt to continue this synthetic approach towards an understanding of the architectonic design of the molecular (A) and the submolecular layers (B) as a whole.

The cerebellar cortex is a marvel of economical use of space with the ultimate aim of achieving maximum connectivity — both divergence and convergence — with the minimum of "dead" or "non-useful" space. Lengths of axons or dendrites not being used for effecting synaptic connexions can be regarded as "dead" space. Undoubtedly, there is little "unused" space in the packing of neuronal elements in any other grey matter; both extracellular space as well as glial and vascular space are kept down to the minimum necessary for the metabolic requirements of the nervous tissue. But there is, nevertheless, a decisive difference between the molecular layer of the cerebellar cortex and other grey matters. While in most cases the dendritic arborizations of neighboring neurons interlace, this occurs only to a very limited degree in the molecular layer. The dendritic arborization of each Purkinje cell has its independent space compartment of roughly $300 \times 225 \times 6\,\mu$, which it does not share, pratically, with other dendritic arborizations. Each Purkinje dendritic arborization shares this space — of course — with a number of axons (parallel, climbing, stellate and ascending basket axon collaterals) and with glial elements. The dendritic arborizations of the stellate, basket and the ascending dendrites of Golgi neurons interlace with each other, but they are confined largely to the thin space of about $2\,\mu$ thickness left free between the arborizations of neighboring Purkinje cells.

It is relatively easy to fill in any space with random interlacing elements, each of which during the development can be visualized as finding its compartments and free niches by trial and error and mutual adjustment and according to some general pattern of arborization inherent in the different types of neurons and processes. But it is by no means simple to fill in the space with a number of separate elements with predetermined sizes and shapes, even if considerable allowance is made for shape changes such as are seen with Purkinje cells in the depth of sulci and at the top of the folia (Fig. 2). The flattening in the transverse plane of the dendritic tree mainly of Purkinje cells, but consequently also of stellate and basket cells, is undoubtedly an ingenious adjustment to the task of filling in the space available with relatively individual cell compartments, i.e. with negligible inter-lacing of the respective dendritic arborizations, without having in between "dead" spaces and "dead" lines of connexions. This would occur obviously if the dendritic trees would be flattened, for example, in the longitudinal direction of the folia.

If it were primarily a question of connectivity, an equally high degree of divergence and convergence could be achieved simply by interlacing arborizations of the dendritic trees, as is seen for example in the hippocampus where the main output elements, the large pyramids, are also arranged in a single sheet, but where the dendrites do interlace. It is, therefore, interesting to speculate about the sig-nificance of the strict separation of the dendritic arborizations of Purkinje cells. The phylogenesis of the cerebellar cortex offers few if any clues, since there are relatively small changes through the entire vertebrate phylum. It can be said — in general — that phylogenetic progress is associated with the tendency of the neurons to extricate themselves from the random interlacing of their dendrites, which is characteristic of primitive and lowly differentiated nerve nets. This trend is more obvious in the phylogenesis of the cerebral cortex, where, simultaneously with a spectacular decrease in neuron density, the dendritic arborizations become pro-gressively more elaborate, complex and increasingly defined: i.e. each dendritic arborization becomes more isolated or independent from that of other neurons. However, this process of "individualization" does not get very far in the cerebral cortex. Probably any center with an over-separation of its neurons would lose its integrative capacities, resulting, in the extreme, in completely linear chains of neurons. But the trend of "individualization" of the various kinds of neurons and the tendency to elaborate specific spaces for their dendritic arborizations are never-theless unmistakable [1].

The cerebellar cortex has achieved a singularly advanced position by the almost complete "individualization" of its most characteristic type of neuron: the Purkinje cells. But what may be the significance of this separation of the dendritic tree, when all the cells — about three hundred and fifty according to Fox and BARNARD (1957) — situated one behind the other in the longitudinal axis of the folium in the length of 2—3 mm (the length of the parallel fibers) have a major common input anyway? Could it be simply on behalf of the climbing fibers, which effect an almost unique one-to-one projection from inferior olive cells to Purkinje neurons? Establish-ment of a selective synapse of this kind can be more easily imagined in neurons having separate dendritic trees than in those with dendritic interlacing. Almost all other known one-to-one synapses are calyciform or brush-like axosomatic contacts, such as the acoustic receptors and nuclei, the ciliary ganglion of birds and reptiles; and these postsynaptic cells are in general adendritic. In fact also the climbing fiber is an axo-somatic type of synapse in earlier stages of its development (CAJAL, 1911).

---

[1] Speculations along these lines have been made independently by several authors (BODIAN, 1952; SZENTÁGOTHAI, 1952, 1962b; YOUNG, 1964). In spite of the wide varia-tions in viewpoint and approach, these speculations have important common elements, but it would be far beyond the frame of this monograph to go into their details.

As can be inferred from the connexions of climbing fibers with basket and stellate cells, the climbing fiber is not absolutely confined to the Purkinje cell on the dendritic tree of which it starts to climb, but has a certain "freedom" to explore its environment and engage in contacts with other closely neighboring nerve elements. If the dendrites of Purkinje cells would interlace with each other, one could hardly imagine such rigid adherence of one climbing fiber to one Purkinje dendritic arborization as that actually observed both anatomically and functionally (Chapter VIII). This reasoning is undoubtedly very teleological, but "faut de mieux" it could stimulate thoughts directed at a better understanding of such meaningful structures.

The abundance of interneuronal connexions arranged in the transverse plane of the folia might also be related to the strict isolation of Purkinje dendritic trees. As described already in Chapters I, VI and IX, and in more detail in Chapter XII A, the major interneuron circuits are organized in the transverse plane of the folium. Most of them — it is true — are operating at a small distance, well inside the limits of the folium. But again the only intercortical association system operating at larger distances — the recurrent Purkinje axon collaterals (Chapter IX) — is organized in the transverse plane of the folia (FREZIK, 1963). Thus interneuronal connectivity on the whole emphasizes the importance of the organization of cerebellar cortical structure in the transverse plane of the folium in minor scale and in larger scale in the sagittal plane, cutting many successive folia transversely. However, the distortions in the hemispheres that are brought about secondarily, are left unconsidered. There may well be an architectural adaptation of advantage in the separation and flattening of the dendritic trees of Purkinje cells that are organized transversely across the individual folia.

In connexion with this strange fact it might be recalled that for several relay nuclei projecting to the cerebellar cortex the separation of dendritic arborizations is characteristic. In some cases the dendritic arborizations are separated only from those of neighboring grey regions: for example in CLARKE's column. In others the cells themselves are more or less completely individualized, e.g. in the inferior olive. It is of particular interest that the climbing fibers, having this unique one-to-one synaptic relation to the completely "individualized" Purkinje cells, are originating from the inferior olive which shows a similar individualization — or "compartmentalization" of the dendritic spaces of the neurones. In the pontine nuclei individualization of dendritic space is less conspicuous, but nevertheless exhibits the same trend. Furthermore in the efferent pathways of the cerebellum the separation of dendritic trees and of axon ramifications into individual cell compartments or cell group compartments is a predominant feature of the structural organization. On account of the intricate and not satisfactorily understood modes of synaptic coupling in these nuclei, the consequences of these structural peculiarities of the cerebellar neuron chains — in the wider sense — are difficult to appreciate. It is the result of a vague feeling rather than a rationally founded inference, when the writer of this Chapter thinks that these peculiarities are a decisive feature of the structural and connectivity design of the cerebellar system, and are tied up in some way or other with its specific manner of information processing.

A. Space Arrangement of Neuronal Elements in the Molecular Layer

The molecular layer is built up of sheets of dendritic arborizations — oriented in the transverse plane of the folium — sheets of Purkinje cell dendritic arborizations alternating with sheets containing the dendritic arborizations of basket, stellate and probably also of Golgi cells. Additionally the axons and the main branches of stellate and basket neurons are also situated in the spaces between the Purkinje dendritic arborizations. According to the calculations of Fox and Barnard (1957), based on the number of Purkinje cells per square mm of surface area and the spread of their dendritic trees, parallel fibers of 3, 2 and 1.5 mm length would traverse the dendritic trees of approximately 460, 310 and 230 Purkinje cells respectively. This would mean that the average distance along the longitudinal axis of the folium — between Purkinje cell dendritic arborizations ought to be 6.4 μ. Since there was no opportunity to study material of the monkey, our own estimates were made on human and cat material. Using Golgi stained longitudinal sections, the average minimum distance between neighboring Purkinje cell arborizations was found to be somewhat less than 10 μ, both in man and the cat[2] (Fig. 26). Another approach makes use of the EM picture. Fig. 110 is from an electronmicrograph of the cerebellar cortex of the cat oriented very carefully in the tangential plane. The cross sections identified as being Purkinje spiny branchlets and their spines are indicated in blue, basket dendrites in red and a third kind of dendrites — possibly of a Golgi neuron — in yellow. All of these dendrites have been identified separately under larger optical magnification, on the basis either of their spines or their synaptic contacts. The EM photomicrograph was taken from a region of the neuropil completely lacking in larger dendrites, and in the lower left corner of the field there is the body of a basket cell. This field is therefore representative only of the true fine neuropil of the molecular layer. The presence of larger dendrites or axons would introduce irregularities that would make measurements impossible. But otherwise this region was not particularly selected. It shows a quite clear transverse stratification of the dendrites. The distances between the rows of Purkinje dendrites are 8 μ on the average, but, in order to get really reliable data, one would need similar investigations on a larger scale with statistical evaluation of the data and careful analysis of possible errors. Such investigations are now in progress in our laboratory. Agreement of these data with the estimate of Fox and Barnard (1957) is reasonably good, and the value obtained is intermediate between the distance measured in Golgi preparations both in man and in the cat and that calculated.

The spaces left free between Purkinje dendritic arborizations are obviously too small to accommodate stellate and basket cell bodies. The round holes seen in completely stained dendritic arborizations have, therefore, correctly been interpreted by Cajal (1911) and Fox and Barnard (1957) as containing the basket and stellate cell bodies. The dendritic arborizations of both stellate and basket

---

[2] Distance were measured from the left side of one P-dendrite to the left side of the next, so that they are comprising the thickness of the P-cell arborization and of the intermediate space.

cells do not seem to interlace with the Purkinje dendrites. Only in the immediate neighbourhood of the large smooth dendrites (recognizable as they protrude from

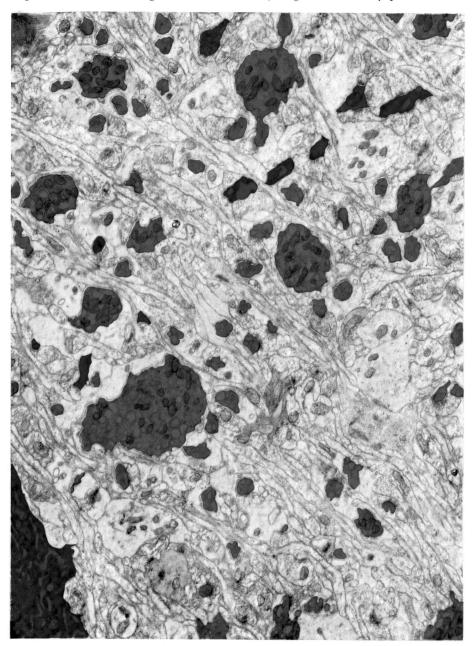

Fig. 110. Tangential — surface parallel — section of the molecular layer in the cat. Various kinds of dendrites have been indicated in colours. Purkinje dendrites and their spines in blue, basket dendrites in red (basket cell body at lower left corner) and probably Golgi dendrite in yellow. Arrangement of dendrites in alternating transversal sheets — here running from right above to left below — can be well recognized. Parallel fibers are left uncoloured and are seen to run in bundles in the longitudinal direction of the folium — here from left above to right below

the flat sheet of the spiny branchlet arborization) are basket dendrites seen to come into the immediate neighbourhood of the Purkinje dendrites when crossing them.

The Purkinje dendrite sheet, containing only spiny branchlets and spines, was found to be 6 µ thick on the average; hence only about 2 µ would remain for the arborization of the non Purkinje dendrites. But, as the thickness of the P-dendritic sheet is calculated with the spines protruding in all directions from the branchlets, the intermediate space is in reality more than 4 µ. According to the planimetric determinations from the same region, using the paper weight method, about 60 % of the space in this fine neuropil is made up by the parallel fibers, 20 % by glia, 15 % by Purkinje dendrites and their spines, 3 % by basket and other non P-dendrites and their spines and finally 2 % by axons other than parallel fibers.

B. Space Arrangement in the Ganglionic and Granular Layer

There is nothing remarkable in the spatial arrangement in the two submolecular layers, excepting the unusually high percentage of space occupied by glial elements in the ganglionic layer by the large cells long known as the Bergmann glia.

The Purkinje cell bodies are arranged at random, so that neither in the transverse, nor in the longitudinal plane can true rows of cell bodies be distinguished. There is a rather exact fitting of the dendritic sheets of Purkinje cells, which are spaced transversely at the average spread of the dendritic arborizations (about 250 µ). Such an isolaminar arrangement leads to the expectation that these 250 µ spaced cells ought to form exact transverse rows. Since the average thickness of the dendritic tree is around 6 µ, whereas the diameter of the cell body is 30—35 µ, it is obvious that slight deviations in their longitudinal direction in the folium could provide sufficient longitudinal separation (8—10 µ) for the dendritic laminae of two cells situated in exactly the same transversal plane and with bodies touching each other. In this way the dendritic trees of such cells could secure ample room for forming two dendritic sheets spaced at the standard longitudinal separation of 8—10 µ and shifted slightly in transversal direction.

A very considerable part of the space surrounding the P-cell bodies is occupied by the preterminal or terminal basket axons and by the thin ascending axons of granule neurons as well as by the myelinated collaterals of P-axons. Quite frequently ascending dendrites can be seen to transverse this layer, densely covered with synaptic contacts. They can be interpreted as Golgi dendrites. It is obvious that in the level below the equators of the P-cells a considerable amount of space ought to remain free of neuronal elements, because the granular layer does not, in general, extend above the level of the axonal poles of the P-cells. These spaces are occupied by the watery profiles of the Bergmann glia (Fig. 111). The ascending processes of these cells will be mentioned briefly in the next section (C). As already mentioned in Chapter VI (Fig. 56), thin finger-like processes of their bodies are engaged in the outer stratum of the Purkinje cell baskets, interdigitating with similar thin processes of the basket endings. These glial processes also appear to wrap around axons that are impressed or embedded into them, in the fashion of axons with Schwann cells, so producing myelin-like circular layers.

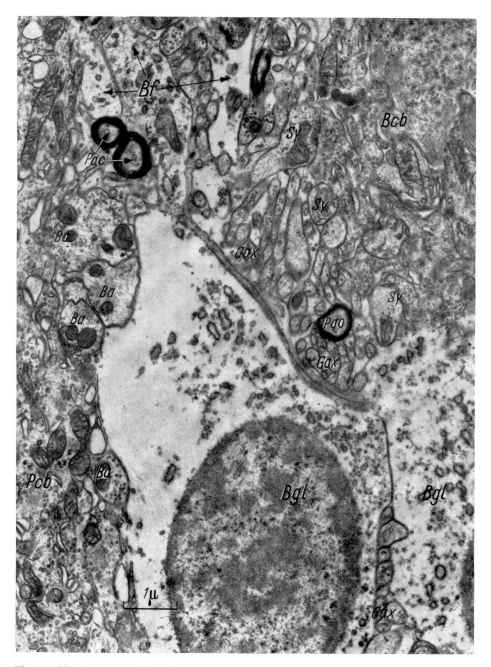

Fig. 111. Two Bergmann glia cells (*Bgl*) are wedged between two Purkinje cell bodies, one of which appears at extreme left (*Pcb*). Process of the Bergmann glia can be followed first along the cell body and principal dendrites of Purkinje cells and later independently as Bergmann fibers (*Bf*) up to the surface of the cortex. Basket cell body appears at upper right (*Bcb*), covered with numerous synaptic terminals (*Sy*). Thin obliquely cut axons are granule axons (*Gax*), small myelinated fibers are Purkinje axon collaterals (*Pac*). Purkinje cell body is covered by basket axons (*Ba*).

The spatial arrangement of tissue elements in the granular layer is determined by the relative amount of space occupied by the cell bodies, about $(70—X)\%^3$, versus that of the glomeruli (about 30%). The individual glomeruli are significantly larger than the individual granule cells and their number relation is 4.5 : 1. Glial elements are found only outside the glomeruli, which are wrapped by thin sheets of their plasma. Even in chronically isolated folia, where a strong hypertrophy of the glial elements accompanies a considerable shrinkage of the glomeruli, the remnants of the glomeruli are devoid of glial elements (Fig. 73).

C. Participation of Glial Elements in the Molecular Layer

This monograph is concerned exclusively with neuronal functions, hence glial architectonics is entirely beyond its scope. It is, therefore, exclusively the spatial arrangement of neuronal and glial elements, mainly on EM level, which is here of interest. No attempts will be made to identify the glial profiles as belonging to one type of glia or the other, although the watery profiles giving the vast majority of glial space either belong to the ascending processes of the Bergmann glia cells or else to the Fañanás glia.

As mentioned already, the amount of glial space is nearly 20% of total space in the true neuropil. This number might change considerably if the molecular layer would be considered as a whole by including both the larger dendrites surrounded by wide glial processes and the larger masses of axons, mainly of basket neurons, that have less glial tissue in their immediate neighbourhood. Only measurements carried out on a large scale and avoiding conscious or unconscious selection of particular kinds of visual fields could furnish reliable data in this respect. The material used for measuring the glial space in the true neuropil, containing only spiny branchlets and parallel axons, was a conventional type of electronmicrograph, having no extracellular spaces with the exception of the usual 200 Å wide interspaces. If it would turn out that this is only an artefact due to swelling of the glial processes as advocated by VAN HARREVELD, CROWELL and MALHOTRA (1965), the amount of interspace would increase mainly at the cost of the glial space.

Fig. 112 shows the glial profiles indicated in full black for the same region of the molecular layer neuropil as Fig. 110. It is obvious from this figure and a comparison with Fig. 110 that glial profiles are concentrated around the dendrites — particularly the Purkinje dendrites — and the spines. Little if any glial space is found between the groups of parallel fibers. The same close relation of the glial elements to the dendrites is even more pronounced in the larger dendrites. As seen from many of the EM photographs (e.g. Figs. 6, 23, 24), these are almost completely wrapped by glial profiles, only the climbing fibers and the terminals of stellate axons as well as ascending basket terminals being admitted to contact the surface of the dendrites. The "watery" character of these glial profiles leaves little doubt about their astrocytic nature. A considerable proportion of the profiles may

---

[3] X equals the fraction of tissue space of undetermined size (probably less than 5%) occupied by elements that are neither granule cell bodies nor glomeruli, i. e. by axons running through, and by Golgi cells, glial cells, and vessels.

belong to the Bergmann glia processes, and this becomes obvious in the most superficial stratum of the molecular layer (Fox *et al.*, 1964). Other profiles of the same kind may be Fañanás glia cells. Oligodendrocytes with denser plasma structure are

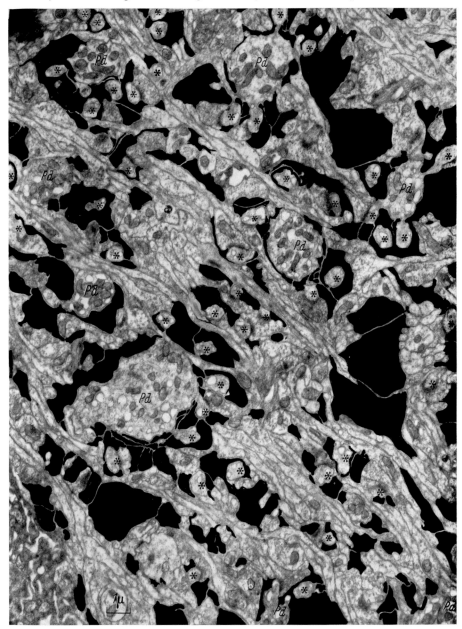

Fig. 112. Same figure as Fig. 110, the glial profiles being shown in black. Glial profiles are accumulated around dendrites, particularly of Purkinje cells (*Pd*) and their characteristic spines (indicated by asterisks) are almost everywhere (with the exception of their contacts with the parallel fibers) "floating" in glial space. The thin bridges left free from black cover correspond to glial double membranes, often running to spines = so called "mesospines". Bundles of parallel fibers are not, in general invaded by glial processes

seen mainly in the deeper stratum of the molecular layer, being related mainly to myelinated axons.

It might be interesting to speculate about the significance of the predominant attachment of glial (astrocytic) elements to the dendrites. The dendrites appear always to be enveloped by a glial cellular layer, blocking them from direct contact with axonal elements. Also the initial parts of the spines are completely surrounded by this glial layer. Occasionally the spines appear simply to pierce this glial layer. In other cases it looks as if the glial processes had secondarily surrounded the stalk of the spine leaving free a duplicate of their surface membrane, which connects the general intercellular space of the neuropil with the thin extracellular layer surrounding the spine. These double membranes have been termed "meso-spines" on analogy to the mesaxons of the unmyelinated nerve fibers in peripheral nerves (HÁMORI and SZENTÁGOTHAI, 1964). The parallel axons, conversely, have no specific relations to glial elements, except in the neighbourhood of dendrites or spines, where the region of the synapse is generally completely surrounded by glial space. Wherever parallel axons have no immediate contacts with dendrites, they are floating free in the intercellular space. This applies particularly to the outer strata of the molecular layer. Only in the deeper strata, containing numerous myelinated axons (the recurrent Purkinje axon collaterals), are there profiles of non-astrocytic character — probably of oligodendrocytes — forming a honeycomb background into which many of the parallel fibers are impressed or occasionally embeded (Fig.101). Does this strange difference in the relations of astrocytic elements to dendrites and spines indicate the specific metabolic dependence of the latter from the glial elements and the relative independence of the parallel fibers – particularly of their nonsynaptic regions? Or is it primarily a question of insulating the dendritic surface, with the exception of the specific synaptic contact regions, from accidental contact with axons, or more specifically for insulation of the synaptic regions? However, these interesting questions have to be left unanswered for the time being.

The question of extracellular space might be touched here very cursorily. It is, of course, beyond the scope of this monograph to enter into the lengthy discussions around this general problem of neurohistology. It appears that the amount of extracellular space encountered in the EM picture of central nervous tissue is largely dependent on the technique employed (VAN HARREVELD, CROWELL and MALHOTRA, 1965). It is today more or less a matter of judgement (or taste), mostly on the basis of some kind of indirect information, whether one accepts the conventional "good" pictures with little extracellular space, the 200 Å interspaces or less, or those with wider extracellular spaces as produced by instantaneous freezing (VAN HARREVELD, CROWELL and MALHOTRA, 1965). Even with conventional EM preparation techniques the amount of interstitial space is different in various regions of the cerebellar cortex. Relatively wide interstitial spaces are found between parallel axons in the outer strata of the molecular layer. Particularly large interstitial spaces occur in the outer part of the baskets surrounding Purkinje cells (Chapter VI), and in the environment of Golgi cell dendrites that descend into the granular layer (Chapter I). Strangely, in both cases larger intercellular spaces occur where axons or dendrites have finger-like processes that are of somewhat smaller size than dendritic spines.

Chapter XII

Operational Features of the Cerebellar Cortex

A. The Geometry of Intracortical Neurone Chains

After the histological information presented in Chapters I and II and the additional details in Chapters III, IV, VI, VII and IX, it will be necessary to give only a brief summary mainly of the geometry of the connexions established over the various chains. While doing so, it is desirable to start with the neurone chains activated by the mossy fiber input because these have such complex and also such extended relations to the neuronal network of the cerebellar cortex.

1. The Mossy Fiber Input

Fig. 113 shows the connexions of a single mossy fiber (*Mf*) having numerous rosettes in two neighboring folia. By stimulating a number of granule cells in both folia, there is activation of parallel fibers, each of which runs in the longitudinal direction of its folium for about 1.5 mm in both directions from its granule cell, i.e. from the site where the stimulus is delivered by the mossy fiber input (see lower diagrams). Fig. 113 emphasizes the fact that, while the dendritic tree of the Purkinje cell (left) has a span of slightly above 200 μ in the transversal plane (outer stellate and basket cells have about the same dendritic span), the Golgi cells have a dendritic spread about three times as much. As seen clearly in the lower part of the diagram, this means that all dendrites of Purkinje cells having their dendritic arborization in a relatively narrow band or beam of parallel fibers are strongly excited, provided that enough parallel fibers of this beam are simultaneously excited. Those other Purkinje cells with dendritic arborizations only partly embedded into this narrow beam (dotted profiles) receive less stimulation. The same considerations would apply also to basket and stellate neurones (*B, Sa* and *Sb* in Fig. 114).

The situation is different for the Golgi cells, because they have sparsely distributed dendrites in a band three times wider. As seen in Chapter I the Golgi cells show little overlap in their arborizations, so that each cell can be visualized (ideally) to be occupying a separate cortical compartment of the shape of a hexagonal prism, or a hexagonal truncated pyramid. In order to have stimuli delivered to all dendrites of any given Golgi neurone, there would, therefore, need to be broader beams of parallel fibers. This is indicated in Fig. 113, lower right, by hatching in the direction right above to left below. As shown in Chapters I and VII the lower dendrites of Golgi cells are also directly contacted by mossy fibers. These dendrites have a somewhat smaller spread than the upper dendrites, so that there is a smaller zone below each Golgi cell — indicated by hatching in the other direction — where each Golgi cell receives an additional direct excitatory input.

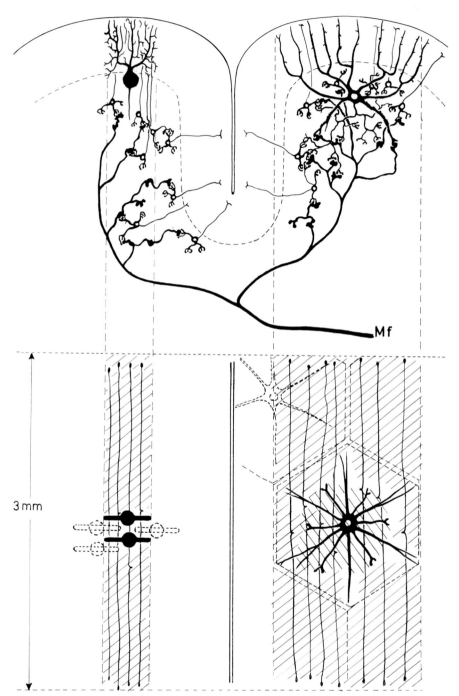

Fig. 113. Diagram illustrating the termination of a single mossy afferent (*Mf*) and some of its connexions in two neighboring folia. Upper part of the diagram in transverse section, lower as viewed from above. In consequence of the smaller spread of the dendritic tree of Purkinje cells (left) a narrow beam of simultaneously excited parallel fibers (hatched zone left below) would have access to all dendrites of a longitudinal row of Purkinje cells (representative examples drawn in full black in left lower part of diagram). Due to larger spread of Golgi dendrites (right upper)

We do not know how large is the fraction of the dendrites of a cerebellar neurone that has to be acted upon by the excitatory synapses of parallel fibers in order to evoke an impulse discharge; yet the thought is close at hand that Purkinje, basket and stellate cells are excited by relatively narrow beams of parallel fibers, whereas Golgi cells are more likely to be activated if the excited beams of parallel fibers are broader. Considering the wide distribution of mossy fibers, one has to admit that an input bringing about relatively narrow beams with many simultaneously excited parallel fibers is unlikely to occur. Nevertheless, as will be seen below, the Golgi cell inhibition will have a focusing action; hence this aspect of cerebellar neurone connectivity is worth considering theoretically, as will be done in the next paragraphs and using Figs. 114, 115 and 116.

The considerations pertinent to the left part of Fig. 113, i.e. on a narrow beam of simultaneously excited parallel fibers, are extended in Fig. 114 to the basket cells and the two main types of stellate cells ("a" and "b") which must be excited under the same conditions as the Purkinje cells. Stellate "a" cells (Fig. 11 A, B) have their axons distributed in their own perikaryal regions, and so can be expected to exercise "on-beam" effects on Purkinje cell dendrites, as is indicated in the lower part of the diagram by horizontal hatching. Stellate "b" type neurones (Fig. 11 C, D) can be expected to exercise "off-beam" effects on both sides of the excited parallel fiber beam to the maximal width of 900 μ, but probably much less, as indicated by oblique hatching in the direction left above to right below. According to the diagram given in Fig. 54 for the matrix of Purkinje cells potentially reached by the axon branches of a basket cell, basket cells would also exercise only "off-beam" effects for as long as 1 mm on each side of the excited parallel fiber beam (oblique hatching from right above to left below). All of these effects can be expected to occur along the entire length of the parallel fiber beam, i.e. for 3 mm; and only close to the end, where some of the parallel fibers have already ended, would one have to expect a "falling off" of these influences.

Fig. 113 and 114 have been constructed on the basis of structural information only, and are completely unbiased by considerations of the possible inhibitory or excitatory functions of the various kinds of neurones. As has been shown already in the previous chapters, all true interneurones of the cerebellar cortex (the basket, stellate and Golgi) are inhibitory in character; thus we may now extend our speculations by taking this information into account. Fig. 115 was constructed by SZENTÁGOTHAI as early as 1963 for illustrating diagrammatically the pattern of basket cell inhibition in the cerebellum. Fig. 54 has already given the pattern of distribution of the inhibitory synapses made by a single basket cell onto the somata of Purkinje cells that are seen to lie across the folium in serially arranged transverse planes (cf. Figs. 32, 110). Any one basket cell is distributed to the Purkinje cells of several transverse planes and to as many as 10 cells in one plane. Such a diagram

a considerably broader beam of parallel fibers is necessary to have stimulation conveyed to all dendrites (hatching right above to left below in lower right part of diagram). The tissue compartments occupied by Golgi cells are indicated by hexagonal pattern of dashed lines. Hatching in opposite direction around Golgi cell body indicates the region where mossy impulses are delivered directly to Golgi cell dendrites. Further explanation in the text implies that axon collaterals from many basket cells (probably as many as 20 to 30) contribute to the basket formed around any one Purkinje cell (Chapter VI A 1).

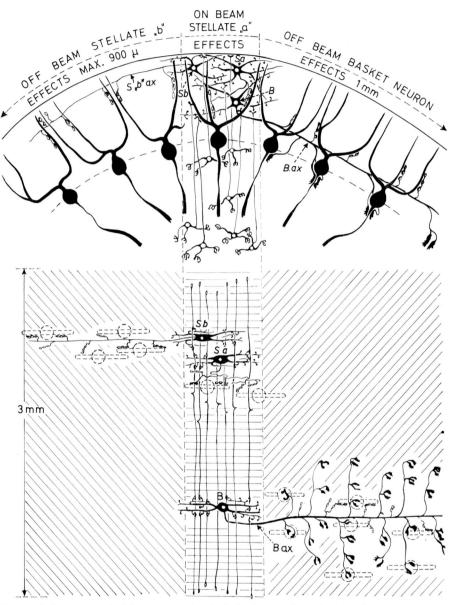

Fig. 114. Influence exercised by a narrow band of simultaneously excited parallel fibers by way of two types of stellate and of basket neurons. As seen in the upper part of the figure, illustrating a transverse section of the folium, stellate "a" type neurons (*Sa*) with short axons exercise an influence on Purkinje cells only within the limits of the excited band, giving thus "on beam effects". As the axons of stellate "b" (*Sb*) type neurons extend to the sides for maximally 900 μ, there are also stellate "off beam influences". The axons (*Bax*) of basket neurons (*B*) extend in lateral direction as far as 1 mm, exercising thus "off beam" effects at this distance. As seen from lower part of diagram — viewing a folium from above — all of these influences occur along the whole length of the parallel fibers, i. e. 3 mm. Further explanation in the text

The operational features of Fig. 115 can be best appreciated by considering the consequence of an input into the folium of repetitive volleys of impulses in mossy fibers that excite the granule cells shown circumscribed by a broken line in Fig. 115 A and D. As a consequence, these granule cells will generate repetitive discharges of

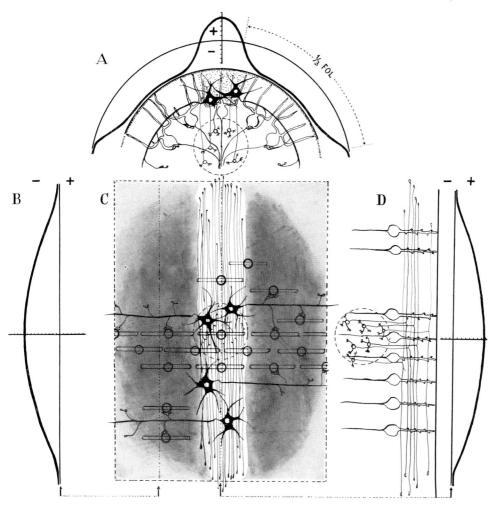

Fig. 115 A—D. Composite diagram of a cerebellar folium (plan in C, transverse section in A and longitudinal sections in B and D) showing that in an ideally simple situation a focal input onto granule cells (outlined by circle in A, C and D) set up an excited band of Purkinje cells along the folium flanked on each side by a deep inhibition. Further description in text. (SzENTÁGOTHAI, 1963)

impulses along the parallel fibers shown as a central band in Fig. 115 C and as a dotted zone of the molecular layer in the transverse section (Fig. 115 A). The impulses in this band of parallel fibers will in turn excite synaptically the Purkinje and basket cells along this band: and, sequentially, the basket cells (shown in black in A and C) will produce a wide zone of inhibition flanking the central excited zone, as is indicated by the dark shading in C and the plotted line on top of A, where + symbolizes a net excitation of Purkinje cells, and — a net inhibition.

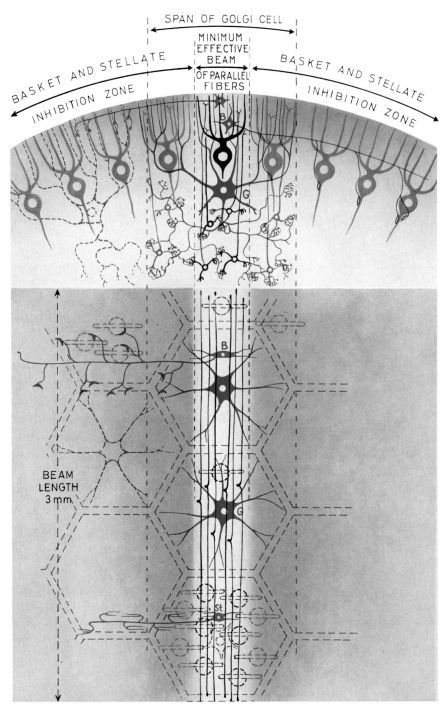

Fig. 116. Diagram illustrating the extension of inhibitory fields (shadowed areas) in the case that a narrow beam of parallel fibers be excited. Developed further from the earlier concept, shown in Fig. 115, in which the Golgi neurons have not been considered. Weak "on beam" stellate "a" inhibition is neglected. As in the diagrams Figs. 113 and 114, also here the upper part of the diagram is a transverse section of the folium and the lower part a view at the folium surface from

B and D give the distribution of the inhibitory and excitatory synaptic actions at the longitudinal sections indicated by arrows below C.

Here we have the first glimpse of an operational pattern for the postsynaptic inhibitory action produced by a circumscribed mossy fiber input. A sharply localized mossy fiber input into the cerebellum is converted into a narrow strip of excited Purkinje cells in the longitudinal axis of a folium, and it steeply grades into a deep and wide zone of inhibition on either side. Thus, an intense localized input via mossy fibers would suppress the Purkinje cell activation produced by all less intense inputs that were distributed laterally thereto.

Fig. 116 combines structural information of Figs. 113 and 114 and further develops concepts deriving from the inhibitory nature of the interneurones. The difference between this diagram and the original structure-functional diagram of this kind (Fig. 115) is that it attempts to explain the significance of the difference in the dendritic arrangement of the Purkinje, basket and stellate cells on the one hand and of the Golgi cell on the other. One could on structural grounds imagine theoretically that there exists a "minimum effective beam" of parallel fibers that can stimulate all the Purkinje, basket and stellate cells that have their dendrites embedded into this beam. This obviously would result in a zone of inhibited Purkinje cells on either side of the excited beam (the shadowed zone of the diagram) and each about 1 mm breadth. For the sake of simplicity we assume here that the size of the minimum effective beam is as wide as the dendritic span of a single Purkinje cell, but it could be much smaller without making any essential difference in the concept.

The functional consequences of an excited narrow beam of parallel fibers appear to be simple. Since the a-type stellate neurones give only weak on-beam connexions and since the basket and b-type stellate neurones give strong off-beam connexions, and at most weak on-beam connexions, the off-beam inhibition of Purkinje cells ought to be much stronger than the on-beam inhibition; and superimposed thereon would be the direct on-beam excitation. But this idealized distribution applies only to a narrow beam of parallel fibers not exceeding the dendritic span of one of these inhibitory neurones. The situation becomes more confused when the excited beam is broader and several rows of Purkinje, basket and stellate cells become simultaneously excited as in Fig. 62 A, C. This would result in a mixture of conflicting excitatory and inhibitory influences upon the Purkinje cells with the ultimate effect that any meaningful spatial pattern would be blurred.

Introduction of the Golgi cell circuits into the picture greatly helps in giving new sense to the model, which otherwise would be in danger of losing its functional coherence. Whenever there is a broad beam of excited parallel fibers as in Fig. 62 A—C, the Golgi cells ranged along this beam would be strongly excited.

above. It is assumed that there is a "minimum effective beam" of simultaneously excited parallel fibers, which is more likely to stimulate a row of Purkinje (black), stellate and basket (blue) cells. Golgi cells (red) having a much larger dendritic spread would be more likely to be excited by broader bands of simultaneously excited parallel fibers. Effective stimulation of the Golgi cells would then in turn tend to stop — as a negative feedback — all mossy input. Thus the Golgi cell system can be considered as a "focussing" device restricting — or giving preference to — granule neuron (parallel fiber) activity in relatively narrow bands

This would then result (Chapter VII C) in a feedback depression of all mossy fiber input into this region, which would be particularly effective on the peripheral less intense zone. Thus, from purely structural considerations, using in addition only the fundamental information of the specific inhibitory function of basket, stellate and Golgi neurones, we develop the concept of the focusing action of the Golgi cells. This action would tend to limit the simultaneous excitation of Purkinje cells to narrow longitudinal strips of about 3 mm length and would tend to suppress all other mossy fiber inputs leading to more diffuse fields of simultaneously excited Purkinje cells.

2. The Climbing Fiber Input

The influence of the climbing fibers can also be conveyed over interneurones and is shown diagrammatically in Fig. 117. As seen from Chapter VIII, there is a very intense direct excitatory action of one climbing fiber on one Purkinje cell. In addition, however, that climbing fiber has connexions probably to all kinds of inhibitory interneurones with cell bodies situated in the near neighborhood of its arborization (Chapter II; Figs. 18, 36). These collaterals presumably are responsible for the weak excitatory action exerted by inferior olive stimulation on Golgi cells (Table 1, Chapter IV) and these Golgi cell discharges would give the observed inhibition of the spontaneous discharge of granule cells (Fig. 107 C). The Golgi cells may receive excitatory synapses from a climbing fiber from a distance of up to half a millimeter. Due to their relatively widespread connexions, the interneurones may exercise a potential influence on a relatively large field of Purkinje neurones.

As appears from Fig. 117, the inhibitory influence of the basket neurone indicated in Fig. 54 potentially corresponds to the matrix of 10×7 Purkinje cells; and, as there are presumably several basket cell bodies localized sufficiently close to any climbing fiber arborization, a similar field of action can theoretically be expected on both sides. Inhibitory influences from stellate neurones can be expected not to exceed two parallel rows of Purkinje cells, as indicated by oblique hatching (left above to right below) at the left side of the lower part of Fig. 117; and again this influence can be assumed to occur at both sides of the climbing fiber arborization on its Purkinje cell.

The potential inhibitory influence that climbing fibers exert via Golgi cells is the most difficult to understand. The effective excitation of a Golgi cell by climbing fiber collaterals would secure an immediate inhibitory influence on the transmission through all glomeruli reached by the axon ramification of that Golgi neurone. This is indicated in Fig. 117, lower part, by vertical hatching with continuous lines. Indirectly, however, this inhibitory influence upon granule cells is extended through the granule axons, and so, by the parallel fibers, to a longitudinal band of about 3 mm length in the molecular layer. This is indicated at lower left in Fig. 117 by vertical hatching using dashed lines. Again, as with the inhibitory influences conveyed by basket and stellate cells, this depression of the potential excitatory action on Purkinje cells may occur on both sides of that Purkinje cell excited by the climbing fiber. The widespread inhibitory influence exercised potentially by a single climbing fiber may be a device to secure a silent background for the Purkinje cells that are directly activated by the incoming climbing fiber volley. However, as

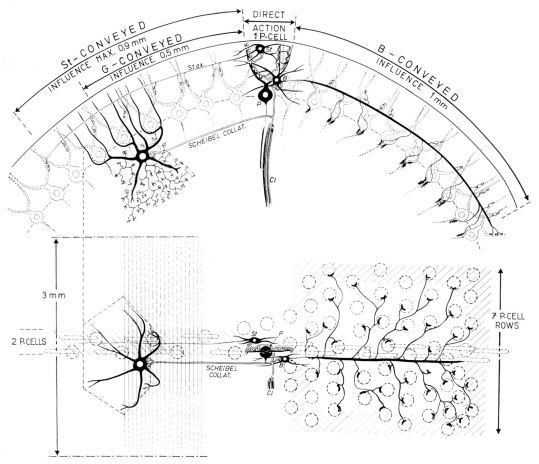

Fig. 117. Fields of neurons influenced *de facto* and potentially by impulse arriving in a single climbing fiber (*Cl*), above in transverse section and below as viewed from above. As seen in Chapter VIII each climbing fiber has by direct action a strong excitatory effect on a single Purkinje cell (*P*). By sending collaterals to basket, stellate and Golgi cells, situated near the terminal arborization of the climbing fibers, it can generate (inhibitory) influences in relatively large fields on both sides (in the transversal plane) of the stimulated Purkinje cell. By reaching a single basket cell a field of 7×10 Purkinje cells can potentially be influenced (oblique hatching from right above to left below). By contacting a stellate "b" type neuron a double row of Purkinje cells, extending as far as 0,9 mm could be reached in the transversal plane (oblique hatching left above to right below). By way of the Scheibel collaterals the climbing fiber can exercise an effect upon the vertically hatched area, corresponding to the axon ramification of the Golgi cell. Indirectly over the granule neuron this (inhibitory effect) is potentially extended as far as 1.5 mm longitudinally in both directions, i. e. 3 mm of the folium (dashed vertical hatching)

indicated in Table 1, a climbing fiber volley evoked by stimulation of the inferior olive exerts at best only a weak excitatory action on the inhibitory interneurones.

There probably is some convergence of climbing fiber axon collaterals on to the various interneurones. In the case of the Golgi cell this can be estimated very approximately on the basis that there are ten times more Purkinje cells and consequently ten times more climbing fibers than Golgi cells. If we assume that each climbing fiber gives one Scheibel collateral on the average — an assumption that

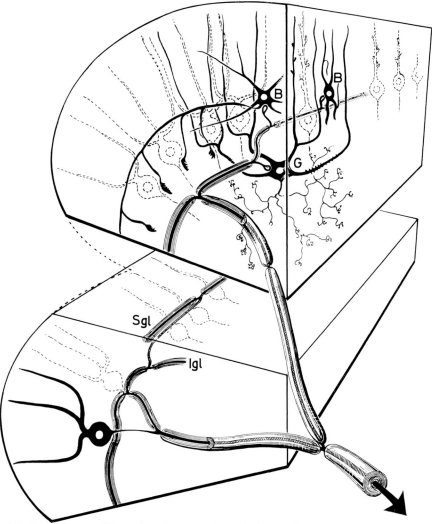

Fig. 118. Stereodiagram illustrating the connexions of the myelinated recurrent branches from single Purkinje axon, to Golgi (G) and basket (B) neurons in neighboring folium. Similar connexions in its own (lower) folium of the Purkinje neuron are omitted for the sake of simplicity. Predominantly transversal course of collaterals in the infraganglionic (Igl) and longitudinal course in the supraganglionic plexus (Sgl) are indicated

can be made with fair probability — we arrive at a convergence of ten climbing fibers on to one Golgi neurone. The convergence may be somewhat smaller for basket cells and considerably smaller for stellate cells.

3. Input via Purkinje Axon Collaterals

Although the connexions established by the recurrent Purkinje axon collaterals have been treated in detail in Chapter IX, they may be mentioned here briefly again. As seen from the drawings of Golgi pictures by CAJAL (1911), and partic-ularly the beautiful photographs of Fox *et al.* (1967), these collaterals are not only numerous but also very richly arborizing. It is, therefore, to be expected that the connexions established by the recurrent collaterals are quantitatively of larger significance than those effected by the side connexions of climbing fibers. On a large scale these connexions are predominantly organized in the sagittal plane of the cerebellum (Chapter IX), which for a large part of the cerebellar cortex cor-responds to the transverse plane of the folia. On a smaller scale the organization of these connexions is also transversal to the folium axis, but with respect to the preterminal arborizations the picture is complicated especially in the supra-ganglionic plexus by the predominant course of the preterminal fibers in the longitudinal direction of the folium, i.e. in parallel with the parallel fibers. This was not observed correctly by CAJAL or any other light microscopist, but it is obvious enough in the EM picture (Fig. 101). Unfortunately, the length of the longitudinal course of the preterminal branches is not known, hence its functional significance cannot be estimated.

The connexions of recurrent Purkinje axon collaterals are illustrated diagram-matically in Fig. 118. This diagram tries to emphasize the fact that these con-nexions go far beyond the border of the folium, so securing an association between corresponding parts of neighboring and even distant folia. The details of the con-nexions are not elaborated in the diagram since they are not yet sufficiently elucidated and since there is some disagreement between the structural and func-tional data (Chapter IX). Structural as well as functional observations are both positive with respect to the action of Purkinje cell collaterals on Golgi cells and basket cells, but there is disagreement concerning the possibility that recurrent Purkinje axons make synapses on Purkinje cells. In general the agreement between structural and functional observations is almost too good in the cerebellar cortex at present! In fact it is so good that it may appear suspicious, but here at last we have some disagreement between the histologist and the physiologist!

B. The Functioning of the Neuronal Pathways

1. Introduction

When attempting to understand the physiological mechanisms of the cerebellar cortex, the most important initial consideration is that the output of the cerebellar cortex is mediated solely by the discharges of Purkinje cells. Therefore, attention must be concentrated on the excitatory and inhibitory synaptic actions on these cells, and also on the frequencies of their spontaneous discharges (cf. Fig. 104). Inhibitory action on Purkinje cells would be exhibited by a reduction or silencing of this discharge. Of great significance also is the fact that there are two quite distinct, even opposed, cerebellar inputs, mossy fibers and climbing fibers, and every Purkinje cell is subjected to these two inputs, either directly, as with climbing fibers, or indirectly. It has long been recognized (DOW, 1942; BRODAL, WALBERG and BLACKSTAD, 1950; DOW and MORUZZI, 1958) that this dual input to Purkinje cells must provide most valuable clues for guiding our attempts to understand the way in which the cerebellar cortex processes information. There will be firstly a survey of the physiological discoveries described in detail in the preceding Chapters, and then the development therefrom of general operational concepts.

In Chapters III to V there have been descriptions of physiological investigations into the responses of functional units of the cerebellar cortex: the parallel fibers, the inhibitory interneurones and the Purkinje cells. Chapter VI introduced the study of geometrical pattern in the operational performance. As discussed in detail in the initial part of this Chapter, this pattern derives from the rectangular lattice construction that is such a remarkable feature of the neuronal architecture: the parallel fibers running strictly longitudinally in the folium and exciting basket and

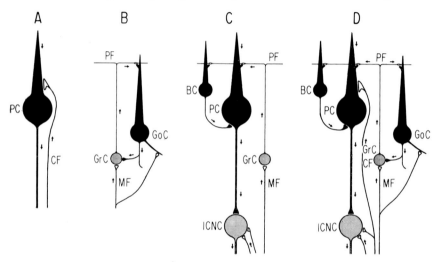

Fig. 119 A—D. *Diagram of the most significant neuronal connexions in the cerebellum, as described in the text.* The component circuits, A, B and C are assembled together in D. All cells in black are inhibitory

type "b" stellate cells that send their axons in one or the other transverse direction across the folium, i.e. orthogonal to the parallel fibers. Since each parallel fiber extends for about 1.5 mm longitudinally in either direction from its origin in the bifurcation of a granule cell axon, and, since the basket cell axon runs for about 1 mm transversely giving inhibitory synapses to Purkinje cells en route, it would be expected that the functional unit for parallel fiber impulses would be a rectangular area about 3 mm along the folium and 2 mm transversely. As shown in Figs. 66, 115 and 116, the longitudinal axis would be a zone of relative excitation of Purkinje cells flanked by deeply inhibited cells on either side. Physiological tests corroborate this prediction from anatomical data, but, with the relatively wide bands or beams of excited parallel fibers, inhibition is dominant even on-beam (Figs. 62, 65).

Fig. 119 summarizes diagrammatically the principal neuronal circuits in the cerebellar cortex. In A there is the highly selective excitatory action by climbing fibers on Purkinje cells (Chapter VIII). In B there is shown for the mossy fiber input the negative feedback circuit via granule cells to Golgi cells and so back to the mossy fiber-granule cell synapses (Chapter VII). Also in B there is the mossy

216

fiber synapse directly on the Golgi cell. C shows the more complicated inhibitory pathways in which basket cells (and outer stellate cells) provide a feed-forward inhibition onto the Purkinje cells (Chapters V and VI) and D shows how these two inhibitory systems lock together in controlling the excitation of Purkinje cells by the mossy fiber and climbing fiber inputs. In Fig. 120, there is a somewhat more

CEREBELLUM

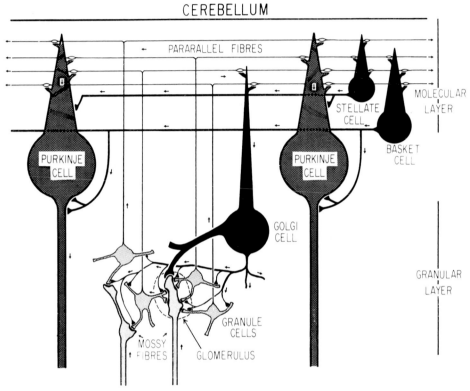

Fig. 120. *Diagram showing the principal features that have been postulated for the mossy fiber input and the cerebellar glomerulus.* The Golgi, stellate and basket cells are all inhibitory in action and are shown by convention in black. The broken line represents the glial lamella that ensheathes a glomerulus. The diagram is drawn as for a section along the folium and the main distribution of the basket and stellate cells would be perpendicular to the plane of the diagram, but they are also distributed as shown to a band of several Purkinje cells along the folium. The arrows indicate the direction of impulse propagation. Further description in text. (ECCLES, LLINÁS and SASAKI, 1966 f)

realistic diagram of part of the synaptic relationships in these inhibitory pathways in the cerebellar cortex. This figure also illustrates the postulated inhibitory synapses from outer stellate cells onto Purkinje dendrites.

2. The Mossy Fiber Input and the Glomerulus

The various investigations described in Chapter VII have led to the development of a fairly comprehensive account of the events produced in the cerebellar cortex by a mossy fiber input. Mossy fiber impulses exert their synaptic excitatory action solely within the cerebellar glomerulus (Chapter VII, section B). The functional relation between the three elements of the glomerulus can be formulated as follows: the mossy fibers exert a synaptic excitatory action on the granule cells (Figs. 77, 78), and impulses discharged along their axons (the parallel fibers) excite, by dendritic spine synapses, all cells with dendrites in the molecular layer, viz. the Purkinje, basket, stellate and Golgi cells. The axons of the Golgi cells end exclusively in the glomeruli of the granular layer (Figs. 13, 68, 71, 75) as inhibitory synapses on the dendrites of the granule cells (Fig. 120). This simple negative feed-back is, however, complicated by the fact that the Golgi cell receives excitatory inputs from other sources. Some of the mossy fibers enter into direct contact with dendrites of the Golgi cells in the superficial levels of the granular layer, and also with the deep Golgi cells at deeper levels (Figs. 41, 72, 75; Sections B and E of Chapter VII).

It is of special interest that there is a physiological correlate for every component of the complex synaptic apparatus, the cerebellar glomerulus (Chapters II and VII). In Fig. 120 a mossy fiber forms the center of the glomerulus and gives excitatory synapses to granule cell dendrites and to the deep dendrite of a Golgi cell. Also in the glomerulus are the axonal terminals of a Golgi cell that exert a postsynaptic inhibitory action on the dendrites of granule cells, but not on the Golgi cell dendrites. As shown by the arrows, the mossy fiber excitation evokes a discharge of impulses from granule cells along their axons that bifurcate to give the parallel fibers in the molecular layer. These parallel fiber impulses in turn form a large number of excitatory synapses with the dendritic spines of Purkinje, Golgi, basket and outer stellate cells, which are all inhibitory cells. Thus a mossy fiber input is completely transformed into inhibition either after the first synaptic relay to a Golgi cell and thence to its inhibitory synapses, or after two synaptic relays — to granule cells and thence, by mediation of basket, outer stellate, Golgi and Purkinje cells, to inhibitory synapses as described in Chapters VI, VII, IX and XIII respectively.

The mossy fiber excitation of granule cells can be quite powerful, as described in Chapter VII, and parallel fiber impulses are powerful exciters of basket, outer stellate, Purkinje and Golgi cells as described in Chapters IV, V and VII, yet suddenly all of this immense excitatory activity in the cerebellar cortex is transformed into inhibitory depression. There is no excitatory action of any kind beyond the second synaptic relay in the cerebellar cortex except possibly the pseudo-excitation of post-inhibitory rebound. This discovery alone places the cerebellum in a quite different category from all other regions of the central nervous system that are concerned in the integration of information, and not simply in its relay.

The most remarkable feature of the mossy fiber input into the cerebellar cortex is the extraordinarily wide dispersion of the branches of any one mossy fiber. Besides the anatomical evidence (Chapter II) there is also good physiological evidence for this wide dispersal. LUNDBERG and OSCARSSON (1960, 1962) and OSCARSSON (1964) find that single fibers in the ventral spino-cerebellar and rostral spino-cerebellar tracts can be activated antidromically by weak stimulation over fairly wide areas of the anterior lobe of the cerebellum, whereas there is a much smaller excitatory area for dorsal spino-cerebellar fibers. These excitatory areas can be taken as a measure of the distribution of the respective single mossy fibers. The activation of mossy fibers by transfolial stimulation in Figs. 77, 80, 82 and 84 provides further evidence for the wide dispersal of the branches from a single mossy fiber.

Fox *et al.* (1967) estimate that each mossy fiber is distributed to as many as 40 glomeruli, and that in each glomerulus the single mossy fiber enters into synaptic relations with the dendrites from about 15 granule cells, i.e. there is a divergence of synaptic excitation to 600 granule cells. Thus, essentially the mossy fiber-granule cell relay is a divergence mechanism giving a large dispersal of the input to the cerebellar cortex by a single mossy fiber. However, as shown in Chapter VII, B 1, by its radiating dendrites any one granule cell participates in several glomeruli (four to five on the average), and hence there is a small but very significant opportunity for convergence of several mossy fibers onto one granule cell. Moreover there is physiological evidence that small mossy fiber inputs fail to set up a discharge from any granule cells in an area under observation (Fig. 77 A, B, G, H), whereas the summed excitatory action of a large volley is effective (I, J). Hence there must be summation between the excitatory synaptic actions exerted on the different dendrites of a granule cell in different glomeruli. Furthermore, with weak excitatory action, all granule cell discharges may be inhibited by a given inhibitory input (Figs. 78, 80 D, 82 K, 83 A—F), whereas inhibition is much less effective against a strong excitatory action of mossy fibers (Figs. 80 B, 82 M), which again indicates summation.

3. The Inhibitory Circuits

Fig. 121 is designed to display the essential features of three quite distinct inhibitory mechanisms in the cerebellar cortex. A shows part of the pathways diagrammatically illustrated in Figs. 114 and 115. The mossy fiber input excites granule cells to discharge impulses along their axons, the parallel fibers, and these in turn throughout their length of about 3 mm excite basket cells that exert a postsynaptic inhibitory action on Purkinje cells for as far as 1 mm in either direction transversely across the folium. The initial stage of the pathway of B is shown diagrammatically to the right of Fig. 113 and is similar to that of A, the mossy fiber input exciting the granule cells to discharge impulses along the parallel fibers; but the further stage is a negative feedback loop: viz. the parallel fiber impulses excite the Golgi cells to discharge impulses which exert a postsynaptic inhibitory action on the granule cell dendrites. In Fig. 121 C the mossy fiber input in addition excites the Golgi cell by synapses on the dendrites in the granular layer (right side of Fig. 113). The inhibitory pathway is then, as in B, by the Golgi cell discharges to inhibit the granule cells; but to the right of Fig. 121 C the inhibitory action of the Golgi cells is of the feed-forward type and not feed-back as in B and to the left of C.

Because of their different circuits of operation, these three inhibitory mechanisms have quite distinctive patterns of distribution. Experimentally it is simplest to investigate the action of parallel fiber volleys directly evoked by LOC stimulation rather than to set up parallel fiber volleys by a mossy fiber input. Fig. 88 illustrates the invariable finding (ECCLES, SASAKI and STRATA, 1967 b) that Golgi cell inhibition evoked in this way (Fig. 121 B) occurs in a much narrower zone along the length of the parallel fiber volley than the basket cell inhibition (A). As pointed out by HÁMORI and SZENTÁGOTHAI (1966 b), the inhibition by a Golgi cell would

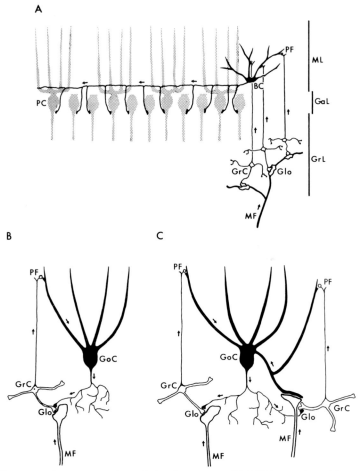

Fig. 121. *Diagrammatic representations of the three types of inhibition activated by a mossy fiber input to the cerebellar cortex.* In a subvariety of A that is not illustrated, the outer stellate cells are the inhibitory neurones instead of the basket cells. *MF*, mossy fiber; *GrC*, granule cell; *PF*, parallel fiber; *PC*, Purkinje cell; *BC*, basket cell; *GoC*, Golgi cell; *Glo*, glomerulus; *ML*, *GaL* and *GrL* are respectively the molecular, ganglionic and granular layers of the cerebellar cortex. Further description in the text

have a lateral spread beyond the edge of the parallel fiber volley because of the extensive spread in all directions both of its dendrites in the molecular layer and of its axonal branches in the granular layer (Chapter I, section 5). Thus Golgi cells with somata as far as 200 µ off-beam with respect to the parallel fiber volleys would have some dendrites in this beam (right lower part of Fig. 113), and by their axons would exert an inhibitory action on glomeruli still further off-beam. Nevertheless effective Golgi cell inhibition extends no further than 200 µ off-beam, whereas basket cell inhibition extends as far as 1000 μ (cf. Figs. 62, 88) by virtue of the transverse axonal distribution of the basket cells that are on-beam to the parallel fiber volley (Figs. 8, 37, 54). The superposition of inhibition of outer stellate cells does not affect the general pattern of Fig. 66 because they are also excited by the parallel fiber volley and type "b" also acts as a lateral distributor of inhibition to Purkinje cells, though probably to a lesser distance than for basket cells (cf. Fig. 11 C; Chapters I and VI). Essentially the Golgi cell inhibition of Fig. 121 B is on-beam with respect to the activating parallel fibers, whereas basket cells are predominantly off-beam in their inhibitory action.

As pointed out by HÁMORI and SZENTÁGOTHAI (1966 b), the inhibitory circuit to the right of Fig. 121 C is of particular significance on account of the strictly localized inhibitory action. The impulses generated in a Golgi cell dendrite (Fig. 41) presumably will propagate to the soma and thence along all the axonal branches of that Golgi cell; hence the inhibitory action is restricted to the glomeruli supplied by that Golgi cell, which would be in an area of the granular layer usually about 600 μ in diameter (Figs. 13, 16, 113; Chapter I, section 5). This inhibitory mechanism is of special significance because of its effectiveness in suppressing the discharges of all the granule cells weakly excited by any given mossy fiber input. This is indicated in Figs. 78, 80 D and 83 B, D, F, whereas those granule cells strongly excited would continue to discharge, as is indicated in Figs. 79 B, C and 80 B.

The wide dispersal in the granular layer of the initial spike of the N_2 wave evoked by a mossy fiber input (Fig. 41) is in agreement with anatomical data (HÁMORI and SZENTÁGOTHAI, 1966 b) in revealing that the direct excitatory action of mossy fibers on Golgi cell dendrites occurs in a considerable proportion of the glomeruli. This inhibitory mechanism can therefore be regarded as sampling very effectively the mossy fiber input and as being distributed to all the glomeruli supplied by that input and to a still wider zone, as indicated to the right of Fig. 113. It was suggested by HÁMORI and SZENTÁGOTHAI (1966 b) that Golgi cell discharge may occur only when it is excited by both parallel fibers and mossy fibers; but physiological investigation shows the effectiveness of parallel fibers alone (Figs. 39 N—Q and 40 A—J) and of mossy fibers alone (Figs. 41 and 82 E—I), and these two regions of excitation of a Golgi cell are usually so distant from each other that summation of subliminal excitatory actions must be very inefficient.

The functional design of the glomerulus, namely the mossy fiber-granule cell relay with the built-in Golgi cell inhibition, will serve to limit the effective range of any one mossy fiber to the zone of its intense granule cell innervation. Of course, this focusing action will occur only when there is a repetitive mossy fiber input, but that would be the situation with natural activation of mossy fibers, as for example the dorsal spino-cerebellar tract by muscle stretch or contraction (LUND-BERG and WINSBURY, 1960; JANSEN and RUDJORD, 1965).

4. The Operational Geometry of the Neuronal Circuits

As a consequence of the focusing action of the Golgi cell inhibition, it is justi-fiable to postulate that repetitive impulse discharge along a small bundle of mossy fibers becomes restricted to an effective excitatory action on a small focus of granule

GRANULE CELL
EXCITATION

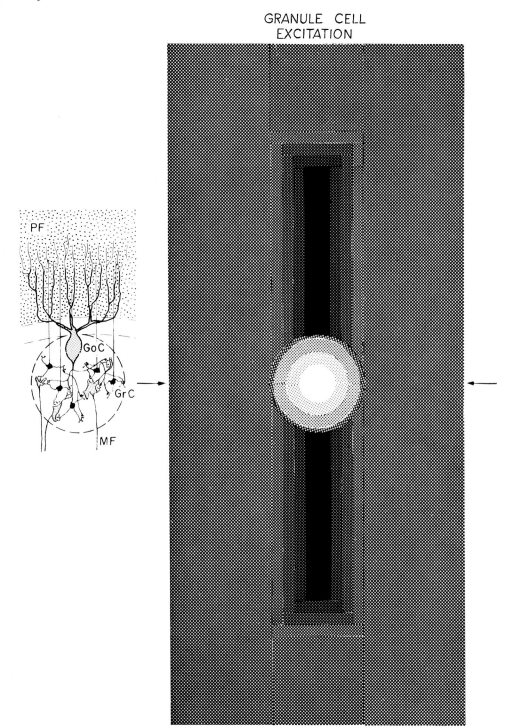

Fig. 122. *Diagram showing the postulated action of impulses in a small bundle of mossy fibers (MF) innervating a focus of granule cells (GrC) as shown in the transverse section beside the larger diagram, where the folium is seen from above. GoC is the Golgi cell distributed to that focus. The parallel fibers (PF) are shown in the cross-section. Further description in text.* (ECCLES, 1965)

222

most axons have numerous initial collaterals that terminate within the nucleus (CAJAL, 1911).

Besides these large and obviously efferent neurons there have been described, particularly in the dentate nucleus (SACCOZZI, 1887; LUGARO, 1894), numerous

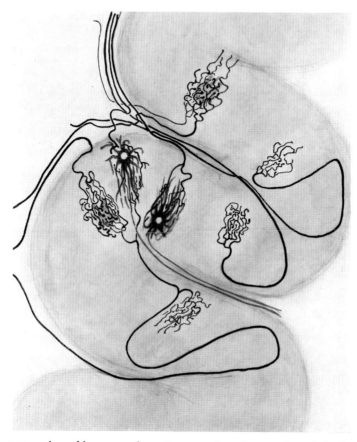

Fig. 125. Dentate nucleus of human newborn, Cox procedure. Outer surface of the dentate is to the left. Terminal arborizations of Purkinje axons. The dendritic arborizations of dentate neurons are relatively short and dense. The dendrites of each neuron are confined to independent pericellular territories with little if any overlap between neighboring arborizations. Although the axonal arborizations are arranged into similar pericellular nests, there is both divergence from a given axon to several cells and convergence from various axons to the same cell.

smaller cells with short axons. These cells are considered by JACOB (1928) as Golgi type II cells, but this is questioned by JANSEN and JANSEN (1955) for the cat because retrograde changes are found in most of these cells after transection of the brachium conjunctivum.

b) Axonal Ramification Patterns and Synapses. The ramification of axons entering the cerebellar nuclei have been described by CAJAL (1911) as a most remarkable and rather unusual type of preterminal arborization. Although the afferent axon ramifications are essentially similar in all the nuclei, those in the lateral (dentate) nucleus are undoubtedly the most specific and elaborate. The

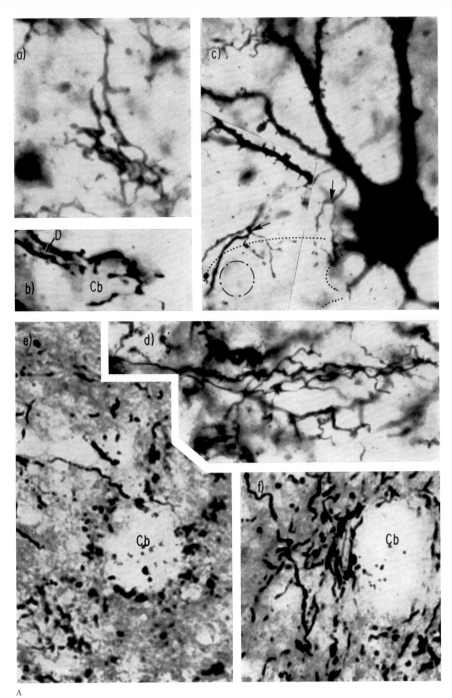

A

Fig. 126 A, B, a—f. Left half (A) of this figure shows details from Purkinje axon terminations in the fastigial nucleus in a young kitten, as seen in the Golgi picture (a—d), and degeneration evidence (e, f), after focal lesions in the vermal cortex, that the dense pericellular arborizations in fact do belong to Purkinje axons. Adult cat, Nauta procedure. — Preterminal axons arborize in brush-like fashion (a, d) and their terminal branches, sometimes running along larger dendrites (D) terminate with end knobs in the cell body (Cb) surface (Photomicrograph b). In picture (c) the preterminal branches indicated by arrows have terminal knob contacts with the surface of cell body, outlines of which are indicated by dotted line. Pale nucleus of this cell is indicated by "dash-dot-dash" line. Neighboring cell is fully stained. — The degeneration pictures (e, f) are showing that degeneration fragments after cortical lesions are concentrated around surface of cell

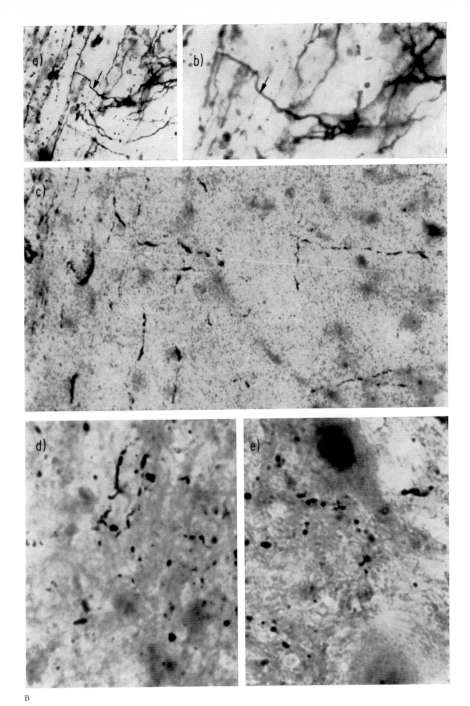

B

body (*Cb*) and of the principal dendrites. — The right half (B) of the figure shows side branches
of ascending fibers (arrows) entering the fastigial nucleus and under larger magnification (b) attachment of one of the collaterals to nuclear neuron dendrite can be recognized. Young kitten, Golgi
rapid stain. The same collaterals can be shown by degeneration (c) to originate from the spino-
cerebellar tracts. Adult cat, 5 days after lateral funiculus lesion in midthoracic level. This Figure
is from the same region and cut with the same orientation as (a) and (b). — (d) Degeneration in the
interpositus nucleus after lesion in ipsilateral inferior olive. — (e) Degeneration in lateral nucleus
after pontine lesion. Adult cat Nauta procedure. Although character of fragments corresponds to
terminal degeneration, few fragments are localized in close contact to the surface of cell bodies
or of larger dendrites. This would indicate that the majority of these synapses are axo-dendritic.

afferent fibers that enter the nuclei mainly from their dorsal circumference break up into a long and intricate brush-like arborization arranged into vertical columns. A similar type of terminal arborization is generally known to occur in the superior olive. The cell bodies of the nuclear neurons are embedded into these columns of terminal arborizations.

From the figures of Cajal (1911) it is difficult to judge the amount of overlap between the columns of neighboring fiber arborizations. The situation is simpler in the human dentate, due to the transformation of the lateral nuclear mass into the wavy thin cellular lamina of the dentate nucleus. Here it becomes apparent that the terminal arborizations are divided up into individual cell territories — as for example in the inferior olive — one afferent contributing numerous tortuous branches enveloping the whole dendritic tree of each individual neuron by dense spheric or ovoid nests (Fig. 125). There is, however, no one-to-one relation between presynaptic afferents and nerve cells, since branches detach themselves from neighboring or even more distant pericellular nests and enter the nests around other cells so joining in with these profuse arborizations. There can be little doubt that these brush-like arborizations are the terminals of Purkinje axons; this becomes apparent also from a comparison of some details of the brush-like axon arborization patterns as seen in the Golgi picture and the corresponding degeneration pattern in the same region (Fig. 126 A) after cortical lesion of the cerebellum. The majority of the synaptic contacts appear to be concentrated around the cell bodies and the principal dendrites.

Although most prominent in the Golgi picture, these arborizations are by no means the only afferents of the cerebellar nuclei. It has been supposed earlier that secondary vestibular afferents are terminating in the fastigial nucleus. Their existence has been substantiated by Brodal and Torvik (1957) who found their origin to be mainly in the lower part of the descendens nucleus and the cell group (X). There are also scattered data about the termination in the cerebellar nuclei of collaterals from other afferent systems. Since they have now gained crucial importance (see below), we have looked for these terminals in our own degeneration material (Fig. 126 B). Although the number of such collaterals is never very large, one can consequently trace collaterals from almost all afferent systems to one or several of the cerebellar nuclei. The spinocerebellar systems contribute quite a number of collaterals to the fastigial nucleus, less but still significant numbers in the interpositus nucleus and even some to the lateral nucleus. The pontocerebellar and olivocerebellar as well as probably the reticulocerebellar systems supply the cerebellar nuclei with quite abundant numbers of collaterals. These

Fig. 127 A—E. Various kinds of synapses on giant neuron of the Deiters nucleus, They are shown in slightly diagrammatic fashion on drawing in the center and one example of each type is shown in inset photomicrograph. — A = "collier type", reaching the cell body (Cb) usually at the basis of one of the dendrites and leaving it at that of another. While passing the cell body 5—7 relatively large end-feet are given arcade-like fashion. — B = "bouquet type" ending, terminating in a group of sometimes larger or smaller end-feet. B might be a terminal ending of a fiber that has A-type terminals on one or several other cells. Both types are mainly axo-somatic. — C = "non-selective" mostly fine preterminal fibers that have numerous short terminal branches,

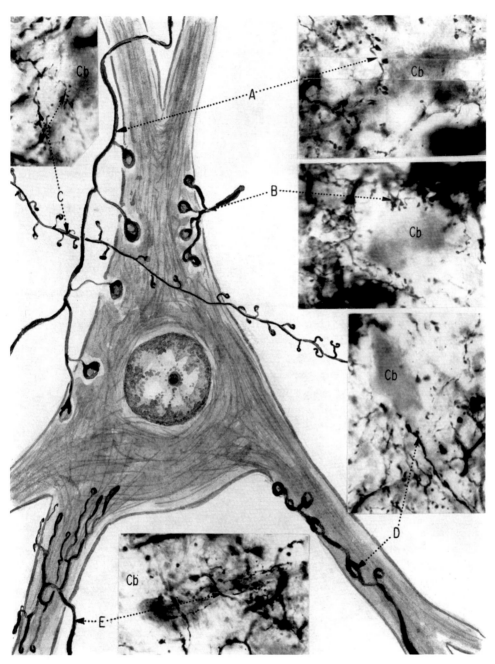

ending in small bulbs, over their entire course. These small terminals appear to get into contact with whatever part of neuron — either cell body or dendrite — they happen to come across hence called "non-selective". — D = large terminal axon creeping along principal dendrite (*D*) and stopping generally at its origin from cell body (*Cb*). This axon terminal appears to have repeated "de passage" synaptic attachments to the dendrite and short side branches increasing the surface of contact. — E = "palisade-type" termination at or close to the root of principal dendrite. — Young kitten, rapid Golgi procedure. — According to the degeneration pictures of WALBERG and JANSEN (1961) types D and/or E are most likely to originate from Purkinje axons.

facts are important because they reveal that the two afferent systems giving rise in the cerebellar cortex to mossy and to climbing fibers both contribute collaterals to the cerebellar nuclei. It is difficult to judge the numbers of such collaterals terminating in the cerebellar nuclei, because some of the afferents are running through the nuclei, however, their synaptic relations to the nuclear neurons can safely be inferred from degeneration fragments found in immediate contact with the surfaces of the dendrites. Cell bodies seem not to be contacted by these collaterals.

It would be quite premature to try to construct any more specific concepts on the mode of synaptic linkage in the cerebellar nuclei. One has, however, to reckon with at least three kinds of synapses on the large projective neurons of these nuclei: 1. endings of the Purkinje cells, 2. endings of afferent system collaterals and 3. terminals of local axons. On analogy with the principal arrangement between recurrent collaterals, interneurons and their axon ramifications, as it appears from many other regions of the central nervous system, one may infer that the recurrent collaterals of the efferent axons enter into contact with the Golgi II interneurons, which then in turn exercise their influence upon the main projective cells, perhaps even presynaptically on their input channels. Much work, however, will have to be done before the synaptic arrangement in the cerebellar nuclei will be understood.

2. Direct Cerebellar Efferents to the Vestibular Nuclei

Direct cerebellar corticofugal efferents to the vestibular nuclei have been first observed by ALLEN (1924) and later by numerous authors. For detailed information on this question the reader is referred to the comprehensive treatment of these connexions by JANSEN and BRODAL (1958). More recently the exact sites of termination of Purkinje cell axons have been shown by WALBERG and JANSEN (1961) to be mainly in the dorsal part of the lateral vestibular nucleus with some expansion into the adjacent dorsal parts of the superior and descending nuclei.

Even more important from the viewpoint of the synaptic architecture of the efferent cerebellar systems is the observation that the degenerating synaptic terminals are situated mainly on the giant cells and particularly along their larger dendrites. Fewer and only smaller degeneration fragments could be observed in the immediate vicinity of the cell bodies. On the basis of Golgi studies five different types of synaptic terminals have been found on the giant Deiters neurons (SZENTÁGOTHAI, unpublished). The degeneration patterns seen in the excellent photomicrographs of WALBERG and JANSEN (1961) would correspond particularly to types D and E shown somewhat diagrammatically in Fig. 127. Obviously further studies are needed before it will be possible to correlate the different kinds of pathways impinging upon the giant vestibular neurons and the various kinds of synapses.

For information about the connexions of the vestibular nuclei and their functional correlates the comprehensive study by BRODAL, POMPEIANO and WALBERG (1962) has to be consulted.

B. The Postsynaptic Inhibition of Cerebellar Subcortical Nuclei

1. Introductory Experiments

Because the Purkinje cell axons project not only to the intracerebellar nuclei but also to the vestibular nuclei, all of these structures will conjointly be referred to as the cerebellar subcortical nuclei. The specific inhibitory action of the Purkinje cells was discovered when a microelectrode was inserted into their target neurones in Deiters' nucleus (ITO and YOSHIDA, 1964 e, 1966 b). These neurones are approached from the ventral surface of the medullary pyramid and identified by their antidromic invasion from the vestibulospinal tract, either from the cervical or lumbar segments (ITO, HONGO, YOSHIDA, OKADA and OBATA, 1964 a, b).

As shown in Fig. 128 A—G, when the anterior lobe of the cerebellar cortex is stimulated on the ipsilateral side, there is very frequently the production of inhibitory postsynaptic potentials (IPSPs) in Deiters neurones. With relatively strong stimuli, successive IPSPs occur and build up a large and prolonged membrane hyperpolarization, there being complete suppression of spontaneous discharges from Deiters neurones for 50—100 msec (Fig. 128 K). The predominance of the IPSPs conforms to the well known inhibitory action of the cerebellar stimulation upon the brain stem postural centers (MORUZZI, 1950; BROOKHART, 1960), which is indicated most vividly by the drastic melting of the decerebrate rigidity during stimulation of the cerebellar anterior lobe (SHERRINGTON, 1897, 1898; LÖWENTHAL and HORSLEY, 1897). The striking finding is, however, that the latencies of the IPSPs are within the monosynaptic range. Much as with IPSPs in spinal motoneurones and the other nerve cells (cf. ECCLES, 1964), the IPSPs in Deiters neurones are reversed to a depolarizing potential by intracellular injection either of hyperpolarizing currents or of chloride ions (Fig. 128 H, I). Superposition of the original and reversed IPSPs gives, by their diverging point, the moment of their initiation (Fig. 128 I, at arrow). From lobule III or the anterior part of lobule IV, the average latency of the IPSP is only 1.06 msec. It is longer (1.23 msec) from the remote lobule V, while it becomes shorter (0.86 msec) when the stimulating electrode is brough into the deep interior of the cerebellum toward Deiters nucleus.

It emerges that the inhibitory impulses travel directly through the cerebellum at a relatively slow conduction velocity of 15—20 m/sec and eventually impinge on Deiters neurones monosynaptically, about 0.5 msec being occupied by the single synaptic delay time for setting up the IPSP. Similar investigations have been performed on the intracerebellar nuclei (ITO, YOSHIDA and OBATA, 1964 f; ITO, YOSHIDA, OBATA, KAWAI and UDO, 1967 h) and have demonstrated an abundance of long inhibitory fibers between the cerebellar cortex and the subcortical nuclei. This is of particular interest from the viewpoint that the inhibitory neurones so far identified in the mammalian CNS are mostly short-axoned (cf. ECCLES, 1964).

2. Evidence for the Monosynaptic Inhibitory Action of Purkinje Cells on Deiters Neurones

The evidence for assigning this monosynaptic inhibitory pathway to the Purkinje cell axons has been obtained in the following two types of experiments.

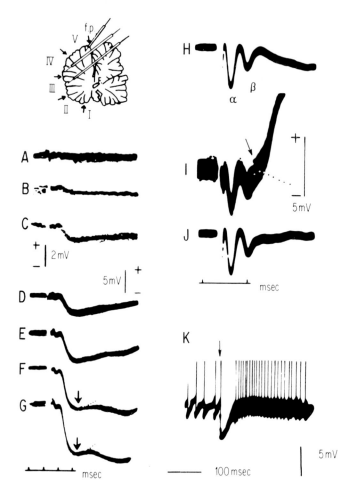

Fig. 128 A—K. *The cerebellar-evoked monosynaptic inhibition of Deiters neurones.* Diagram shows arrangement of stimulating concentric electrodes on a sagittal plane through the cerebellar vermis. I—V refer to LARSELL's (1953) lobular divisions. *f.p.*, fissura prima. Arrows indicate the interlobular sulci. A—G, H—J and K, intracellular recording from three Deiters neurones, respectively. In A—G 0.2 msec pulse stimuli were applied to the vermal cortex of lobule IV at intensities of 1.9 volts (A), 2.1 (B), 3.2 (C), 5 (D), 10 (E), 20 (F) and 30 (G). Note the different voltage scales for A—C (2 mV) and D—G (5 mV). Dotted lines in F and G indicate the possible time course of the monosynaptic IPSPs if they were similar to that in D. Vertical arrows indicate the diverging points between the dotted lines and actual potential curves. H, initial part of the potential changes following 30 volt stimulation of lobule III. α and β denote the two spiky peaks of the field potential. I, same as in H but reversed during passage of hyperpolarizing currents of 2×10^{-8} A through the KCl-filled microelectrode. Dotted line indicate the time course of the potential curve of H. Arrow marks the diverging point of the two curves before and during current passage. J, extracellular record taken just after withdrawal. K shows spontaneous spike discharges from a Deiters neurone, and its suppression and later facilitation by the cerebellar stimulation. 0.2 msec pulses of 30 volts were applied at the time indicated by arrow to the ipsilateral lobule III. Time constant of the recording amplifier was 200 msec for A—J, while there was d. c. recording in K. The records in this as well as in the succeeding figures of Chapters XIII and XIV were formed by 10 to 40 superimposed traces unless otherwise stated. Note that K in this figure was taken in a single sweep. (ITO and YOSHIDA, 1966 b)

First, the cerebellar area which gives rise to the monosynaptic inhibition of Deiters neurones is localized on a longitudinal medial zone that covers the ipsilateral vermis and also the medial portion of the paravermis in both the anterior and posterior lobes of the cerebellum (Fig. 129; Ito and Kawai, 1964 c; Ito

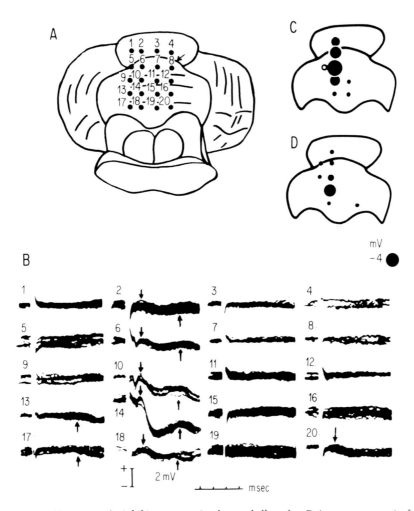

Fig. 129 A—D. *Monosynaptic inhibitory zone in the cerebellum for Deiters neurones.* A, frontal view of the cerebellum. Black dots Nos. 1—20 indicate the sites of stimulation provided by four multipolar stimulating electrodes. Each of these electrodes was made of 5 pieces of enamel wire stuck on a shaft of steel needle. They were mounted on a micromanipulator and inserted into the culmen in the caudo-dorsal to rostro-ventral direction. B, intracellular records taken in a Deiters neurone during stimulation at each spot of A. The figure attached to each record refers to the position of cathode, while the anode was served by the caudal partner except when spots Nos. 1—4 were used as cathode against anode at their rostral partners. Pulse duration was 0.2 msec and pulse amplitude was 10 volts. Downward arrow indicate the onset time of the monosynaptic IPSPs. Upward arrows point to the delayed onset of IPSPs. C and D plot for two Deiters neurones, respectively, sizes of the monosynaptic IPSPs at the sites of stimulation. In C an open circle indicates the size of the depolarization produced by monosynaptic EPSP. (Ito and Kawai, 1964 c; Ito, Kawai and Udo, 1967 b)

237

KAWAI and UDO, 1965 a, 1967 b). The frequency with which the monosynaptic inhibition is obtained in impaled Deiters neurones is much reduced when the stimulating electrode is shifted from the anterior to the posterior lobe — to about 50% for the lobulus simplex, and actually it is zero for the pyramis or the caudal surface of the uvula. This is in excellent agreement with the histological observations that Deiters neurones receive Purkinje cell axons from the ipsilateral vermal (WALBERG and JANSEN, 1961) and paravermal (EAGER, 1963 a) cortices — predominantly from the anterior lobe and much less from the posterior lobe. Also in good accord with the histological data is the finding that the monosynaptic inhibition is absent in neurones of the relatively ventral portion of Deiters nucleus, which is the portion not impinged upon by Purkinje cell axons from the anterior and posterior lobes (WALBERG and JANSEN, 1961).

Secondly, there is excellent temporal correlation between the inhibitory events in Deiters neurones and the activity of Purkinje cells in the anterior lobe of the cerebellum (ITO, OBATA and OCHI, 1964 d; 1966 a). Stimulation of the cerebellum either in its white matter or in the deep lamellae of the cortex excites the Purkinje cells not only antidromically through their axons, but also orthodromically through the cerebellar afferent fibers, particularly through the climbing fibers (Chapter VIII; ECCLES, LLINÁS and SASAKI, 1964; 1966 d). Correspondingly, in Deiters neurones IPSPs are induced not only monosynaptically, directly from Purkinje cell axons, but also polysynaptically via these axons, either in isolation or in addition to the monosynaptic IPSPs (Fig. 130 A—D). It is surprising that the latency of the delayed IPSPs varies over a wide range from 1.5 to 9 msec, but this again corresponds to the similarly wide latency variation observed in the activation of Purkinje cells by the climbing fiber impulses (Fig. 130 E—G), as described in Chapter VIII (see also below). The climbing fibers can be stimulated very effectively at their site of origin in the inferior olive (Chapter VIII). There is a powerful activation of the cerebellar Purkinje cells at 3 msec after olivary stimulation, as indicated by the large spiky potential deflection extracellularly recorded in the cerebellar cortex (Fig. 131 A at arrow). Intracellular recording reveals that there are climbing fiber responses in many Purkinje cells at this phase of the cerebellar potential (ITO et al., 1966 a). In Deiters neurones, on the other hand, an EPSP appears in advance of the cerebellar Purkinje cell activation (upward arrow in Fig. 131 B), which in turn is succeeded by large and prolonged IPSPs, there being a delay of about two milliseconds between the onsets of the EPSP and the IPSP (Fig. 131 B, upward and downward arrows respectively). It appears that the impulses originating from the inferior olive produce first an EPSP in Deiters neurones, presumably monosynaptically, and then activate Purkinje cells, which in turn send back the inhibitory impulses to Deiters neurones (ITO et al., 1966 a). Similar activation of Purkinje cells and associated postsynaptic events in Deiters neurones can also be induced by stimulating the spino-olivary tract at the ventral surface of the spinal cord, either at the cervical (Fig. 131 D—F) or lumbar segments. From the second cervical level (C_2), there is activation of Purkinje cells at 6 msec latency, and from the first lumbar level (L_1) the latency is about 16 msec. The EPSPs and IPSPs of the Deiters neurones (Fig. 131 E, upward and downward arrows) begin respectively about 1 msec before and about 1 msec after the Purkinje cell activation (Fig. 131 D, downward arrow).

3. *Evidence for Monosynaptic Inhibitory Action of Purkinje Cells on Neurones of the Intracerebellar Nuclei*

Similar situations hold for neurones of the intracerebellar nuclei (ITO *et al.*, 1964 f; 1967 h). These cells were approached also from the ventral surface of the

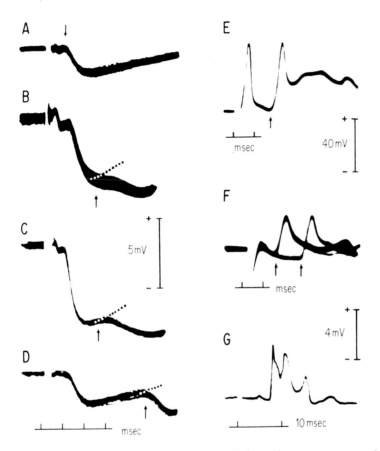

Fig. 130 A—G. *Delayed IPSPs in Deiters neurones and climbing fiber responses in Purkinje cells.* A—D, intracellular records from two Deiters neurones. In A the stimuli given to lobule IV were of 0.2 msec duration and of 5 volt amplitude. Downward arrow marks the onset of IPSP. In C the stimulus intensity was increased to 30 volts for the same cell as in A. In D 30 volt stimuli were given to the other electrode placed laterally to that in A, C by 2 mm. B was taken from the other Deiters neurone by stimulating at the same site as in A, C. Dotted lines indicate the probable time course of the monosynaptic IPSPs and upward arrows mark the points where they deviate from the actual potential curves. E—G, intracellular records from Purkinje cells. Pulse currents of 0.2 msec duration and 30 volt amplitude were applied to the concentric electrode inserted into the deep lamellae of lobule III. In E antidromic spike was first induced by direct excitation of the axon of the impaled Purkinje cell, and then there was a characteristic climbing fiber response, its onset being marked by upward arrow. F, climbing fiber response in another cell. The stimulus intensity was adjusted so that the climbing fiber response occurred at two alternative latencies. Arrows point to their onset times. G, a very late climbing fiber response in a Purkinje cell sampled at remote region from the stimulating electrode. (ITO, OBATA and OCHI, 1966 a)

medullary pyramid and were identified by their antidromic invasion from the regions of the red nucleus or thalamus or by their location in histological sections. When surveyed with a multipolar assemblage of stimulating electrodes, it is apparent that each neurone in the lateral nucleus has its own monosynaptic inhibi-

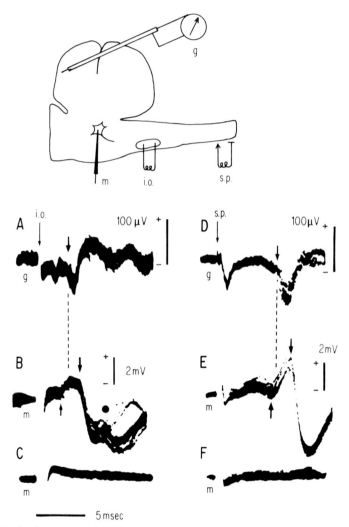

Fig. 131 A—F. *Evoked potential in the cerebellar cortex and postsynaptic potentials in Deiters neurones induced by the olivary and spinal stimulation.* Diagram shows arrangement for recording and stimulation. g, differential recording from the internal and external poles of the concentric electrode in lobule IV. m, microelectrode inserted into a Deiters neurone. i. o., stimulating electrodes in the inferior olive. s. p. those placed on the ventral surface of the cervical segments. A, D, evoked potentials recorded with g. Vertical thin arrows indicate the moments of stimulation, the site of stimulation being indicated on their tops. Thick arrows point to the onset of large spiky deflections. + sign on the voltage scales of 100 μV refers to the positivity in the internal pole of g. B, E, intracellular potentials taken in a Deiters neurone under the same stimulating conditions as in A, D, respectively. Upward arrows point to the onset of EPSPs and downward ones that of IPSPs. Dot in B indicates the delayed onset of IPSP. C, F, extracellular control for B, E, respectively. (ITO, OBATA and OCHI, 1966 a)

tory zone in the hemispheral cortex (Fig. 132 A, B, C). Likewise, interpositus neurones are inhibited monosynaptically from the overlying intermediate part of the anterior lobe, and those in the fastigial nucleus from the vermal cortex. Much

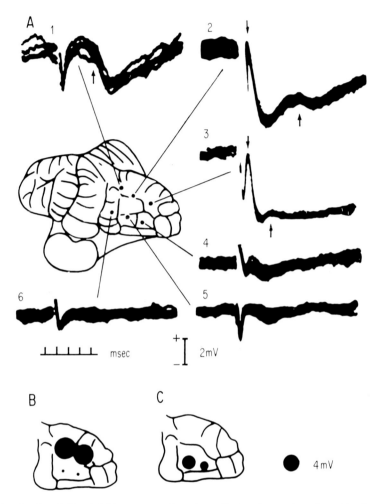

Fig. 132 A—C. *Cerebellar inhibitory zone for the cells in the nucleus lateralis.* A, potential changes recorded from a cell of lateral nucleus. The inset diagram shows the dorso-caudal view of the cerebellum. Dots Nos. 1—6 represent the sites stimulated with concentric electrodes. These electrodes were implanted with the edges of their external poles placed on the cortical surface and the internal poles inserted into 1 mm depth. Downward arrows indicate the onset of mono-synaptic IPSPs and the upward ones that of delayed IPSPs. B, C plot sizes of the mono-synaptic IPSPs for two cells of lateral nucleus on the sites of stimulation. Note that the line drawing of B and C represents only the right hemisphere of the cerebellum shown in A. (ITO, YOSHIDA, OBATA, KAWAI and UDO, 1967 h)

as in Deiters neurones, these neurones are inhibited not only monosynaptically but also polysynaptically. This is indicated by the delayed onset of IPSPs either in isolation, when the cerebellar area outside of the inhibitory zone is stimulated

(Fig. 132 A, No. 1 spot), or in superposition upon the monosynaptic IPSPs, as occurs in the records from spots No. 2 and 3 where downward and upward arrows mark respectively the onsets of monosynaptic and polysynaptic IPSPs. Corresponding to these delayed IPSPs, the Purkinje cells around the stimulating electrode in the overlying cortex are found to be activated at 2 to 8 msec after the stimulation.

The cells of the cerebellar nuclei are also inhibited by stimulation of the inferior olive. Much as with Deiters neurones, this inhibition occurs just after the time of the Purkinje cell activation, which is indicated by the cerebellar evoked potential or by climbing fiber responses in individual Purkinje cells. With stimulation of the spinal cord as in Fig. 131 D, E there is also spino-olivo-cerebellar activation that eventually results in the inhibition of fastigial neurones.

4. Comment

In view of these clear experimental demonstrations it is appropriate to make the general postulate that cerebellar Purkinje cells are all inhibitory. The original idea of the cerebellar efferent system seems to have been as follows: The cerebellar cortex synthesizes various input signals and thereby generates its own signals which are transferred to the cerebellar nuclei and successively to the brain stem neurones, the cerebellar nuclei being relay stations. It should now be considered that the subcortical nuclei are reflex centers by themselves, which receive excitatory signals from extracerebellar structures and thereby generate out-going signals for the brain stem neurones, and that the cerebellar cortex controls them by inhibition (ITO et al., 1964 f; ECCLES, 1965). This view will further be developed when the input sources to the subcortical nuclei are considered (section D of this chapter and chapter XIV).

There are some histological data that can be integrated with the physiological observations. According to measurements on the human cerebellum (SZENTÁGO-THAI-SCHIMERT, 1941), the Purkinje cell axons, being medullated (JACOB, 1928), are of small diameter (3—5 μ), which agrees well with the relatively slow conduction velocity calculated above for the inhibitory fibers, 15—20 m/sec, which is equivalent to 3 μ diameter (HURSH, 1939). Anatomically, Purkinje cell axons form a powerful bundle of corticofugal fibers which pass through the region of the deep nuclei and finally terminate in Deiters nucleus, making abundant synaptic contacts mainly on the stems of the large dendrites (section A 2 of this chapter; WALBERG and JANSEN, 1961; EAGER, 1963 a). Within Deiters nucleus there is usually a remarkable field potential with two peaks, the α and β spikes (Fig. 128 H—I), which represent two groups of impulses travelling down from the cerebellar cortex at different velocities. In their time course and amplitude, the later β spike can be related to the monosynaptic IPSPs, as representing the presynaptic inhibitory volley (ITO and YOSHIDA, 1966 b), while the significance of the α spike will be discussed below. On passing dorsoventrally through Deiters nucleus (Fig. 138 B), the β spike turns from a predominantly negative to a predominantly positive wave (ITO and YOSHIDA, 1966 b), which indicates the closed end formation of the fibers, much as occurs in the terminal region of a motor nerve fiber (KATZ and MILEDI, 1965).

5. Properties of the IPSPs Produced by Purkinje Cell Axons

Because of the large size of Deiters neurones and the consequent ease in their impalement, they have been mostly used in investigating the properties of the IPSPs induced by impulses in Purkinje cell axons. Since the stimulation of Purkinje cell axons is usually contaminated by activation of climbing fibers (Fig. 130 E) and also by the disinhibitory process (see below and Fig. 134), there are only a few cases in which the monosynaptic IPSPs are seen in virtual isolation (Figs. 128 C, D and 130 A). Such IPSPs attain the summit at about 1 msec and decay approximately exponentially with a half time of about 3 msec. These values are comparable with those obtained for the IPSPs in spinal motoneurones (cf. ECCLES, 1964). By fine adjustment of the stimulus intensity, the least distinguishable size of the IPSP is revealed to be as small as 0.2 mV (see Fig. 128 A, B).

The size of the IPSPs can be increased, though reversed to the depolarizing direction, when chloride ions are passed into the cell by intracellular injection of hyperpolarizing currents from a KCl-filled microelectrode (Fig. 133 E, F). Under these conditions, the unitary IPSPs can more easily be recognized as depolarizing potentials of relatively large size. For example, in Fig. 133 A—D the stimulus intensity was increased continuously from 1.8 to 5.0 volts, and there was increase of the reversed IPSPs in unit steps of about one millivolt, as shown in the superposed tracings of G. Comparison of the mean unitary size of the IPSPs with the IPSP obtained with supra-maximal stimulation yields the number of inhibitory fibers which pass by the stimulating electrode and impinge on a single Deiters neurone. The assessed figures with stimulation in relatively deep lamellae of the anterior lobe range from 22 to 30, which gives the lower limit for the convergence number of Purkinje cells on Deiters neurones. On the basis of histological investigations (sections A), a lower figure would be expected for the cerebellar nuclei.

The ionic mechanism generating the IPSPs in Deiters neurones appears to be the same as in spinal motoneurones (ITO, MATSUNAMI, NOZUE and SATO, 1967 e), even when tested with anions of critical size such as formate and bromate ions (ARAKI, ITO and OSCARSSON, 1961; cf. ECCLES, 1964). In contrast, there is a large discrepancy between Deiters neurones and motoneurones in respect of the pharmacology of their inhibition (OBATA, 1965; OBATA, ITO, OCHI and SATO, 1967). In motoneurones, but not in Deiters neurones, strychnine and tetanus toxin (ITO, MATSUNAMI and NOZUE, unpublished) prevent inhibition.

When applied to the vicinity of Deiters neurones through coaxial microelectrodes by currents of about 500 nA, GABA produces a membrane hyperpolarization of several millivolts (3—8 mV) in association with a large increase in the membrane conductance, thus mimicking the natural transmitter action (OBATA et al., 1967). The effects of the blocking agents of GABA transaminase were also examined during their iontophoretic application. Passage of hydroxylamine by currents of 500—1000 nA sometimes enhanced the inhibitory action of Purkinje cells on Deiters neurones. The intracellularly recorded IPSPs increased sometimes in amplitude by 50—100% and the inhibitory postsynaptic current that is indicated by the positive extracellular field potential was also sometimes increased by 10 to 15%. However, there was no change in the time course of these postsynaptic currents or potentials. The effects by hydroxylamine may be interpreted as due to the increase produced in the GABA content in the presynaptic terminals. Since GABA transaminase appears to exist in the pre-

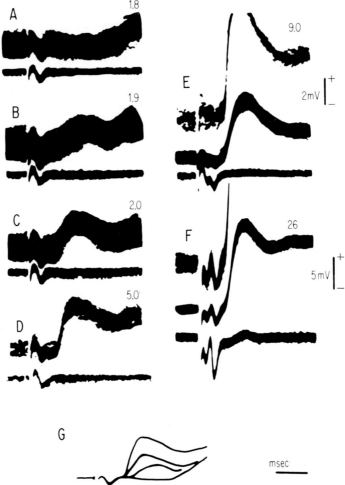

Fig. 133 A—G. *Unitary composition of the cerebellar-evoked monosynaptic IPSPs in Deiters neurone.* Upper traces of A—D and uppermost ones in E, F, intracellular recording during passage of hyperpolarizing currents of 5×10^{-8} A through the impaled KCl-filled microelectrode. A pair of needle electrodes with bare tips of 1 mm long (interpolar distance, 1.5 mm) were inserted into deep lamellae of the anterior lobe for stimulation. Figure attached to each record indicates the stimulus intensity in volts. Lower traces in A—D and lowermost traces in E, F are extra-cellular control taken after withdrawal. Middle traces in E and F are same as in uppermost ones but taken with reduced amplification. Voltage scale of 2 mV applies to the upper in A—D and uppermost traces in E, F. The voltage scale of 5 mV applies to the middle traces in E, F. G, super-imposed tracing of the upper traces of A—D. (ITO, KAWAI, UDO and SATO, 1967 d)

synaptic terminals (SALGANICOFF and DE ROBERTIS, 1965), but not in the synaptic cleft like cholinesterase, inhibition of GABA transaminase would not be expected to prolong the time course of the IPSPs. However, the possibility is not excluded that hydroxylamine influences the inhibition secondarily to its action upon other enzymic system or systems, for this drug at relatively high concentration inhibits a rather wide variety of enzymes. Another inhibitor of GABA transaminase, amino-oxyacetic acid, was also examined, but no definite action has yet been detected (OBATA et al., 1967).

The action of GABA has recently been shown to mimic also the inhibitory transmitter for cerebral cortical neurones (KRNJEVIĆ, RANDIĆ and STRAUGHAN, 1966), both in its effects upon the membrane potential and conductance as well as in its ionic mechanism. It is interesting that this cortical inhibition is also resistant to strychnine and tetanus toxin. On the other hand, GABA action is not identical with the inhibition in spinal motoneurones, for it does not induce membrane hyper-polarization (CURTIS, PHILLIS and WATKINS, 1959). This inhibition in spinal moto-neurones is sensitive to strychnine and tetanus toxin, and therefore the transmitter could be different from that in Deiters and cortical neurones.

The GABA content in Purkinje cells was measured for their isolated cell bodies (OBATA, quoted by CURTIS and WATKINS, 1965; OBATA, personal communication) and also with the dissected Purkinje cell layer (KURIYAMA, HABER, SISKEN and ROBERTS, 1966). As measured by OBATA (personal communication) the GABA concentration per unit volume of Purkinje cells is five times as high as that in moto-neurones and ten times that of spinal ganglion cells. The latter two cell species are known to be excitatory. According to KURIYAMA et al. (1966), the Purkinje cell layer has a GABA concentration about twice that in the molecular or granular layers of the cerebellar cortex. In these measurements, however, it is not possible to discriminate whether the GABA is present at high concentration in the postsynaptic cytoplasm or in the profuse inhibitory presynaptic terminals that the basket cells give to cell bodies (Chapter V). A discriminative method should be developed for finding the exact location of GABA in Purkinje cells.

The criteria for identification of the transmitter substance have been discussed by several authors (cf. ECCLES, 1964). In the Crustacean inhibitory system on muscle fibers, they are now shown to be very well satisfied: GABA mimics the natural inhibitory mechanism (KUFFLER and EDWARDS, 1958; BOISTEL and FATT, 1958); GABA exists almost exclusively in the axons (KRAVITZ, KUFFLER and POTTER, 1963) as well as in the cell bodies (OTSUKA, KRAVITZ and POTTER, 1965) of the inhibitory neurones; the enzymic system for GABA metabolism is also present in the inhibitory nerves (KRAVITZ, MOLINOFF and HALL, 1965); moreover, stimulation of the inhibitory nerve increases GABA liberation from its terminal regions (OTSUKA, IVERSEN, HALL and KRAVITZ, 1966). The evidence in mammalian central nervous system is still incomplete. Nevertheless, the above-mentioned results on Deiters and cortical neurones strongly point to the possibility that GABA acts as a natural transmitter in the mammalian central nervous system, as has been proposed for Crustacea. However, there is one discrepancy in that picrotoxin does not influence the inhibition of Deiters and cortical neurones, which is in contrast to its blocking action upon invertebrate inhibitory synapses. It can be anticipated that the wealth of clearly identified inhibitory cells and synapses in the cerebellum will greatly facilitate neurochemical and pharmacological inves-tigations into the transmitters for postsynaptic inhibition.

C. Disinhibitory Phenomena

While postsynaptic inhibition of Deiters neurones is effected by impulses in the Purkinje cell axons, there is also a prominent disinhibitory phenomenon arising from depression of the tonic discharges from Purkinje cells. Stimulation of the cerebellum within either the cortex or the white matter usually builds up in a

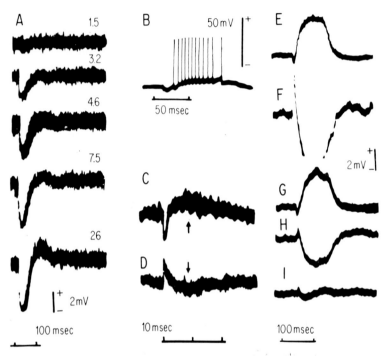

Fig. 134 A—I. *Disinhibitory depolarization in Deiters neurones after cerebellar stimulation.* Intracellular d. c. recording from Deiters neurones. In A pulse stimuli of 0.2 msec duration were given to the anterior lobe of the cerebellum at intensities indicated (in volts). B, double shock to the anterior lobe of the cerebellum (interval, 1 msec; intensity, 30 volts). C, similar to A but in another cell. Stimulus intensity was 30 volts. D, same as in C but during passage of hyperpolarizing currents (3×10^{-8} A). Arrows in C and D points to the direction of the disinhibitory potentials. E, same cell and same double shock as in B but at different trial where there was no spike initiation. F, same as in E but during passage of hyperpolarizing currents (5×10^{-8} A) through the KCl-filled microelectrode. G, same as in E but at different trial. H, same as in G but after intracellular injection of sodium ions by passage of depolarizing currents (5×10^{-8} A for 30 sec). I, at 2 min after sodium injection. (ITO, KAWAI, UDO and SATO, 1967 d)

Deiters neurone a prolonged hyperpolarization by both the direct and the transsynaptic activation of Purkinje cells (Figs. 128 D—G and 130 B—D), which in turn reverses to a late depolarization lasting several hundred milliseconds (Fig. 134 A). The late depolarization is often powerful enough to trigger the discharge of a train of impulses from a Deiters neurone (Fig. 134 B).

The nature of this late depolarization is obvious when it is reversed by the intracellular injection of hyperpolarizing currents and/or chloride ions, the equilibrium potential being at the same level as for the IPSPs (Fig. 134 C, D). It follows that the depolarization is due to removal of background IPSPs, much as has been observed in spinal motoneurones following stimulation of the ventral roots (WILSON and BURGESS, 1962). Double shocks at brief intervals (around 1 msec) potentiate very effectively the late depolarization (Fig. 134 E). It is rather surprising that, as revealed by injection of hyperpolarizing current (Fig. 134 F) or of ions (G, H), the whole depolarization amounting up to 4 mV is shown to be produced by disinhibition. An abundant inhibitory bombardment must be spontaneously acting upon Deiters neurones. This view is in keeping with the old idea that the cerebellar cortex exerts a tonic inhibition upon the brain stem postural centers. This was based on the enhancement of decerebrate rigidity or emergence of the so-called alpha rigidity (GRANIT, 1955), which occurs after partial or total ablation of the anterior lobe. It also occurs after cooling or deprivation of the blood supply to the cerebellum (BREMER, 1922; POLLOCK and DAVIS, 1930). Small spontaneous IPSPs are actually seen in Deiters neurones (Fig. 135 B). Normally they are of small size (about 0.2 mV), but they can be transformed into large depolarizing potentials by current and/or chloride injection (Fig. 135 D). As would be expected, the spontaneous IPSPs are depressed during the phase of disinhibition following the cerebellar stimulation (Fig. 135 F, G).

This disinhibitory phenomenon must be ascribed at least partly to inhibition of Purkinje cells which has been shown to occur through the basket and stellate cells (Chapters V and VI). However, there should also be a contribution by Golgi cell inhibition of the spontaneous discharges from the granule cells up the parallel fibers to Purkinje cells (Fig. 107 A—D). There is also evidence that the cerebellar stimulation produces a prolonged IPSP in the olivary neurones (ITO, OCHI and OBATA, 1967 f) which activate Purkinje cells spontaneously (Chapter VIII). The disinhibition has not been studied in detail in the neurones of the intracerebellar nuclei, but its existence is shown indirectly in the brain stem neurones which they innervate (Chapter XIV). To this extent, Deiters neurones represent quite well the behavior of all first stage target neurones in the cerebellar efferent system. The disinhibition is particularly significant in relation to the following two phenomena.

Firstly, it provides at least a partial explanation (there is also another excitatory process, described in section D below) of the excitatory effect of cerebellar stimulation that has been observed in the muscle tonus (BREMER, 1922; DENNY-BROWN et al., 1929; POMPEIANO, 1958) or upon the discharges from Deitersian (DE VITO, BRUSA and ARDUINI, 1956; POMPEIANO and COTTI, 1959) and fastigial units (ARDUINI and POMPEIANO, 1957). In the older experiments stimulation of the anterior lobe induced a prominent postinhibitory rebound in muscle tonus (BREMER, 1922; cf. BROOKHART, 1960). Correspondingly a small slow depolarization is seen regularly in Deiters neurones following repetitive cerebellar stimulation (Fig. 136 A, open arrows). Because the polarity is reversed with a high intracellular concentration of chloride ions (Fig. 136 B at arrows), this slow depolarization also appears to be of disinhibitory origin. The well-known dual effect of the cerebellar stimulation, i.e. conversion of inhibition to facilitation by lowering the stimulus frequency (MORUZZI, 1950), may well be understood as due to predominance of the disinhibitory depolarization at relatively low frequency.

This could occur because it lasts longer than the initial inhibition (see Fig. 134 A); hence in the total integration on the membrane of subcortical neurones the facilitation may surpass the inhibition. At higher frequencies, the IPSPs are summated to sustain the membrane hyperpolarization and the disinhibitory depolarization arises only after cessation of stimuli (Fig. 136 A).

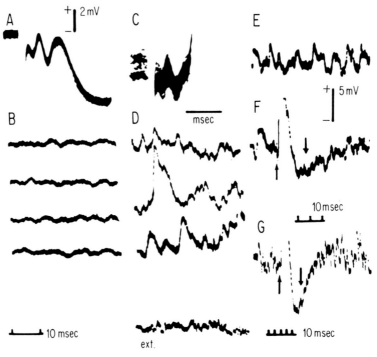

Fig. 135 A—G. *IPSP noise in Deiters neurones and its suppression during disinhibition.* Intracellular recording with time constant of 200 msec. A, IPSP produced by stimulation of lobule IV. B, base lines taken without stimulation. C, same as in A but during passage of hyperpolarizing currents $(8 \times 10^{-8}$ A) through the impaled KCl-filled microelectrode. D, base lines under the same conditions as in C. ext., extracellular control taken after withdrawal by applying the same currents as in C, D. E, reserved IPSP noise in another Deiters neurone recorded during passage of Cl-injecting hyperpolarizing currents $(5 \times 10^{-8}$ A). F, reversed IPSP and disinhibitory potential produced by stimulation of lobule IV under the same conditions as in E. G, similar to F, but recorded at slower sweep velocity. Upward arrows in F, G mark the moment of stimulation. Downward arrows point to the disinhibitory phase, where the IPSP noise was reduced markedly. (ITO, KAWAI, UDO and SATO, 1967 d)

Secondly, the disinhibition provides the way in which the purely inhibitory projection from Purkinje cells can control its target in the direction not only of inhibition but also of facilitation. Under normal operative conditions the membrane potential of subcortical neurones is biassed so that variations in the level of discharge of Purkinje cells can cause potential changes in either direction. In Chapter XIV, a similar situation will be seen with the purely excitatory projection from the nucleus interpositus to the red nucleus, where withdrawal of excitation produces an inhibitory effect in the manner of disfacilitation. It has thus to be realized that, in the analysis of the neurone circuitry, the end effect of a certain system cannot be related immediately to the nature of the neurones at its final output stage. In this connexion it should also be pointed out that, for the Purkinje cells to exert their inhibitory control effectively, the subcortical nuclei must receive some excitatory input in addition to the tonic inhibition demonstrated in Figs. 135 and 136. There would thus be tonic facilitation in balance with, and presumably surpassing, the tonic inhibition. This situation will be discussed further in the next chapter.

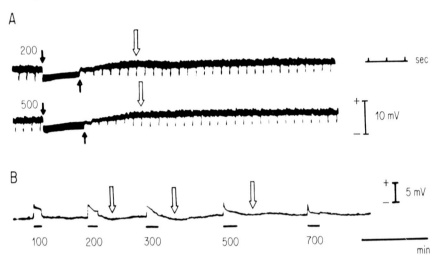

Fig. 136 A and B. *Disinhibition following repetitive stimulation of the cerebellar cortex.* Intracellular d. c. recording from two Deiters neurones. In A stimuli were given to lobule IV at the frequencies indicated. Solid downward and upward arrows indicate the onset and cessation of stimuli, respectively. Horrow arrows point to the later depolarizing potential changes. Stimuli were also given on the background at a rate of 2/sec, and the downward potential deflection represent the IPSPs thereby induced. B, similar to A but registered in another cell by a pen recorder. Horizontal bars signal the periods of stimulation at frequencies indicated. The IPSPs were reversed to the depolarizing direction by diffusion of chloride ions from the KCl-filled microelectrode. Horrow arrows point to the reversed later slow potential changes. Note the different time and voltage scales for A and B. (ITO, KAWAI, UDO and SATO, 1967 d)

D. Axon Reflexes through the Collaterals of Cerebellar Afferents

Though inhibition and disinhibition are the predominant events in Deiters neurones, stimulation of the cerebellar cortex also evokes monosynaptic excitatory postsynaptic potentials (EPSPs) (ITO and YOSHIDA, 1966 b). It is not necessary to postulate excitatory action by some Purkinje cells because a satisfactory explanation is provided by an axon reflex through the collaterals of the cerebellar afferent fibers (ITO, KAWAI and UDO, 1965 a), which is a unique feature of the cerebellar afferent-efferent organization.

The neurones located in the ventral portion of Deiters nucleus do not receive Purkinje cell axons either from the anterior or from the posterior lobe (WALBERG and JANSEN, 1961). In these cells stimulation of the cerebellar cortex usually produces an EPSP, as exemplified in Fig. 137 B. The EPSP is often large enough to excite the cell orthodromically (Fig. 137 B e). There are two points of clear discrimination between the pathways for the monosynaptic IPSPs and EPSPs; firstly, the EPSPs are induced usually bilaterally from a wide area of the anterior

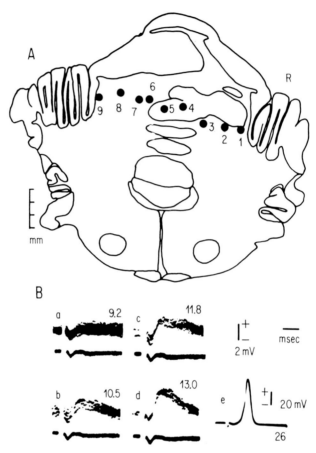

Fig. 137 A—D. *Monosynaptic EPSPs induced in Deiters neurones by cerebellar stimulation.* A shows electrolytic marks made by stimulating needle electrodes on a transverse plane through the anterior lobe of the cerebellum. R, right side. Deiters neurones were inpaled at right side. C, upper traces, intracellular potentials recorded in a ventral Deiters neurone by stimulating at spots Nos. 1—9. The figure attached to each record refers to the position of cathode, the anode being served by the left side partner except for No. 9 against which the spot 8 formed anode. Lower traces, extracellular records taken after withdrawal. D, similar series to C, but recorded in a dorsal Deiters neurone. Dotted lines in the records 2—4 indicate the time course of the extra-cellular potentials given in the lower traces. B, in another experiment. Stimuli were given to the ipsilateral anterior lobe at the intensities indicated in volt. Voltage scale of 2 mV applies to a—d and that of 20 mV to e. (ITO, KAWAI, UDO and MANO, 1967 c)

and posterior lobes of the cerebellum (Fig. 137 C, from spots 3, 4, 5, 6, 7) while the IPSPs arise only from a localized area in the ipsilateral side (Figs. 129 and 137 D, spots 2, 3, 4). This wide origin of the EPSPs is important because it provides a crucial discrimination between the monosynaptic excitatory fibers on the one hand and on the other the Purkinje cell axons which have a well-defined origin (WAL-

BERG and JANSEN, 1961; EAGER, 1963a). Secondly, the latency of the EPSPs is usually shorter than that of the IPSPs. From the lobules IV and V the mean values for the EPSPs and IPSPs are respectively 0.85 msec and 1.15 msec. This

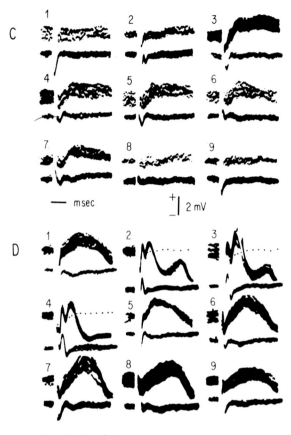

Fig. 137 C and D

latency differential indicates that in the excitatory fibers there is a significantly faster conduction velocity, and hence they would be expected to have a diameter larger than the 3—5 μ derived for Purkinje cell axons (section B, 4).

Even in the dorsal Deiters neurones, the monosynaptic EPSPs are often induced either in isolation, with stimulation of cerebellar cortical areas extraneous to the inhibitory zone, or in superposition on the monosynaptic IPSPs (Fig. 137 D). In the latter case, the EPSPs are detected by comparing the intracellular with the extracellular records, being thus recognized as a brief period of depolarization before the IPSP develops, as is illustrated in Fig. 137 D, records 2—4.

This dual, excitatory-inhibitory action of the monosynaptic pathways from the cerebellar cortex to Deiters nucleus has its counterpart in the presynaptic field potential with the characteristic double peak, the α and β spikes (Fig. 128 H—J). Systematic exploration reveals that the β spike represents the inhibitory presynaptic volley, while the α spike indicates the excitatory one (ITO and YOSHIDA, 1966 b). Like the IPSPs, the β spike can be evoked only from the ipsilateral anterior and posterior lobes, while the α spike is evoked from the whole width of these lobes (Fig. 138 A). When the recording microelectrode is moved dorso-ventrally through Deiters nucleus, as shown in Fig. 138 C, the β spike changes from a predominantly negative to a predominantly positive wave and eventually disappears in the ventral portion of the nucleus, thus conforming to the termination of the Purkinje cell axons within its dorsal component (ITO and YOSHIDA, 1966 b). The α spike, on the other hand, persists throughout Deiters nucleus as a dominantly negative wave (ITO and YOSHIDA, 1966 b).

The monosynaptic excitatory pathway to Deiters nucleus would be provided by the cerebellar afferents if they innervate both the cerebellar cortex and Deiters nucleus, there being an axon reflex pathway along their axon collaterals. There was originally a suggestion by LORENTE DE NÓ (1933) that the dorsal spino-cerebellar tract fibers send their axon collaterals into the vestibular nuclei, though BRODAL et al. (1962) suggest that the fibers are specifically spino-vestibular rather than axon collaterals of spino-cerebellar fibers. However, further evidence is given in section A, 1 of this chapter that numerous axon colleterals arise from the various cerebellar afferents that terminate in the cerebellar cortex either as mossy or climbing fibers.

It may also be recalled that the primary vestibular fibers innervate both a part of the lateral nucleus and the cerebellar cortex at the flocculus and nodulus (cf. BRODAL et al., 1962, and personal communication). Similarly, the secondary vestibular fibers which originate mainly from the descending vestibular nucleus pass both to the fastigial nucleus and to the flocculus and nodulus (cf. BRODAL et al., 1962). It is possible that these cortical and nuclear structures are innervated commonly by the axon collaterals of the same afferent fibers.

Actually, monosynaptic EPSPs are induced in Deiters neurones by stimulating various extracerebellar structures which give rise to the cerebellar afferents: the ventral and lateral funiculi of the spinal cord (ITO et al., 1964 a); the vestibular nerve, though the effect was limited to a few ventral Deiters neurones (ITO et al., 1964 a; 1967 a); the inferior olive (Fig. 131 B; see the EPSP preceding the IPSP) (ITO et al., 1966 a); and the external cuneate nucleus (ITO et al., 1967 c).

The afferent pathways to the anterior lobe of the cerebellum can be stimulated in the restiform body at the level of the external cuneate nucleus. Thus in Fig. 139 Bb stimulation of the external cuneate nucleus induced initially a spiky negative field potential (n_1) indicating synchronized impulses in fibers passing through Deiters nucleus and later there was a slow negativity (n_2) which may represent the synaptic excitation of Deiters neurones. As would be expected, when the external cuneate is stimulated shortly before the cerebellum, there is blockage of the descending impulses from the cerebellum, as shown by the diminution of the α spike (Fig. 139 B b—f). This interference occurs at such a short interval that the stimuli at the external cuneate region and the cerebellar cortex must be exciting the same line of fibers, there being collision of impulses generated from the two sites. This collision of impulses also accounts for the observations of Fig. 139 C where there is occlusion of the EPSPs evoked from the cerebellar cortex and the external cuneate region.

The monosynaptic excitatory pathways from the whole width of the anterior lobe (Fig. 138 A) are very effectively depressed by stimulation at the external cuneate region. Hence, it can be concluded that the cerebellar-evoked monosynaptic EPSPs are produced via the axon collaterals of fibers arising in the

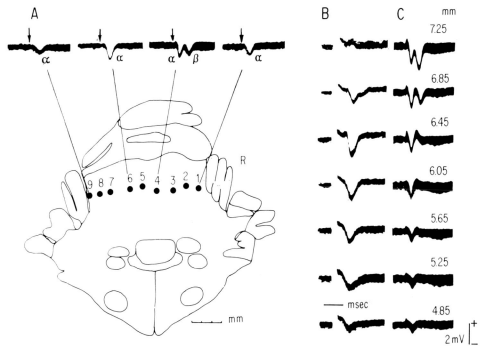

Fig. 138 A—C. *Origins of the presynaptic volleys induced by cerebellar stimulation.* A, field potentials recorded at a point within right Deiters nucleus during stimulation at the spots indicated in the diagram. Arrows mark the moment of stimulation. α and β denote the early and delayed spike fields, respectively. B, antidromic field potential recorded along a track through Deiters nucleus during stimulation of the vestibulospinal fibers at C_2 level. C, field potentials induced by stimulating the ipsilateral anterior lobe at the spot No. 3 of A and recorded at the same points as in B. Figure attached to each record indicates the depth of recording in both B and C, as measured from the ventral surface of the medullary pyramid in mm. (ITO, KAWAI, UDO and MANO, 1967 c)

external cuneate nucleus or of those cerebellar afferents which pass through the restiform body near the external cuneate nucleus, and which would include spinocerebellar, reticulocerebellar, cuneocerebellar and olivo-cerebellar fibers.

There is evidence indicating that the axons from inferior olive cells innervate Deiters neurones monosynaptically (ITO *et al.*, 1966 a). As seen in Fig. 131 B, E after stimulation of either the inferior olive or the spinal cord, EPSPs appear in Deiters neurones about a millisecond in advance of the excitation of Purkinje cells by the olivo-cerebellar impulses in the climbing fibers. Besides this temporal correlation the special features of the spino-olivary transmission illustrated in Fig. 140 indicate a causal relationship between the olivary impulses and the EPSPs

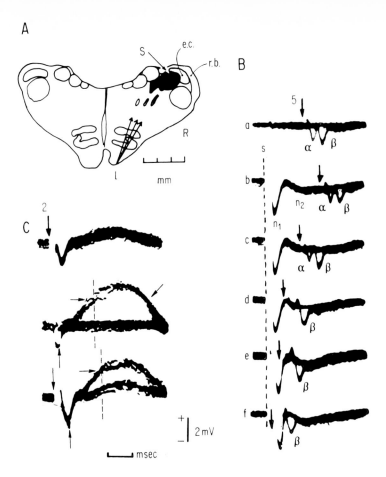

Fig. 139 A—C. *Impulse collision along the cerebellar afferents which innervate Deiters neurones by axon collaterals.* A shows the location of stimulating electrode on a transverse plane of the medulla oblongata. R, right side. r. b., restiform body. e. c., external cuneate nucleus. Arrow (s) points to the position of the stimulating needle electrode which formed cathode. Anode was served by the other electrode located at 1.5 mm rostral to the cathode. Three arrows (*l*) indicate the tracks of the stimulating electrode. Black mark indicates the electrolytic lesion. B, field potentials recorded within Deiters nucleus. In a, pulse stimuli (0.2 msec, 30 volts) were given to the spot No. 5 of Fig. 138 A at the moment indicated by downward arrow. α and β denote two negative spiky peaks of the field potential. The stimuli were switched off in about half of the trials. In b—f pulse stimuli of 0.2 msec duration and of 10 volt amplitude were given to the external cuneate region indicated in A (arrow s) at the moment indicated by vertical interrupted line. n_1, early spike component of the field potentials. n_2, slow negativity. Downward arrows in b—f point similarly to a. C, intracellular recording from a Deiters neurone. Uppermost traces, EPSP produced by stimulation at spot No. 2 of Fig. 138 A. Arrow marks the moment of stimulation. Middle traces, stimulation at the external cuneate nucleus region (s in A). Upward arrow points to the moment of stimulation. The stimuli were switched off in about half of the trials, giving the base line. — The small hump on the rising phase of the EPSP at the time indicated by vertical broken line is probably caused by superposition of delayed EPSPs on the early monosynaptic ones. The relatively quick fall of the EPSPs (marked by oblique arrow) may be caused by superposition of delayed IPSPs. Lowermost traces, combined stimulation at spot No. 2 and external cuneate nucleus region, as indicated by both downward and upward arrows. Similarly to the middle traces, the external cuneate stimulation was turned off in about half of the trials. The EPSPs are compared between the middle and lowermost traces at the same interval from the external cuneate stimulation, as indicated by vertical interrupted lines. Horizontal arrows indicate the points where the amplitudes of EPSPs were measured from the zero base line obtained before stimulation and were virtually the same between the middle and lowermost tracese. (ITO, KAWAI, UDO and MANO, 1967 c)

induced by the reflex activation of olivary neurones via the mossy fiber collaterals or the excitatory interconnexions which appear to be formed by the axon collaterals of the cells of the inferior olive (OCHI, 1965; ECCLES et al., 1966 d; ITO et al., 1967 f), as illustrated in Fig. 142 D. With the direct olivary stimulation, the climbing fiber responses can be induced at a latency as brief as 3 msec (Fig. 131 A; Chapter VIII). Therefore, it should take more than 6 msec for an impulse to travel back along an olivary axon to the inferior olive and then by excitatory axon collaterals to evoke a discharge from an olivary neurone and so back to a Purkinje cell by a climbing fiber (Fig. 142 D). It will also take 5 msec or so even if the impulse propagates antidromically along the fast conducting mossy fibers to activate inferior olive cells by axon collaterals (Fig. 142 D). Therefore, the climbing fiber activation of Purkinje cells at latencies of 2 to 5 msec should not include a recurrent pathway through the inferior olive, but it should be caused directly by a climbing fiber, which may be excited by an impulse along one of its collateral branches (Fig. 142 C). The IPSPs which appear in Deiters neurones at 2—6 msec (Fig. 130 B—D) thus would be included in the group of disynaptic IPSPs. This inference is confirmed by the observation that these IPSPs persist after acute destruction of the contralateral inferior olive, and even of both inferior olives (ITO, UDO and SATO, unpublished). The more delayed IPSPs at 6—10 msec would be caused by the reflex connexions through the inferior olive shown in Fig. 142 D. For example in Fig. 143 A, C five components are discriminated from the potentials evoked by cerebellar stimulation. h_1 and h_2 refer to the monosynaptic and disynaptic IPSPs, respectively, while d_1 denotes the delayed EPSPs which probably arise disynaptically (see below). These relatively early components are further followed by a sequence of delayed EPSPs (d_2) and IPSPs (h_3). When the contralateral inferior olive was damaged electrolytically, these late IPSPs (h_3) disappeared together with the preceding EPSPs (d_2) (Fig. 143 B). These IPSPs resemble those produced by the spinal stimulation (Fig. 131 E, 140 B, C) in being preceded by EPSPs and in being very variable in size (Fig. 143 C); hence they have the properties that would be expected for a reflex activation of the inferior olive through the cerebellar afferent collaterals.

Delayed EPSPs have also been seen in Deiters neurones during stimulation of the cerebellar cortex (Fig. 143 E, F; oblique arrows) or the region of the deep nuclei (Fig. 150). As will be shown in the next chapter, the efferent fibers from the fastigial nucleus excite Deiters neurones monosynaptically. Hence transsynaptic excitation of fastigial neurones would result in disynaptic EPSPs in Deiters neurones. The former would be induced via the axon collaterals of the cerebellar afferents, just as is assumed for Deiters neurones, and it is illustrated in Fig. 142 E. Similar polysynaptic excitation would occur through the axon collaterals of the inferior olive cells, and probably through the other excitatory sources for Deiters neurones (cf. section D above).

The disinhibitory depolarization could be induced also from the whole width of the anterior and posterior lobes of the cerebellum. The inhibition of Purkinje cells that causes disinhibition of Deiters neurones may be induced through the pathway — mossy fibers to granule cells to basket cells (Fig. 142 F). Though the parallel fibers extend for no more than 3 mm along the transverse folia, inhibition of the Purkinje cells located within the monosynaptic inhibitory zone might be induced by stimulation of mossy fibers that, by means of their collateral branches,

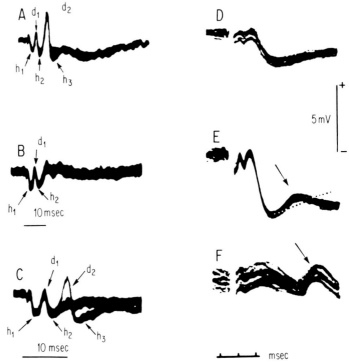

Fig. 143 A—F. *Reflex activation of the inferior olive and fastigial nucleus after cerebellar stimulation.* A, PSPs recorded in a Deiters neurone after stimulation of lobule IV. Pulse duration was 0.2 msec and intensity 30 volts. h_1, h_2 and h_3, IPSP components. d_1, d_2, EPSP components. B, same cell and same stimulating conditions as in A but after electrolytical damage of the contralateral inferior olive. d. c. currents of 2 mA were passed for 1 min through the needle electrode inserted into the contralateral inferior olive. C, similar to A but in another Deiters cell. Intermittent disappearance of d_2 and h_3 components is indicated by superimposing the sweeps at a repetition rate of 1/sec. Symbols indicate similarly to A. (Ito, Udo and Sato, unpublished). D—F, in another experiment. D, monosynaptic IPSP induced from lobule III with pulses of 0.2 msec duration and of 1.1 volt strength. E, same cell and same stimulating site as in D but with stronger pulses of 21 volts. Dotted line superposed on E indicates the possible time course of the potential change if it were similar to that in D. Oblique arrow points to the deviation of the actual potential curve from the dotted line in the depolarizing direction. F, potential changes in another cell of the same preparation as in D, E. 10 volt pulses of 0.2 msec duration were applied to the same stimulating electrode as for D, E. There was first depolarization followed by a delayed hyperpolarization, upon which, at 4 msec after stimulation, a further delayed depolarization was superposed. Arrow marks the delayed depolarization. Time scale of 10 msec under B applies to A and B, and that of msec under F to D, E, F. (Ito and Yoshida, 1966b)

extend far beyond this zone. The disinhibition, however, would be induced also by the inhibition of the granule cells through Golgi cells which would depress the excitatory bombardment from granule cells to Purkinje cells (Fig. 107 A—D). It should also be considered that reflex activation of the olivary neurones or their antidromic excitation from the cerebellar cortex would produce a prolonged inhibition in this nucleus (Fig. 142 G, see section C) and so would depress the spontaneous climbing fiber activation of Purkinje cells.

The total effect of the cerebellar stimulation is the sum of the various events mediated through the pathways of Fig. 142 A—G. When the stimuli are given repetitively, complication will further be introduced by summation of the post-synaptic potentials and/or alteration of the transmission efficacy at different cells and synapses included in the circuits of Fig. 142. Whether the integrated end effect is inhibitory or excitatory should depend on the spatial location of the stimulating electrode in the cerebellar cortex, on the temporal parameters of stimulation and upon the phase which is looked at — whether early or later during or after the stimulation.

Chapter XIV

Excitatory Signals from the Intracerebellar Nuclei

A. The Nuclear Efferents of the Cerebellum

A general survey of the nuclear efferents of the cerebellum is given by the summarizing diagrams of JANSEN and BRODAL (1954 Fig. 71; 1958 Fig. 187). Considering the extreme multiplicity of these connexions, and that the scope of this monograph is limited to the general neuronal mechanisms of the cerebellum, there would be no point in embarking on a detailed discussion of these connexions. Everything known about them has been so well documented by JANSEN and BRODAL (1954, 1958) that nothing could be added to these masterpieces of functional anatomical analysis. The principal nucleofugal projections are schematically illustrated in Fig. 124 and only a very brief description will be given below of the synaptic relation of cerebellar efferents in the red nucleus and in the ventralis lateralis (VL) nucleus of the thalamus.

1. Synaptic Articulations in the Red Nucleus

According to CAJAL (1911) the fibers originating from the cerebellar nuclei and running towards the red nucleus do not give any collaterals before crossing and before reaching the posterior margin of the red nucleus. They penetrate through this nucleus, giving off numerous collaterals that arborize between the nerve cells. However, the fibers themselves do not terminate here, but leave the nucleus on its anterior border and enter into the thalamus. The nerve cells of the red nucleus are thoroughly enveloped by a very dense feltwork of rather coarse preterminal fibers (see CAJAL, 1911: Fig. 94). If this feltwork is well stained in Golgi preparations — as it often is in material taken from younger animals — it is not possible to recognize the true nature of synaptic contacts (Fig. 144 A and C). The dense feltwork surrounding each cell is only the outer preterminal layer of the presynaptic fibers. As can be judged from the large size of the preterminal degeneration fragments after lesions of the sensorimotor cortex, the coarser fibers may probably be the descending cortical fibers, whereas the cerebellar ones and especially their collaterals are rather delicate. Occasionally when part of the pericellular feltwork remains unstained, can one observe — emerging from axons running through the nucleus in the anteroposterior direction — collaterals that upon reaching the cell bodies arborize in an almost brush-like manner (Fig. 144 B). The delicate branches are beaded and more closely attached to the cell body surface than the coarse pericellular feltwork. Also, from tangential sections of the cell bodies with both the pericellular feltwork and the brush-like terminals stained, one can recognize clearly that the latter are situated inside the coarse feltwork. The branches of the brush-like arborizations terminate in very delicate terminal knobs (Fig. 144 D).

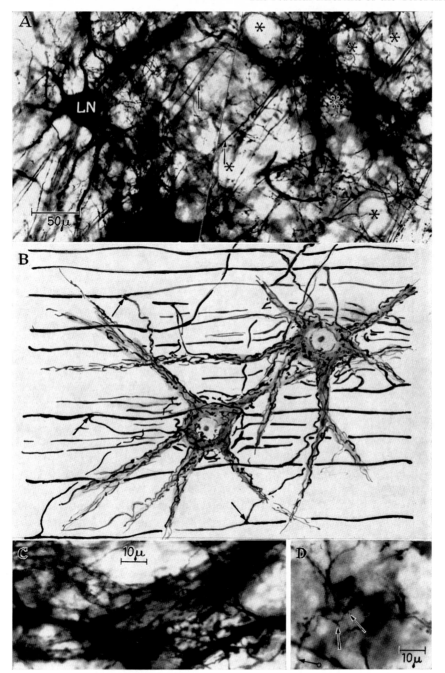

Fig. 144 A—D. Synaptic structure in the red nucleus as revealed in the Golgi picture. One week old kitten. Valverde modification of the rapid Golgi procedure. A. Overall view with one large neuron (LN) stained at left. Arrows point to cerebellofugal fibers running through. The holes indicated by asterisks correspond to unstained cell bodies embedded into the coarse neuropil. — B. Drawing made from another part of the same material showing the terminal ramifications of collaterals branching off (arrows) from the brachium conjunctivum fibers. — C. Pericellular dense neuropil of red nucleus neurons, originating mainly, although not exclusively, from the collaterals of cerebellar efferents (compare with drawing of CAJAL, 1911, Fig. 94). — D. Incompletely stained pericellular feltwork showing single collateral of cerebellar efferent (ringed arrow) to terminate on cell body with numerous very delicate boutons (arrows)

It frequently occurs that only that part of the neuropil is stained in the Golgi picture, which is in contact with the cell body and the larger dendrites (Fig. 144 C). It can be deduced from such pictures that both cell body and dendrite surface of red nucleus neurons are densely covered by terminal branches of the collaterals of the cerebellofugal pathways. Many of the collaterals seem to reach the cell bodies directly, although quite a number approach the larger dendrites.

A detailed investigation of the synaptic systems of the red nucleus, using combined degeneration and EM techniques, might be worth while and might provide better understanding of the function of this nucleus, the pathways of which have been so thoroughly analysed recently by the Oslo group (POMPEIANO and BRODAL, 1957; RINVIK and WALBERG, 1963). From the degeneration pictures resulting from lesions of the motor region one gets the impression that the majority of their contacts is at the dendrites, perhaps even of the smaller ones, of the red nucleus cells.

2. Synaptic Arrangement of Efferent Cerebellar Pathways in the (VL) of the Thalamus

The question of whether the majority of ascending cerebellofugal fibers of the brachium conjunctivum are terminating within the red nucleus or whether most of them ascend further to the thalamus is still controversial among histologists. As mentioned previously, Golgi pictures are rather suggestive of the latter. JANSEN and BRODAL (1958) on the basis of a detailed discussion also arrive at the conclusion that the majority of ascending brachium conjunctivum fibers ascend to the VL of the thalamus. Moreover the claim that the majority of fibers from the interpositus nucleus terminate in the red nucleus is difficult to reconcile with the extreme wealth of degeneration fragments in VL after lesions of the interpositus nucleus. The recent physiological studies (see below) also indicate that the majority of the interpositus axons extend up to VL after impinging upon red nucleus neurones by axon collaterals.

The structure of the VL nucleus of the thalamus corresponds in cell types to that of most other specific nuclei, particularly of the lateral group. The *projective cell* that has an axon ascending to the motor cortex is a large multiangular cell with the characteristic "tufted" dendritic arborization (Fig. 145 A), i.e. the main dendrites break up into a whole tuft of secondary dendrites. The dendritic arborization tree is a sphere of about 150 μ radius. Another cell group are Golgi II type cells having the characteristics recently discussed by TÖMBÖL (1967): smaller cell body of rounded shape, 3—4 main dendrites that are longer and have a less regular often "wavy" character, and the smaller dendrites have drum-stick shaped side branches that look like spines (Fig. 145 B). The axon has a typical Golgi second type arborization, generally in the close neighbourhood of the cell body. Whether all branches of the axon terminate in the neighbourhood, or whether some of the larger branches reach more distant regions as in the similar although somewhat larger cell type, described recently by SCHEIBEL and SCHEIBEL (1966) as the integrator cell of the thalamus, cannot be judged from our own adult material.

Most of the neuropil in the VL has a rather diffuse "non specific" character. It is built up of delicate fibers of generally straight course giving short side branches

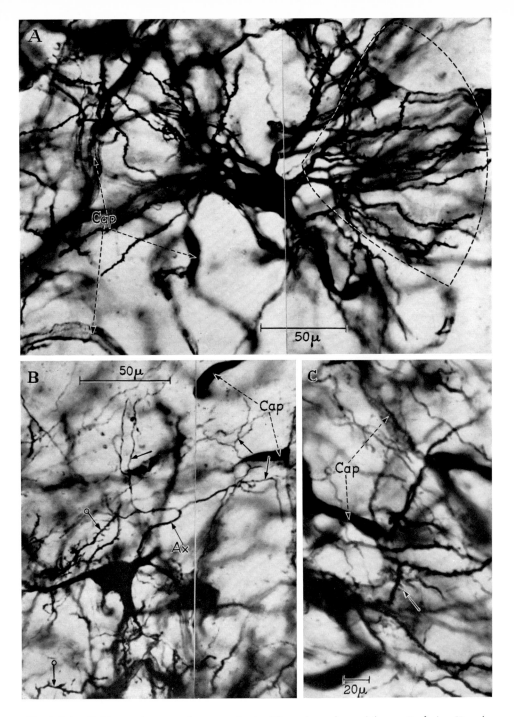

Fig. 145 A—C. Two main types of neurons in the VL nucleus of an adult cat. Perfusion Kopsch procedure. Part of the capillary network (*Cap*) is also stained unfortunately. — A. Projective (relay) cell with characteristic "tufted" dendritic arborization. Conic space occupied by one of the tufts brought into focus is marked by dashed outlines. — B. Golgi 2nd type neuron having an axon (*Ax*) that arborizes in characteristic manner in the neighbourhood of the cell body. Only small part of the dense arborization (arrows) could be brought into focus in this photograph. Typical smaller dendrites, with their short spine-like side branches, of this cell are indicated by ringed arrows. — C. Part of the general neuropil in this nucleus, showing the termination of very delicate boutons (arrow) on secondary dendrites of projective cell, giving the appearance of spines

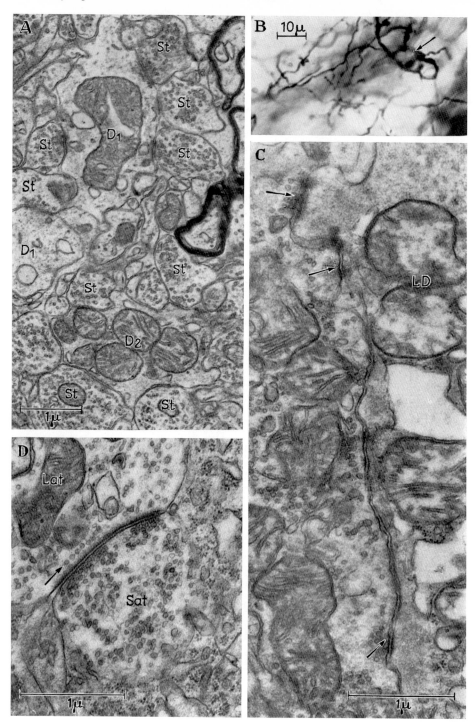

Fig. 146 A—D. Some EM information on the synapses in the VL of the thalamus. Adult cat. — A. Secondary dendrites (D_1 and D_2) are almost completely covered by relatively small synaptic terminals (St) that obviously correspond to the small spine-like boutons seen in the Golgi picture (Fig. 145 C) and arise from the general neuropil of the nucleus. The two different kinds of

along the nucleofugal pathway towards the VL (Fig. 148 Bb to a). This reduction of the EPSP latency can be related to the continuous conduction of impulses at a relatively low velocity of 10—20 m/sec. Extrapolation to zero distance, i.e. to VL, indicates that the impulses monosynaptically induce EPSPs in VL cells with a synaptic delay time of about 0.5 msec.

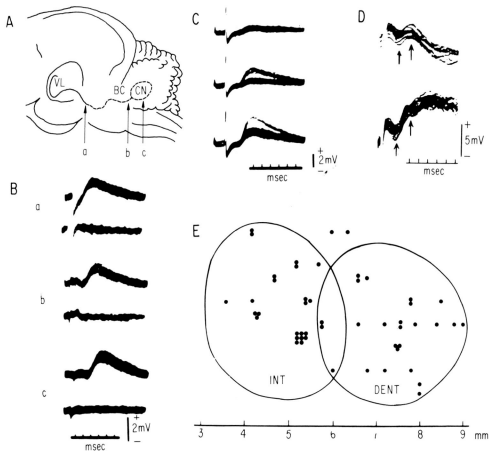

Fig. 148 A—E. *Potential changes produced in VL cells during stimulation of cerebellar nuclei and their fibers.* A shows a sagittal section through the cerebrum and cerebellum. *CN*, cerebellar nuclei. *BC*, brachium conjunctivum. Dotted line connecting CN and VL represents the course of nucleofugal fibers. Arrows, a, b, c, indicate the position of stimulating electrodes. B, Upper traces, monosynaptic EPSPs recorded from a VL cell after stimulation at a, b and c, as indicated. Lower traces, extracellular controls. C, unitary steps in the EPSPs. In the uppermost traces the stimulus intensity was just at threshold for producing a small EPSP of 0.9 mV amplitude. The stimulus intensity was increased in the middle traces to 1.3 times the threshold and in the lowermost traces 1.5 times. D, upper traces, IPSP induced in another VL cell from a spot within interpositus nucleus. Second arrow marks its onset. First arrow points to the onset of the initial EPSP. Lower traces, same as in D but during passage of hyperpolarizing currents (5×10^{-8} A) through the KCl-filled microelectrode. There was reversal in the IPSP. Note that the initial EPSP was also increased slightly by the hyperpolarizing currents. E plots with one dot for each VL cell the positions of the stimulating electrodes with which monosynaptic EPSPs were induced with lowest threshold. *NT*, interpositus nucleus. *DENT*, lateral nucleus. Figures on the abscissa indicate the distance from the sagittal midplane through the cerebellum. (UNO, YOSHIDA and HIROTA, 1967)

A unique feature in VL cells is the large unitary size of the nuclear-induced EPSPs (Fig. 148 C). Fine adjustment of the stimulus intensity reveals a prominent step-wise change in the size of the EPSPs, even by as much as 2—3 mV. Synchronized impulses along fewer than ten fibers is thus sufficient to discharge the VL cells. The site of origin of these nucleofugal fibers is determined in experiments where eight stimulating electrodes are implanted over the nuclei interpositus and lateralis. The point with the lowest threshold for inducing the EPSPs is thus derived for each VL cell. For about half of the sampled VL cells it lies within the nucleus interpositus (INT) and for the other half within the lateral nucleus (DENT) as plotted in Fig. 148 E. These two groups of VL cells did not appear to occupy distinct regions within the VL nucleus.

A further interesting finding is that some VL cells also receive delayed IPSPs from some points within the nucleus interpositus (Fig. 148 D). Such IPSPs are seen in the VL cells excited monosynaptically from certain loci within the nucleus interpositus, as plotted in Fig. 148 E but never from the lateral nucleus. When the stimulating electrode is brought closer to the VL, the latency of the delayed IPSPs is reduced in parallel with that of the monosynaptic EPSPs, there remaining a difference of about 1 msec between them when extrapolated to zero distance, i.e. to the VL nucleus itself. Consequently it can be postulated that at least one inhibitory neurone is interposed in this inhibitory pathway, presumably within the VL. The presence of Golgi type II cells in the VL is indicated histologically (see above), and these could be the inhibitory neurones. The neuronal connexions in the VL found in these studies are summarized in Fig. 124.

The finding of a disynaptic inhibitory pathway does not contradict the general statement that the nucleofugal projection is purely excitatory because the action of the impulses in the interpositus axons would be excitatory also on the inhibitory neurones in the VL. This inhibitory pathway would make possible a reciprocal innervation; impulses in the interpositus axons could activate the red nucleus and one group of VL cells, while inhibiting another VL group. Since the VL cells project to large pyramidal tract neurones in the cerebral cortex (YOSHIDA, YAJIMA and UNO, 1966), the possibility can be suggested that the interpositus impulses inhibit a part of the pyramidal tract system, while the rubrospinal system is activated. This problem would be relevant to the coordination between the pyramidal and extrapyramidal motor systems.

3. From the Fastigial Nucleus to Reticular Formation

The neurones in the reticular formation of the medulla and the caudal level of the pons have been penetrated and identified by their antidromic invasion from (a) the spinal cord, (b) the midbrain tegmentum, or (c) the cerebellum (ITO, UDO and MANO, 1967 g; cf. MAGNI and WILLIS, 1963). There are also a number of cells (d) which are identified not by antidromic invasion but by the appearance of their postsynaptic potentials, either inhibitory or excitatory, following the stimulation of one or other of these regions.

Stimulation of the deep nuclear region of the cerebellum induces in the reticular neurones EPSPs with monosynaptic latencies (0.8 msec on the average). In the case of Fig. 149 B the effect is most prominent in the fastigial nuclei on both sides (spots 5 and 6). The EPSPs could also be induced by stimuli applied to the ipsilateral interpositus region (Fig. 149 B, spot 2), but is found to be due to stimulation of the fastigial axons which originate from the contralateral fastigial nucleus and pass by

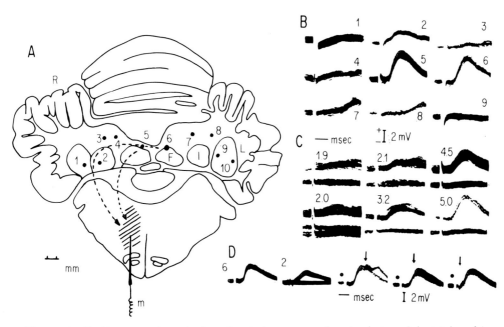

Fig. 149 A—D. *Monosynaptic excitation of reticular neurones by stimulation of fastigial nuclei.* A, transverse section of the cerebellum and medulla. Black dots labelled by 1—10 indicate the electrolytic marks produced by the stimulating needle electrodes. R, right side. F, fastigial nucleus. I, interpositus nucleus. L, lateral nucleus. Interrupted curves with arrows on top indicate the course of fastigiofugal projections. m, microelectrode. Shaded is the reticular formation from which the cells were sampled. B, Potential changes recorded from a reticular neurone during fastigial stimulation. Figure attached to each record indicates the position of cathode in A. Anode was served by the left partner except when the spot No. 9 was made cathode against anode at 8. Pulse duration was 0.2 msec and intensity 5 volts. C, upper traces, in the same cell as in B. Stimuli were given to the spot No. 6, and their intensity was increased gradually as indicated (in volts). Lower traces, extracellular records. D, interference between the EPSPs induced from the spots Nos. 2 and 6. The moments of stimulations are indicated by dots and arrows. (ITO, UDO and MANO, 1967 g)

the ipsilateral interpositus nucleus, forming the hook bundle (cf. BRODAL, 1957). This is demonstrated by the refractoriness experiment in which stimulation at the interpositus nucleus fails during a short period after the contralateral fastigial stimulation (Fig. 149 D). EPSPs are produced also from the contralateral interpositus region, but at a longer latency (Fig. 149 B, spots 7, 8), and hence presumably there is a disynaptic pathway. It is possible that this effect arises because the fastigial neurones are being excited orthodromically by impulses along the cerebellar afferents, which may pass lateral to the fastigial nucleus and may send axon collaterals into it (Chapter XIII).

On the basis of degeneration experiments, the reticular formation appears to receive fibers also from the nuclei interpositus and lateralis (cf. BRODAL, 1956), in addition to those from the fastigial nuclei. However, among the reticular neurones sampled mainly in the medullary reticular formation, there was no case where the nuclei interpositus and lateralis of the ipsilateral side were the exclusive source of monosynaptic EPSPs. Stimulation of the fastigial nuclei always produced EPSPs that were at least as large (ITO et al., 1967 g). It was also found that monosynaptic EPSPs were never evoked from the nuclei interpositus and lateralis of the contra-lateral side. It is possible that the axons from the nuclei interpositus and lateralis impinge upon the midbrain reticular neurones, or, even in the medulla, upon rela-tively small cells which may not be included in the microelectrode sampling. Pos-sibly also the EPSPs evoked monosynaptically from the fastigial nuclei may, at least in part, be produced by an axon reflex pathway resembling that assumed for the EPSPs evoked in Deiters neurones after stimulation of the cerebellar cortex (Chapter XIII). The reticular formation and the fastigial nucleus of the cerebellum may receive common innervation from the cerebellar afferents through their axon collaterals, for the reticular formation receives a wide variety of afferent inflows. Nevertheless, the excitatory influence from the fastigial neurones is indicated by the disfacilitation phenomenon which occurs in reticular neurones during stimula-tion of the cerebellum; there is a membrane hyperpolarization due to removal of tonic EPSPs, as will be described in detail in the next section. This phenomenon suggests that the reticular neurones are subjected to a tonic bombardment from the fastigial neurones and that this bombardment is under the inhibitory control of Purkinje cell axons.

In comparison with the EPSPs in RN and VL, the minimum unitary size of the fastigial-induced EPSPs in reticular neurones is relatively small (0.5 mV at the most), as revealed by finely graded stimulation at threshold (Fig. 149 C, see below).

4. From the Fastigial Nucleus to the Vestibular Nuclei

Stimulation of the neurones in the fastigial nucleus is usually contaminated by excitation of Purkinje cell axons which pass by this nucleus on the way to Deiters nucleus and which induce large IPSPs in the majority of Deiters neurones (Chapter XIII). These IPSPs usually mask any effect that impulses in the fastigial axons induce in Deiters neurones. Careful adjustment of the stimulus intensity, however, sometimes enables one to discriminate between the excitatory and inhibi-tory fibers. In Fig. 150 monosynaptic EPSPs are thus shown to be produced in Deiters neurones by relatively weak fastigial stimulation. In the ventral region of Deiters nucleus the monosynaptic EPSPs are found in isolation because these neu-rones receive no synapses from Purkinje cell axons that project through the fastigial region (Chapter XIII). Similarly EPSPs are recorded also from the neu-rones within the descending vestibular nucleus (KAWAI, ITO and NOZUE, 1967), and these are explicable by the histologically defined fastigiofugal projection to this nucleus (BRODAL et al., 1962).

In the vestibular neurones the effect of stimulation is not restricted to the fastigial nuclei, but it arises also from a rather wide area surrounding these nuclei

(Fig. 150). This extension may be due to contamination by axon reflexes through collaterals of the cerebellar afferents, as was shown to occur with stimulation of the cerebellar cortex (Chapter XIII). Nevertheless the disfacilitation phenomenon (see next section) seen in vestibular neurones is indicative of tonic impingement by the fastigial impulses. It is also illustrated in Fig. 150 (trace 4) that the stimulation of the fastigial nucleus evoked a delayed EPSP (marked by oblique

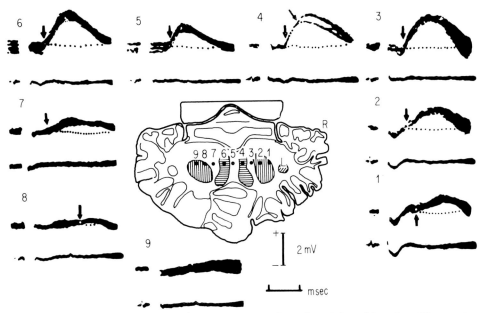

Fig. 150. *Monosynaptic excitation of Deiters neurone from fastigial nuclei region.* Diagram in the center shows a horizontal section of the cerebellum. *L,* lateral nucleus. *R,* right side. Spots Nos. 1—9 represent electrolytic marks made by the stimulating electrodes. Records were taken from a Deiters neurone with pulses of 0.08 msec duration and 10 volt strength. Figure on each record indicates the site of cathode. Anode was formed by the left side partner except when the spot No. 9 was used as cathode against anode at No. 8. Lower traces, extracellular records. Dotted lines superposed on the upper traces indicate the time course of the lower traces. Vertical arrows point to the moment of onset of EPSPs. Oblique arrow in the record 4 indicates the diverging point of the two sets of the potential curves which were separated spontaneously during stimulation with constant pulses. (ITO, KAWAI, UDO and MANO, 1967 c)

arrow) superposed upon the monosynaptic EPSP (downward arrow). On account of the small difference (0.4 msec) of the onset times of these EPSPs, the delayed EPSPs can be ascribed to the trans-synaptic activation of some fastigial neurones. As in the reticular neurones, the unitary size of the fastigial-induced EPSPs is relatively small — less than 0.5 mV.

5. Comment

The nucleofugal impulses thus appear to be excitatory for all the brain stem neurones so far examined. It is of interest to compare the unitary sizes of the EPSPs which are produced in these various neurones by single nucleofugal impulses. It is as large as 2—3 mV in VL cells, 0.75 mV in RN cells and less than

0.5 mV in the reticular and vestibular neurones. These excitatory synaptic trans-missions thus seem to be designed for converging and integrating in the reticular and vestibular neurones and for impulse generation with less convergence in VL cells, with the RN cells lying in between. This change seems to follow the phylogenetic development from the paleo- to the neocerebellum.

These different synaptic potencies would depend not only on the properties of the presynaptic terminals liberating the transmitter substance but also on the electrical properties of the postsynaptic membrane. For example, because of their larger total membrane impedance the relatively small VL cells would be expected to have larger unitary EPSPs than the large Deiters neurones or RN cells, the assumptions being made that the membranes have similar specific imped-ance and that, when activated, single synaptic knobs evoke the same ionic con-ductance changes in the subsynaptic membranes. However, the pharmacological properties of the synapses on VL and RN neurones seem to be different (DAVIS, 1965), which suggests that there are different synaptic transmitter substances. Evidently, further investigation is needed to explain the different efficacies ob-served for the various nucleofugal synaptic transmissions.

It may be recalled in this context that the climbing fibers on Purkinje cells are an extreme form of the relay type of synapse which occurs also in the sym-pathetic ganglia and in the motor endplate. On the other hand, the synapses on the motoneurones are typical of the converging type, which conforms with the function of these neurones as the final common pathway. The sensory relay cells in cuneate nucleus (ANDERSEN, ECCLES, OSHIMA and SCHMIDT, 1964; ANDERSEN, ECCLES, SCHMIDT and YOKOTA, 1964) may be ranked with VL cells as lying between the above two extreme examples.

C. Disfacilitation

The inhibitory control by the Purkinje cell axons presupposes that there is a tonic excitatory state in the subcortical nuclei; otherwise, there is no background to be depressed by the inhibitory action of the corticofugal impulses from the Purkinje cells. It follows that the neurones at the second stage of the cerebellar efferent system are affected by the decrease or increase in the discharge of excita-tory impulses from the subcortical nuclei.

This situation is most clearly demonstrated in the RN cells, for in them stimu-lation of the cerebellar cortex induces a prolonged hyperpolarization of the membrane potential (Fig. 151) (cf. MASSION, 1961; MASSION and ALBE-FESSARD, 1963), which is usually followed by a slow depolarizing potential. The hyper-polarization is produced most effectively from the contralateral paravermal cortex of the anterior lobe. Fibers from here pass to the underlying interpositus nucleus, which in turn projects to the RN cells under examination (Fig. 151 B, spots 11—13). The pecular nature of this membrane hyperpolarization is indicated by the demonstration that in Fig. 151 C (upper traces) it increases during intra-cellular application of hyperpolarizing currents and decreases during depolarizing currents. These changes parallel those simultaneously observed in the EPSPs induced from VL (lower traces). The equilibrium potential of the membrane hyperpolarization is thus shown to be at the same level as that of the EPSPs. Therefore, the hyperpolarization is not due to IPSPs, but caused by a decrease of background EPSPs, i. e. by a disfacilitation, as it may be called. A similar phenomenon has been reported in spinal motoneurones after cerebellar stimulation (TERZUOLO, 1959; LLINÁS, 1964).

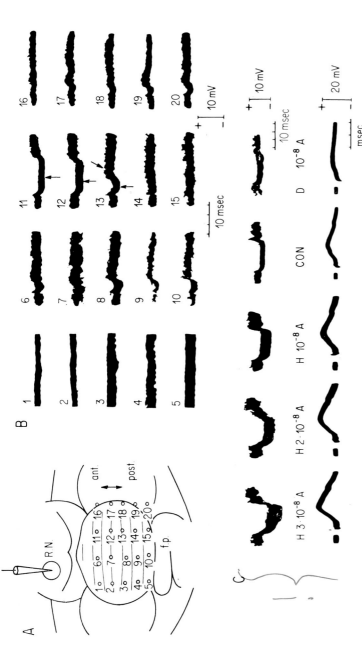

Fig. 151 A—C. Potential changes produced in red nucleus neurones during stimulation of the cerebellar cortex. A shows dorsal view of the midbrain and the cerebellum. RN, red nucleus into which a microelectrode was inserted. ant., anterior. post., posterior. f. p., fissura prima. Open circles represent the positions of stimulating electrodes which were placed mainly on the surface of culmen. B, intracellular potential changes in a RN cell produced by stimulating at the spots Nos. 1—20. Figures attached to these records indicate the sites of cathode, anode being served by their rostral or caudal partner electrodes. Upward arrows in records 11—13 point to the hyperpolarizing potential changes. Downward oblique arrow in 13 marks the later depolarization. C, upper traces, intracellular records from another RN cell during stimulation of the contralateral paravermal cortex of the cerebellum. CON, control. The others were taken during passage of currents in the directions and at the intensities indicated. H, hyperpolarizing. D, depolarizing. Lower traces, EPSPs induced by stimulation of VL in the same cell and under the same polarizing conditions as for the upper traces. Note different voltage and time scales for the upper and lower traces. (TOYAMA, TSUKAHARA and UDO, 1967b)

277

Excitatory Signals from the Intracerebellar Nuclei

The origin of this disfacilitation has been revealed by observing the simultaneous changes produced by cerebellar stimulation in the following three kinds

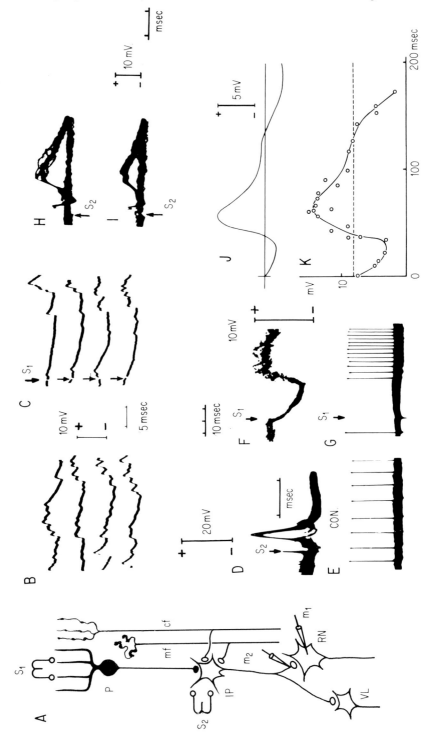

to the anterior part of the contralateral interpositus nucleus (COURVILLE and BRODAL, 1966) which is the source of the fibers innervating the red nucleus. This positive feedback is mediated probably by the axon collaterals of the rubrospinal fibers (COURVILLE and BRODAL, 1966), which are known to be excitatory (Section F, 1). Thus there will be a closed circuit of excitatory impulses between the red nucleus and the nucleus interpositus. However, the number of these rubro-interpositus fibers is rather small (COURVILLE and BRODAL, 1966), and, correspondingly, with intracellular microelectrode sampling from the red nucleus, only a few cells (two) out of many were found to be invaded antidromically after stimulation of the contralateral interpositus nucleus (TOYAMA, personal communication). Obviously much more work is needed on this presumed reverberation and on its contribution to the spontaneous nucleofugal discharges.

Abundant local axon collaterals have also been identified histologically as arising from the neurones of the intracerebellar nuclei (Chapter XIII, Section A, 1). If these collaterals link the neurones by excitatory synapses, possibly through interneurones, there will be positive feedback loops which would enhance the rhythmic discharges from these neurones. Such a positive feedback connexion has been postulated in the thalamus (ANDERSEN, ECCLES and SEARS, 1964) and also in the inferior olive (OCHI, 1965; ECCLES, LLINÁS and SASAKI, 1966 d; ITO, OCHI and OBATA, 1967 f). However, this postulate of intrinsic excitatory loops has yet to be tested experimentally.

D. Late Facilitation

The disfacilitatory hyperpolarization produced by cerebellar stimulation is followed by a slow depolarization, as shown in Figs. 151 B and 152 F for RN cells and in Fig. 153 C, D (arrows) for a reticular neurone. In its time course the slow depolarization corresponds to the phase of disinhibitory depolarization observed in Deiters neurones (Fig. 134). The slow depolarization in these brain stem neurones has been demonstrated to be produced by excitatory synapses and not a disinhibition due to removal of IPSPs, for the equilibrium potential of the slow depolarization is the same as that characterizing EPSPs. It decreases when the membrane is depolarized and increases under hyperpolarization (Fig. 151 C, upper traces; Fig. 153 B). This slow depolarization will be referred to as a late facilitation.

The late facilitation in RN cells is attributable to an increase in the spontaneous discharges along the axons of interpositus neurones (Fig. 152 G) which reflects an enhanced excitability in the interpositus neurones (Fig. 152 K). The membrane potential in the RN cells, during both the disfacilitation and the late facilitation, is thus reflecting closely the postsynaptic events in the interpositus neurones. Besides this temporal correspondence, the causal relationship between the disinhibition in the subcortical nuclei and the late facilitation in the brain stem neurones is suggested by the following two observations. First, the late facilitation is evoked from a wide area of the cerebellar cortex as with the disinhibition in Deiters neurones (see Fig. 142 F, G). Secondly, both potentials can be potentiated very effectively by double shock stimulation of the cerebellar cortex at brief intervals of around one millisecond (ITO et al., 1967 d).

It may be noted in this context that the cerebellar stimulation induces rhythmic oscillatory potential changes in the brain stem neurones. These oscillations follow the initial phases of disinhibition and late facilitation (Fig. 153 D). A similar type of oscillation is also seen at the level of the subcortical neurones (Fig. 134 A, see the records at stimulus intensities of 4.6, 7.5 and 26 V). These phenomena have yet to be investigated both with respect of the synaptic mechanisms and the pathways concerned.

E. Signal Transfer in the Cerebellar Efferent System

The essential features in the transmission of signals in the cerebellar efferent system are summarized diagrammatically in Fig. 155. It is assumed that the cells of the subcortical nuclei are receiving excitatory influences through the collaterals of the cerebellar afferents, both the climbing and the mossy fibers. It is also assumed

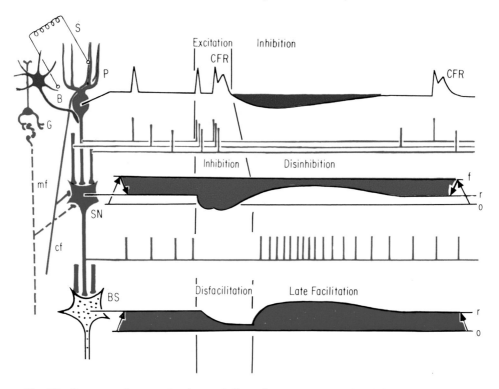

Fig. 155. *Sequence of events in the cerebellar efferent system produced by stimulation of the cerebellar cortex.* The pricipal neuronal connexions are indicated to the left. P, Purkinje cell. B, basket cell. G, granule cell. SN, subcortical neurone. BS, brain stem and spinal neurone. mf, mossy fiber. cf, climbing fiber. S, stimulating electrode. To the right are shown intracellular potentials at successive stages of the cerebellar efferent system. Left vertical line indicates the moment of stimulation with S. Horizontal lines marked by r show the intracellular potential level. Lines labelled by o indicate the resting potential level if there were no synaptic bombardment. The line f for SN represents the potential level which would obtain by the background facilitation if there be no inhibition. Arrows indicate the directions of the membrane potential shift by synaptic bombardment. CFR, climbing fiber response. Blue and green colours represent inhibition and red excitation or facilitation

that the Purkinje cells are driven tonically by the mossy fiber and/or climbing fiber pathways. As a consequence, the neurones of the cerebellar nuclei receive both excitatory and inhibitory bombardments. It is assumed that in these neurones the tonic facilitation dominates the inhibition and therefore that there is a maintained tonic discharge of impulses directed toward the brain stem neurones.

As emphasized in the preceding Chapter (Section E), it is important to recognize that stimulation of the cerebellar cortex will excite all sorts of neuronal elements under the stimulating electrode and that other structures will be indirectly excited by the impulses generated at the site of stimulation. Thus there will be a direct stimulation of the Purkinje cells and their axons, followed by an orthodromic excitation of the Purkinje cells through the climbing fibers (Chapter VIII; see also Fig. 130). There will also be excitation of Purkinje cells by the mossy fiber-granule cell pathway (ECCLES, LLINÁS and SASAKI, 1966c). The impulses thus set up in the

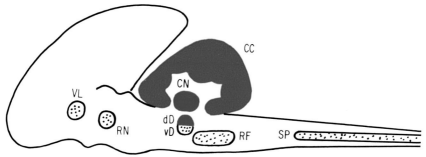

Fig. 156. *Distribution of the cerebellar efferent targets in the central nervous system.* CC, cerebellar cortex. CN, cerebellar nuclei. *dD*, dorsal part of Deiters nucleus. *vD*, vestibular nuclei except *dD*. RN, red nucleus. *VL*, nucleus ventralis lateralis of the thalamus. *RF*, reticular formation. *SP*, spinal neurones, particularly extensor motoneurones and the inhibitory neurones which inhibit flexor motoneurones. Different colours indicate similarly to Fig. 155

Purkinje cell axons will induce IPSPs in the cells of subcortical nuclei, which in turn will cause a disfacilitatory hyperpolarization in the brain stem neurones.

Stimulation in the cerebellar cortex will also induce by the pathways through basket and stellate cells inhibition of the Purkinje cells (Chapters VI and VII). There will also be inhibition of the inferior olive cells which spontaneously activate the Purkinje cells (Chapter XIII, Section E). As discussed above, the resulting depression of the tonic inhibitory bombardment to the subcortical neurones will cause a disinhibition in the subcortical neurones and correspondingly a late facilitation in the brain stem neurones.

These events are summarized in the diagram of Fig. 155. For simplification, the axon reflex through the cerebellar afferent collaterals (see Fig. 142 B) and the inhibition within the inferior olive (Fig. 142 G) are omitted from this diagram. It will be appreciated that the complex features of cerebellar stimulation are here spelled out to some extent. It is important to recognize that the nature of the synaptic mechanisms varies at different stages of the cerebellar efferent system. The language spoken at the first stage (Purkinje cell output) is mainly IPSPs, while in the second stage it is EPSPs. Yet the same effects are transferred — inhibition becomes disfacilitation and disinhibition becomes the late facilitation. The cerebellar cortex would thus control very effectively a wide area of the brain stem including the vestibular nuclei, reticular formation, red nucleus and thalamus. The dorsal Deiters neurones form the first stage target for Purkinje cell innervation and on the other hand project into the spinal cord, making direct excitatory connexions with extensor motoneurones and with the interneurones which inhibit flexor motoneurones (POMPEIANO, 1962; LUND and POMPEIANO, 1965; and personal communication). Therefore, the second stage of the cerebellar efferent system can be extended to cover these extensor motoneurones and inhibitory neurones in the spinal cord. Disfacilitation phenomenon was indeed seen in motoneurones during stimulation of the anterior lobe of the cerebellum (TERZUOLO, 1959; LLINÁS, 1964). The location of these first and second stage targets of the cerebellar efferent system is diagrammatically illustrated in Fig. 156.

F. Integration in the Brainstem Neurones

The cerebellar nucleofugal signals are integrated in the brain stem neurones with the inputs from other sources. The final outcome is then transferred into the spinal cord through the vestibulospinal, reticulospinal and rubrospinal tracts or into the cerebral cortex through the thalamocortical projection. The details of this final integration are beyond the scope of this monograph, and only a few characteristic features will be described. These have been obtained mainly in recent intracellular studies on brain stem neurones.

1. Red Nucleus

In addition to the interpositus axons, the RN cells receive abundant synaptic connexions from the ipsilateral sensorimotor cortex (RINVIK and WALBERG, 1963; POMPEIANO and BRODAL, 1957; MABUCHI and KUSAMA, 1966). When the cerebral cortico-rubral fibers are stimulated at the cortex (Fig. 157 A $[S_1]$ and B) EPSPs appear in RN cells with a latency of about 2 msec (TSUKAHARA and KOSAKA, 1966). They have a characteristically slow rising phase and a similarly prolonged falling phase (Fig. 157 C, D). When the stimulating electrode is inserted into the internal capsule to excite the cortico-rubral fibers on their way to the red nucleus (S_2 in Fig. 157 A), the latency of the EPSPs shortens to 1 msec (E, F). It is calculated in this experiment that the cortico-rubral fibers conduct impulses at a velocity of less than 20 m/sec and induce EPSPs in RN cells monosynaptically. The slow time course of the EPSPs occurs even with stimulation of the internal capsule. This implies that the slow time course of these EPSPs is not only due to a temporal dispersion of the cortico-rubral impulses. In keeping with this view, it is interesting to observe that applied intracellular currents have little influence on the EPSPs evoked from the cerebral cortex. These same currents, on the other hand, influence very profoundly the interpositus-induced EPSPs (Fig. 157 G, H). Similarly, two types of EPSPs with this same differential sensitivity to applied currents were shown to be evoked in frog motoneurones by the dorsal root afferents on one hand and by the lateral column fibers on the other (BROOKHART and FADIGA, 1960; FADIGA and BROOKHART, 1960; KUBOTA and BROOKHART, 1963). Thus the fibers from the cerebral cortex appear

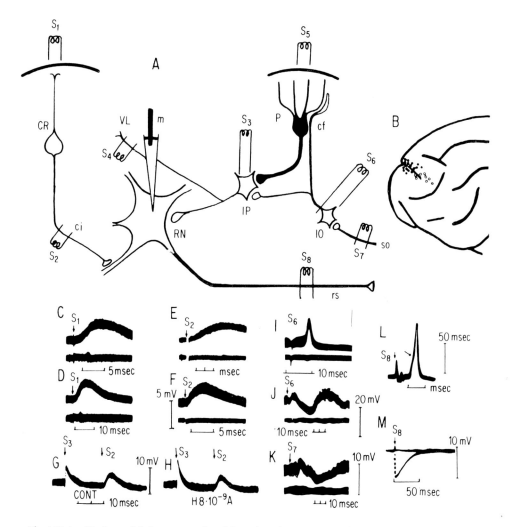

Fig. 157 A—M. *Potential changes produced in red nucleus neurones through various neuronal connexions.* A shows principal neuronal connexions and arrangement of recording and stimulating electrodes. *m*, microelectrode. *RN*, red nucleus neurone. *CR*, cell of origin of corticorubral projection. *ci*, capsula interna. *VL*, nucleus ventralis lateralis of thalamus. *IP*, nucleus interpositus neurone. *P*, Purkinje cell. *cf*, climbing fiber: *IO*, inferior olive. *so*, spino-olivary fiber. *rs*, rubrospinal fiber. S_1—S_8, stimulating electrodes placed on the various structures as indicated. B, shows lateral surface of the anterior part of the cerebrum. Closed circles indicate the effective spots for inducing EPSPs in RN cells which send axons down to the lumboscaral segments. Open circles are for the RN cells whose axons innervate only the cervicothoracic segments. C—M, intracellularly recorded potentials in RN cells. Lower traces in C—F, I—K are extracellular controls. C, slow EPSPs produced by stimulation of the sensori-motor cortex. D, same as in C but recorded with slower sweep velocity. E, slow EPSPs evoked by stimulating the capsula interna. F, same as in E but at slower sweep velocity. G, simultaneous recording of the EPSPs from the nucleus interpositus and from the capsula interna. H, same as in G but during passage of hyperpolarizing currents through the impaled microelectrode (current strength is indicated). I, disynaptic EPSPs evoked from the inferior olive. J, similar to I but recorded in another cell with slower sweep. K, stimulation of the C_4 spinal segment. L, antidromic spike. Oblique arrow indicates the inflection on the rising phase of the spike. M, afterpotential following the antidromic spike. Dotted line is drawn to indicate the time couse of development of the afterhyperpolarization. (TSUKAHARA, TOYAMA and KOSAKA, 1967 a; TSUKAHARA and KOSAKA, 1966; TOYAMA, TSUKAHARA and UDO, 1967 b)

to produce the EPSPs remotely on the dendrites of RN cells, while the interpositus axons impinge upon their somas, as illustrated in Fig. 124. The peripheral origin of the cerebral-evoked EPSPs is supported by the histological observation that the cortico-rubral fibers end in the neuropil of the red nucleus where abundant axo-dendritic synapses exist (RINVIK and WALBERG, 1963).

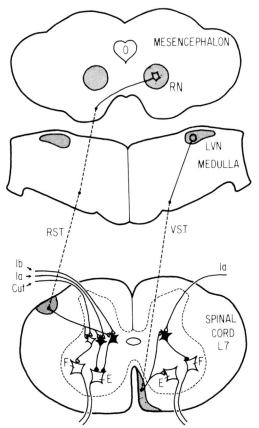

Fig. 158. *Diagram showing the course and destinations at the spinal segments of the rubrospinal and vestibulospinal projections. RN, red nucleus. LVN, lateral vestibular nucleus of Deiters. RST, rubrospinal tract. VST, vestibulospinal tract. L_7, seventh lumbar segment. F, flexor moto-neurones. E, extensor motoneurones. Ia, Ib, group Ia and Ib muscle afferents respectively. Cut, cutaneous nerve fibers. Cell some and synaptic terminals filled black are inhibitory in nature and hollow ones excitatory. Composed according to the histological observations by* NYBERG-HANSEN *and* MASCITTI *(1964) and* NYBERG-HANSEN *and* BRODAL *(1967) and physiological findings by* LUND *and* POMPEIANO *(1965, personal communications) and* HONGO, JANKOWSKA *and* LUNDBERG *(1965)*

Various other brain tissues have been stimulated while recording from RN cells in order to reveal their influence (TOYAMA *et al.*, 1967 b). Stimulation of the inferior olive was found to evoke EPSPs in RN cells at latencies of 4 msec or more (Fig. 157 I; TOYAMA *et al.*, 1967 b), which were depressed when conditioned by stimulation of the cerebellar cortex. Presumably these EPSPs were produced by the transsynaptic excitation of the interpositus neurones by the olivo-cerebellar fibers

the pathway by which it is activated. In addition, OSCARSSON and ROSÉN (cf. OSCARSSON, 1967) have discovered another very effective spino-olivary path that ascends up the dorsal columns to the dorsal column nuclei and presumably reaches the contralateral accessory olive by collaterals from the medial lemniscus.

Electrophysiological investigation with microelectrode tracks through the inferior olive has shown that afferent volleys in muscle nerves very effectively excite the DAO (ARMSTRONG, ECCLES, HARVEY and MATTHEWS, 1967). It has been a quite regular finding that a brief burst of 3 to 4 quadriceps afferent volleys restricted to group I powerfully excite the DAO. However, increase of the stimulus through the group II range always intensified the response. Furthermore, such brief tetani at group II strength in a variety of muscle nerves also are very effective, but the action of I b impulses is still doubtful. There is general agreement on the excitatory action of even low threshold cutaneous impulses (MORIN, LAMARCHE and OSTROWSKI, 1957; GRANT and OSCARSSON, 1966; OSCARSSON, 1967; ARMSTRONG et al., 1967; SEDGWICK and WILLIAMS, 1967) and joint impulses are particularly powerful (ARMSTRONG et al., 1967).

However, a disconcerting feature has been the extreme convergence of muscle afferents on to small foci of the DAO and even on to the same neurone, which can be made to discharge by afferent volleys from a variety of muscles of the contralateral and even also of the ipsilateral hindlimb (ARMSTRONG et al., 1967). This extreme convergence contrasts with the unique specificity of action of a single inferior olive cell on to a Purkinje cell by virtue of the climbing fiber synaptic action (SZENTÁGOTHAI and RAJKOVITS, 1959; ECCLES, LLINÁS and SASAKI, 1966 d). There would seem to be no point in this specific connexion if the single olive cell itself receives excitation from such a wide field of muscle input. A possible way out of this paradox may be given by the powerful postsynaptic inhibitory actions also exerted by afferent fibers to the DAO (ARMSTRONG et al., 1967). Certainly, this inhibitory action would greatly limit the effectiveness of repetitive trains of all excitatory inputs except the strongest, and so it would sharpen the focus of action upon any particular DAO cell. In parenthesis it may be stated that there is much circumstantial evidence that the afferents from tail and midline musculature of the body project via the medial accessory olive (MAO) to the medial part of the anterior lobe (cf. BRODAL, WALBERG and BLACKSTAD, 1950). The limb nerves do not project at all to the MAO (ARMSTRONG and HARVEY, unpublished observations).

C. Synthetic Operations in the Cerebellar Cortex and in the Projections therefrom

1. The Background Conditions

Usually there are continuous discharges in the afferent inputs into the cerebellar cortex via mossy fibers and climbing fibers. For example, in the anesthetized preparation there is a spontaneous discharge in most DSCT fibers even when the muscles are completely relaxed, the frequencies being about 10/sec for the I a DSCT fibers (LAPORTE and LUNDBERG, 1956; JANSEN, NICOLAYSEN and RUDJORD, 1966) and 20/sec for the I b DSCT fibers (JANSEN and RUDJORD, 1965). The VSCT fibers also are often spontaneously active, particularly in the unanesthetized animal (OSCARSSON, 1957), where the frequencies may be as high as 20 to 30/sec. There is also spontaneous activity in fibers conveying exteroceptive information, for example, 1 to 100/sec for the reticulocerebellar fibers with a mean of about 20/sec (OSCARSSON and ROSÉN, 1966). The background activity in climbing fibers is lower, the frequencies being not higher than 1 to 2/sec (GRANIT and PHILLIPS, 1956; GRANT and OSCARSSON, 1966; Chapter VIII).

As described in Chapter X, background activity is also common with the neurones of the cerebellar cortex. In particular, Purkinje cells exhibited a fairly high and regular rhythmic discharge, usually at 20 to 50/sec (Fig. 104). The background input by mossy fiber impulses must contribute to the continuous spontaneous discharges of granule cells (Fig. 107 A—D), of inhibitory interneurones (usually 7—30/sec; Fig. 107 E—L) as well as of Purkinje cells. However, in the chronically isolated cerebellum there is perforce no input by mossy or climbing fibers, yet the Purkinje cells still continue to discharge spontaneously (Fig. 104 B, C). One possible explanation is that discharges from granule cells provide a continuous synaptic excitatory action on the Purkinje cells, this spontaneous activity being possibly attributable to the hypersensitivity induced in granule cells as a consequence of the degeneration of mossy fibers, which provide their total excitatory synaptic input (Chapters II and VII). Alternatively, it can be postulated that impulse discharge occurs spontaneously in Purkinje cells, being independent of the excitatory action of the parallel fibers at the spine synapses.

The background climbing fiber bombardment gives brief bursts of repetitive discharge of a Purkinje cell (Fig. 85 K, 108 P—S), which is quite distinctive from the fairly regular background discharge of single impulses that was considered above.

The background activity of all elements of the cerebellar cortex is of course a resultant of all the interacting excitatory and inhibitory mechanisms described in earlier chapters. For example, the frequency of discharges of granule cells would be dependent not only on the background input by mossy fibers, but also on the inhibitory feed-back by the spontaneously active Golgi cells. Likewise, the frequency of Purkinje cell discharge is dependent not only on the background excitation by the granule cell-parallel fiber pathway, but also on the background inhibition by the spontaneously active basket and stellate cells. Thus, we must envisage that, even under conditions of minimal sensory input, there is a state of dynamic poise in the level of activity of the various types of cerebellar neurones, which discharge at a frequency determined by the net balance of excitatory and inhibitory synaptic actions upon them. The background conditions on which an input signal is superimposed are provided by the dynamic situation arising from the continuously operating excitatory and inhibitory synaptic actions on every neurone, and this is usually signalled by their continuous discharge.

2. Synthetic Operations Generated in Response to a Mossy Fiber Input

In the first place it will be assumed, in conformance with the well established neurophysiological principles, that information in nerve pathways is coded so that the frequency signals the intensity of input, and of course that in turn this frequency evokes a synaptic action in which likewise frequency is transformed into intensity. This coding of intensity by impulse frequency in transmitting lines occurs both for excitatory and inhibitory pathways.

As shown by JANSEN and RUDJORD (1965) a brief stretch of a muscle or its contraction will greatly intensify the discharges along the I a and/or I b fibers of the DSCT and so evoke in the topographically related area of the anterior lobe the mossy fiber response reported in Chapter VII. As already described, the focus of this response will be sharpened by the Golgi cell inhibition of all weakly excited granule cells, but, even so, the branching of each mossy fiber would result in a considerably wider action than the unitary area of inhibitory action depicted in Figs. 66, 114 and 115 for an ideally sharp mossy fiber input; and of course the assemblage of mossy fibers excited by the stretch or contraction of a single muscle would have a much more extensive zone of action, with perhaps some central zone with dominant excitation and a much wider inhibitory surround.

However, the task of the cerebellum is not just to respond to some such ideally simple input, but to integrate and organize the information from the muscles, not only of one limb, but of all limbs and the body, and to use for this purpose the information, not only from the muscle receptors, but also from the skin, fascia, and joints — in fact all of the information that flows to the cerebellum along all the pathways described above. It will be appreciated that the cerebellar cortex can be thought of essentially as a neuronal machine designed to utilize the complex inflow of information for the purpose of producing complex interacting patterns of Purkinje cell excitation and inhibition, because the only outflow from the cortex is by impulses discharged from Purkinje cells. The various mossy fiber pathways will make quite diverse contributions to this creation of activity patterns. Thus, the DSCT and CCT fibers must be specially concerned in creating patterns with modality and space specific information, whereas the VSCT, RSCT and the spino-reticulo-cerebellar paths would be specially concerned with much more extensive patterns that integrate information derived from the whole of the limbs and body and with but little in the way of detailed contours. The distribution of the RSCT (Fig. 165) certainly shows that the input via this pathway from the fore-limb muscles would be integrated with all the more regional and specific information conveyed by the DSCT. The spino-reticulo-cerebellar pathway likewise must function in the overall correlation of exteroceptive information.

It does not seem expedient here to build upon the differences in laminated distribution to the granular and molecular layers between the DSCT and VSCT on the one hand, and the reticulo-cerebellar paths on the other (SZENTÁGOTHAI, 1965 a) because it has not been possible to discover a physiological correlation for this distribution (Chapter VII; SASAKI and STRATA, 1967).

It is recognized that this account is merely a sketch of the manner of operation of the cerebellar cortex, but it indicates that the anatomical and physiological knowledge provides a basis for the integrative and coordinative function of the cerebellum. From a synoptic viewpoint, the Purkinje cell excitatory levels could be represented as a kind of animated cartoon of patterns, as so felicitously described by SHERRINGTON (1940) for the cerebral cortex, "an enchanted loom where millions of flashing shuttles weave a dissolving pattern, always a meaningful pattern though never an abiding one; a shifting harmony of subpatterns".

We now come to the problem of how these patterned excitability levels of the Purkinje cells achieve expression first by impulse discharges along Purkinje cell axons, and ultimately as effective motor control. Since the Purkinje cells are discharging spontaneously in the resting state, their excitability level will, of course, achieve expression as an increase or decrease of this background discharge. However, Figs. 104 A and 106 indicate that this background excitation is at such a low level that even a small inhibition often suppresses it completely. Hence, in its expression of the level of inhibition, the background discharge of the Purkinje cell may be over-loaded. On the other hand, an increased excitatory level is, of course, well expressed by a raised frequency of discharge. The Purkinje cell is well fitted for a wide range in its signalling of such excitatory levels because it receives such an intense excitatory convergence from the parallel fibers on its spine synapses (about 200,000 synapses) and because it is capable of a wide range in its maintained frequency of firing, which can exceed 400/sec. The background level of resting discharge is a great advantage in this frequency coding of its excitatory convergence; there is no threshold barrier to overcome so that even the smallest input achieves expression as raised frequency.

3. The Climbing Fiber Input

Evidently it is desirable to have some additional device for allowing the Purkinje cells to signal their inhibitory levels more effectively. It is here postulated that this is the special function of the climbing fibers.

The investigations described in Chapters V and VI have revealed how intense and widespread is the inhibitory action exerted by basket and stellate cells on Purkinje cells (Figs. 51, 52, 61, 62, 66). It seems that an input of mossy fiber impulses has a much greater inhibitory than excitatory potency. Yet a climbing fiber impulse so powerfully excites a Purkinje cell that it evokes the discharge of one impulse even during the deepest inhibitory depression. For example, in Fig. 98 B, at the testing interval for maximal inhibition there was a reduction of the CF-evoked response from four discharges to one. With lesser intensities of inhibition the CF-evoked response exhibited all gradations from this single discharge to the control response of four discharges. Evidently the CF response provides the requisite mechanism for enabling the Purkinje cell to signal all levels of its inhibitory depression entirely without distortion by inhibitory overload. Furthermore, this climbing fiber sampling of Purkinje cell inhibition has an amazingly fine spatial discrimination, each Purkinje cell being individually sampled by its own unique climbing fiber (Chapter VIII).

Since the climbing fiber samples the inhibition generated by a mossy fiber input, it is important to examine the spatial and temporal relationships of actions produced by mossy and climbing fiber inputs that stem from some sensory input that is sharply localized in space and time. As already pointed out, relative to the mossy fiber input there is an in-built delay of an additional 10 to 20 msec on the pathway leading to the cerebellar climbing fibers (Eccles, Llinás and Sasaki, 1966 d, Fig. 12 F). This additional delay is presumably an important feature of functional design, for the Purkinje cell IPSP generated by some mossy fiber input into the cerebellar cortex takes 10 to 20 msec to attain its maximum (Figs. 85, 86); hence this inhibition is sampled at its most effective phase by the climbing fiber input derived from that same sensory input, e. g. by discharges from cutaneous or muscle stretch receptors.

In order to study the specific connections made by afferent fibers to the anterior lobe of the cerebellum, relatively weak stimuli were applied to muscle and to cutaneous nerves, being no more than six times threshold (Eccles, Provini, Strata and Táboříková, unpublished observations). Under such conditions it can be assumed that the responses are produced by the group I and II afferent fibers from muscle and the alpha fibers of the cutaneous nerves. Systematic microelectrode tracking was employed in order to investigate the distribution of climbing fibers throughout the whole depth and transverse extent (ipsilaterally) of the anterior lobe. Two responses were employed in locating the climbing fiber synapses on Purkinje cells: the response of individual Purkinje cells as revealed either by the characteristic extracellular spike responses or intracellular EPSPs, and the extracellular negative field potential observed nearby at the location of the active climbing fiber synapses (cf. Eccles, Llinás and Sasaki, 1966 d). In parenthesis it can be stated that positive field potentials were found to be unreliable for localization since quite large positive fields could be observed even several millimeters from the active synaptic foci.

Using these criteria it was surprising to find that the climbing fiber responses were distributed widely (up to 5 mm) in a transverse direction across the lateral zone of the vermis and the intermediate part of the ipsilateral anterior lobe; however, the fore limb distribution was concentrated in lobule V, and the hind limb distribution very largely to lobule IV and anterior thereto. It was also remarkable to find that there was a considerable degree of specificity in the distribution of the climbing fiber responses evoked from the different muscle and cutaneous afferents. Evidently there is a complex patterned distribution of the information both from muscles subserving different functions in joint movement and from afferents from various skin areas. These results are apparently at variance with the recent finding by Oscarsson and Uddenberg (1966) that muscle and skin nerves from both fore and hind limbs evoke climbing fiber responses that are in narrow sagittal bands running through lobules V and IV of the anterior lobe and that are restricted to the lateral vermis and the adjacent intermediate zone. However, it should be pointed out that Oscarsson and Uddenberg used very strong stimuli to relatively few limb nerves and employed as indices of climbing fiber activity the surface positive waves.

4. Purkinje Cell Projection to the Subcerebellar Nuclei

The only output from the cerebellum is via the impulses discharged down Purkinje cell axons, and in Chapters XIII and XIV it has been shown that they are all inhibitory and that this inhibition is exerted on the cells of the various subcerebellar nuclei — fastigii, interpositus and lateralis — as well as Deiters nucleus. As a consequence the cerebellar output represents a kind of negative image of the excitatory and inhibitory patterns resulting at any instant from the processing of information in the cerebellar cortex. This pattern achieves expression solely by the Purkinje cell discharge which impresses this negative image upon these various nuclei — the more the excitation of a Purkinje cell, the more intense the inhibitory depression of the subcerebellar neurones to which it projects. As a consequence there arises again the disability in signal reception which would derive from inhibitory overload on these subcerebellar neurones.

This contingency makes of great significance the recent demonstration that axon collaterals of both climbing and mossy fibers very effectively excite the subcerebellar neurones (Figs. 131, 137, 139, 140, 141). The pathway is presumably by the collaterals described in Section A of Chapter XIII. For example, in Fig. 131 the EPSP evoked by a CF input is developed about 2 msec before the IPSP produced by the Purkinje cell discharge evoked by that same CF input. Presumably the interval would be a little longer for CF inputs to more superficially lying areas of the cerebellar cortex. There may be functional meaning in this sequential relationship because, by the timed relation of excitation and inhibition, the circuit has the properties of a noise-reducing device. Likewise the Purkinje cell discharge evoked by a mossy fiber input has its inhibitory action on subcerebellar neurones measured against the EPSPs produced therein by collaterals of the mossy fibers (Figs. 139 and 141). These separate accounts of the CF-evoked and the MF-evoked discharges from Purkinje cells are adopted as a provisional description. Actually the Purkinje cells have no such selectivity in their responses to CF and MF inputs. The same Purkinje cells are responding to both inputs. For any one cell the frequency of the discharges from instant to instant gives in coded form the synthesis of all the excitatory and inhibitory actions converging onto it as a consequence of the immediately preceding MF and CF input into cerebellar cortex.

Besides the excitation of the subcerebellar neurones by impulses in the CF and MF axon collaterals, there are also many other excitatory pathways. WILSON, KATO, THOMAS and PETERSEN (1966) have shown that in the decerebellectomized animal most Deiters cells discharge at frequencies ranging from 10 to 80 impulses per second and that this frequency is increased by stimulation of peripheral nerves, volleys in both low and high threshold cutaneous nerve fibers being particularly effective both ipsilaterally and contralaterally. Similar observations had previously been made in animals with intact cerebellum (POMPEIANO and COTTI, 1959). This on-going excitatory activity of Deiters neurones provides the background upon which is expressed the inhibitory patterns created by the Purkinje cell discharges. The negative image of the integrated output from the cerebellar cortex is, as it were, formed by a process analogous to sculpturing in stone. Spatio-temporal form is achieved from moment to moment by the impression of a patterned inhibition upon the "shapeless" background discharges of the subcerebellar neurones, just as an infinitely more enduring form is achieved in sculpture by a highly selective chiselling away from the initial amorphous block of stone. As shown in Chapter XIV this direct inhibitory action of Purkinje cells on the subcerebellar neurones is transmitted as a disfacilitation to the next relay station in the outflow from the cerebellum, and this disfacilitation can of course be transmitted sequentially through any number of excitatory synaptic relays.

D. Properties of Cerebellar Circuitry of Special Relevance to the Operational Performance of a Computer

1. After one or two synaptic relays all inputs into the cerebellum are transformed into inhibition. It has been shown in Chapter VII that, in the cerebellar cortex, impulses in mossy fibers excite only the granule cells and Golgi cells. The latter are purely inhibitory in action, while by the impulses discharged along their axons, the parallel fibers, the granule cells excite only inhibitory cells — Golgi, stellate, basket and Purkinje cells (Figs. 119, 120, 121). All of these cells exert purely inhibitory actions within the cerebellar cortex. This inhibition is exclusively the task of the first three of these cell types; and it is, via the axon collaterals of the Purkinje cells, also a subsidiary task for them (Chapter IX), whose main inhibitory action is exercised via their axonal projections out of the cortex to the subcerebellar nuclei (Chapters XIII and XIV). The situation is even more striking with impulses in climbing fibers, because these fibers excite only inhibitory cells — the Purkinje cells, and by collaterals the inhibitory interneurones of the cerebellar cortex, namely the stellate, basket and Golgi cells. This exclusive transformation of all input into inhibition with at most two synaptic relays gives the cerebellum a "dead-beat" character in its response to input. There is no possibility of the dynamic storage of information by impulses circulating in complex neuronal pathways such as occurs within the cerebral cortex and along the various circuits between it and the basal ganglia. Within at most 30 msec after a given input, there will be no further evoked discharges in the cortical neurones. By 100 msec even the EPSPs and IPSPs will have faded and that area of the cerebellar cortex will have been cleared of all disturbance by the initial input and be in an unbiassed state for the computing of a new input.

This elimination in the design of all possibility of reverberatory chains of neuronal excitation is undoubtedly a great advantage in the performance of the cerebellum as a computer, because what the rest of the nervous system requires from the cerebellum is presumably not some output expressing the operation of complex reverberatory circuits in the cerebellum, but rather a quick and clear response to the input of any particular set of information. For example, in the cerebello-cerebral interactions it is sufficient that the dynamic spatio-temporal patterns of reverberatory circuits be in the cerebral cortex and basal ganglia and that there be virtually no short-term dynamic memory in the cerebellum.

2. It has already been suggested that the inhibitory action of Golgi cells is important in sharpening the field of action of mossy fiber inputs to the zone of intense activation. This simple concept would of course be particularly applicable to the pathway of direct action of mossy fibers on Golgi cell dendrites in the granular layer (Chapter VII), for the Golgi cell inhibition is distributed to the same general area as the activating mossy fiber input (Fig. 113). It has not yet been possible to develop a satisfactory functional meaning for the activation of Golgi

cells in a band 3 mm in length along the beam of parallel fibers (Figs. 113 and 116) with the consequent elongated zone of inhibition of the mossy fiber-granule cell relay (Fig. 122), which presumably would extend far beyond the distribution of the mossy fiber input evoking this reaction; hence inhibition by Golgi cells cannot simply be given the functional meaning of a focussing action on the mossy fiber input.

3. Perhaps the most remarkable feature of design in the cerebellar cortex is the rectangular lattice construction that was particularly emphasized by BRAITENBERG and ATWOOD (1958). An ideally localized mossy fiber input gives a parallel fiber activation for about 3 mm along the length of a folium, exciting all neurones with dendrites in the molecular layer. The basket cells so excited distribute inhibition to Purkinje cells for as far as 1 mm transversely on either side of this beam (Figs. 114 and 115). Hence there arises an intense competition between the inputs of mossy fibers projecting to adjacent areas of the cerebellar cortex, as is depicted very schematically and inadequately in Fig. 123. It must be recognized that it is this competitive struggle for Purkinje cell activation that gives the mechanism of operation of the cerebellar cortex in the coordination and integration of the immense and diverse information that is continuously pouring into it along the various mossy fiber pathways. It can be best envisaged by imagining that the cerebellar cortex is spread out as in Fig. 123 and is a liquid-gas interface that is continuously troubled by microwave production; each wave is a little ridge 3 mm long of Purkinje cell activation and has an inhibitory trough on either side. These waves do not propagate, but of course they competitively interfere, so greatly modifying the pattern of wave forms, and furthermore, even apart from such interference, a wave subsides in less than 100 msec. This competitive patterned operation must be a key feature of the action of the neuronal machinery of the cerebellar cortex.

E. A Component of Cerebellum Oriented to both Spinal Cord and Cerebrum

WALBERG (1956) has found that there is a very dense distribution of the cerebro-olivo-cerebellar pathway to the intermediate part of the anterior lobe; but, by a synthesis of the olivo-cerebellar projections determined by BRODAL (1940) with their own work on the spino-olivary projections, BRODAL, WALBERG and BLACK-STAD (1950) conclude "that in the anterior lobe the vermis only will receive direct spinal impulses through the spino-olivo-cerebellar pathway". However, they stress the necessity of physiological experiments; and already SNIDER and STOWELL (1944) had shown that limb stimuli evoked surface positive potentials (now recognizable from their latency and general configuration as climbing fiber responses) very laterally in the intermediate part of the anterior lobe. As mentioned above, in our very recent experiments the whole depth of the anterior lobe has been systematically explored for the first time, and it has been discovered that the climbing fiber projections from fore limb and from hind limb nerves are very largely restricted respectively to lobule V and to lobules IV and anterior thereto. Superimposed on these responses from the limbs via the accessory nuclei of the olive are the very powerful climbing fiber (CF) responses evoked in the intermediate part of the anterior lobe by stimulation of the contralateral sensorimotor cortex (ARMSTRONG, personal communication; ECCLES, PROVINI, STRATA and TÁBOŘÍKOVÁ, unpublished observations). It has been found that the CF response of the same Purkinje cell in the intermediate zone can be evoked from the sensori-motor cortex and from a limb nerve. Since the latencies of the CF responses evoked from fore limb nerves and from cortex are virtually identical, it can be assumed that both are mediated by pathways relaying in the inferior olive. It is, however, possible that the small and delayed CF response sometimes evoked from fore and hind limb nerves may be mediated by a pathway to the sensori-motor cortex and thence to the inferior olive.

In all cases it is evident that in the intermediate part of the anterior lobe there is every opportunity for the integration of information from the cortex with that ascending from limb nerves.

The intermediate zone of the anterior lobe projects by the interpositus nucleus to the red nucleus and so down the rubrospinal tract and also to the VL nucleus of the thalamus and so to the cerebrum (Fig. 124). The pathway from the interpositus nucleus to the VL nucleus has feed-forward inhibitory connexions. Evidently this intermediate part of the cerebellar cortex has a dual role and may be thought of as mediating some kind of coordinative function between that part of the cerebellum solely oriented to the spinal cord and that part solely oriented to the cerebrum. Furthermore, in this connexion there are collaterals from the interpositus axons spreading into the pontomedullary reticular formation (Fig. 10 of BRODAL, 1957) and also output paths from the fastigial nucleus to the reticular formation (Fig. 124). The reticular neurones send axons either down the reticulospinal fibers or up to the thalamus and to higher centers such as caudate, lentiform nuclei, hypo-thalamus, septal and preoptic regions (cf. BRODAL, 1957). Doubtless, the reticular influences are also directed into many complexities of organization in the brain stem. It appears that the cerebello-VL-cerebral pathway has been developed in special connexion with the sensori-motor cortex, while the cerebello-reticular system may have a much wider relationship with the whole cerebrum.

F. The Cerebro-Cerebellar Loops

The cerebrum may be related to the cerebellum in the following two lines of communication. First, there is convergence of signals from both the cerebrum and the cerebellum onto the brain stem nuclei from which the spinal descending tracts originate. It appears that the cerebellar efferents control these brain stem nuclei directly, while the cerebral influences provide their background levels of activity (Chapter XIV). Second, the cerebrum interacts with the cerebellum by feeding back to it information derived from the signals reaching it through some cerebellar afferents. In general we can say that the MF input occurs via the cerebro-ponto-cerebellar pathway and that this has a wide origin from the cerebral cortex as shown by anatomic investigations and is distributed widely to the cerebellar hemi-sphere of the opposite side. However, it should be recognized that the physiological investigations on these pathways are still at a very early stage. More is known now about the CF input from the cerebrum, there being a monosynaptic activation of cells in the principal olive that in turn projects to the cerebellar hemisphere of the opposite side (ARMSTRONG and HARVEY, 1966). One can presume that the MF and CF information from similar areas of the cerebrum flows through the cerebellum for integration and coordination with inputs of visual, auditory and vestibular information as well as from the general body and limb receptors. In any case, we have to develop the idea of cerebro-cerebellar-thalamo-cerebral loops that are operated by both MF and CF input, and that information flows from the cerebellum via the dentatus or lateral nucleus to the VL thalamus and so back to the cerebrum. The timed relations of this loop should be investigated and also its relation to the pyramidal outflow from the cerebrum because it seems that this pyramidal outflow is responsible for the input to pons and the principal olive. In this way it seems we have already the suggestion of the operation of a computer loop for the cerebellum in relation to the cerebrum.

G. Learning in the Cerebellum

The immense computational machinery of the cerebellum with a neuronal population that may exceed that of the rest of the nervous system gives rise to the concept that the cerebellar cortex is not simply a fixed computing device, but that it contains in its structure the neuronal connexions developed in relationship to learned skills. We have to envisage that the cerebellum plays a major role in the performance of all skilled actions and hence that it can learn from experience so that its performance to any given input is conditioned by this "remembered experience". As yet, of course, we have no knowledge of the structural and functional changes that form the basis of this learned response. However, one can speculate that the spine synapses on the dendrites in the molecular layer are especially concerned in this and that usage gives growth of the spines and particularly the formation of the secondary spines that HÁMORI and SZENTÁGOTHAI (1964) described on Purkinje dendrites. One can, therefore, imagine that in the learning of movements and skills there is the microgrowth of such structures giving increased synaptic function and that as a consequence the cerebellum is able to compute in an especially adapted way for each particular learned movement and thus can provide appropriate corrective information that keeps the movement on target.

H. Experimental Investigations Relating to these New Concepts of Cerebellar Function

1. In the first place, it is essential to investigate the Purkinje cell discharges because the total output of these cells contains all the computed output from the cerebellar cortex. More information is required on the background firing of Purkinje cells and on the changes in frequency produced by controlled inputs, e.g. from muscle stretches or joint movements. It will be necessary to investigate the Purkinje cell discharges arising from all manner of such inputs, and in this way gradually to come to understand how the cerebellum integrates meaningfully the information that flows to it. Of particular importance is a detailed and systematic study of the distributions of the various inputs to the cerebellar cortex, which would be a development of the pioneer work of OSCARSSON and UDDENBERG (1966), and which is

now being actively pursued (ARMSTRONG and HARVEY; ECCLES, PROVINI, STRATA and TÁBOŘÍKOVÁ; unpublished observations).

2. At the further stage of analysis it is essential to record intracellularly from the first stage neuronal relay from the cerebellar cortex, such as occurs in Deiters nucleus and in the various intracerebellar nuclei; and a closely linked study concerns the second stage of the neuronal relay to the red nucleus and to the VL nucleus of the thalamus. This work represents a further development of the pioneer investigations described in Chapters XIII and XIV. In this way one will come to understand the manner in which the cerebellum controls the discharges in the various tracts down the spinal cord and also to the cerebrum.

3. In this connexion it is of special importance to study the cerebellar influences on motoneurones because this represents the final outcome of the integrational and coordinative activity of the cerebellum, not only of that part oriented to the spinal cord, but also of the cerebrally oriented parts. It must be recognized that all parts of the cerebellum are concerned in the control of movement, and hence that all parts ultimately achieve expression through motoneurones, and in no other way.

4. It has been the theme of this chapter and the guiding principle of the whole book that the cerebellum is a part of the brain with a design of neuronal connexions especially adapted for its function in the rapid and effective computation of information fed into it. In attempting to gain insight into the way in which its neuronal structure can function as a computing machine it is essential to be guided by the insights that can be achieved by communication theorists and cyberneticists who have devoted themselves to a detailed study of cerebellar structure and function. We are confident that the enlightened discourse between such theorists on the one hand and neurobiologists on the other will lead to the development of revolutionary hypotheses of the way in which the cerebellum functions as a neuronal machine; and it can be predicted that these hypotheses will lead to revolutionary developments in experimental investigation.

References

[Numbers in square brackets at end of each entry indicate the pages on which it is cited.]

ADRIAN, E. D.: Discharge frequencies in the cerebral and cerebellar cortex. J. Physiol. (Lond.) **83**, 32 P—33 P (1935). [188, 304]
— Afferent areas in the cerebellum connected with the limbs. Brain **66**, 289—315 (1943).
ALLEN, W. F.: Distribution of fibers originating from the different basal cerebellar nuclei. J. comp. Neurol. **36**, 399—439 (1924). [234]
AMASSIAN, V. E., and J. L. DE VITO: La transmission dans le noyau de Burdach. Microphysiologie compareé des éléments excitables. Coll. inter. centre nat. rech. sci. **67**, 353—393 (1957). [165]
ANDERSEN, P., J. C. ECCLES, and Y. LØYNING: Location of postsynaptic inhibitory synapses on hippocampal pyramids. J. Neurophysiol. **27**, 592—607 (1964). [109]
— — T. OSHIMA, and R. F. SCHMIDT: Mechanisms of synaptic transmission in the cuneate nucleus. J. Neurophysiol. **27**, 1096—1116 (1964). [276]
— — R. F. SCHMIDT, and T. YOKOTA: Identification of relay cells and interneurones in the cuneate nucleus. J. Neurophysiol. **27**, 1080—1095 (1964). [276]
— —, and T. A. SEARS: The ventro-basal complex of the thalamus: Types of cells, their responses and their functional organization. J. Physiol. (Lond.) **174**, 370—399 (1964). [283]
— —, and P. E. VOORHOEVE: Postsynaptic inhibition of cerebellar Purkinje cells. J. Neurophysiol. **27**, 1138—1153 (1964). [55, 58, 63, 64, 68, 82, 84, 85, 86, 91, 93, 102, 146, 187, 189]
—, and T. LØMO: Mode of activation of hippocampal pyramidal cells by excitatory synapses on dendrites. Exp. Brian Res. **2**, 247—260 (1966). [144]
ANDRES, K. H.: Über die Feinstruktur besonderer Einrichtungen in markhaltigen Nervenfasern des Kleinhirns der Ratte. Z. Zellforsch. **65**, 701—712 (1965). [11, 182]
ANGAUT, P., and D. BOWSHER: Cerebello-rubral connexions in the cat. Nature (Lond.) **208**, 1002—1003 (1965). [268]
ARAKI, T., M. ITO, and O. OSCARSSON: Anion permeability of the synaptic and nonsynaptic motoneurone membrane. J. Physiol. (Lond.) **159**, 410—435 (1961). [243]
—, and C. A. TERZUOLO: Membrane currents in spinal motoneurones associated with the action potential and synaptic activity. J. Neurophysiol. **25**, 772—789 (1962). [109]
ARDUINI, A., and O. POMPEIANO: Microelectrode analysis of units of the rostral portion of the nucleus fastigii. Arch. ital. Biol. **95**, 56—70 (1957). [247, 280]
ARMSTRONG, D. M., J. C. ECCLES, R. J. HARVEY, and P. B. C. MATTHEWS: Responses in the dorsal accessory olive of the cat to stimulation of hind limb afferents. J. Physiol. (Lond.) (in press, 1967). [164, 167, 305]
—, and R. J. HARVEY: Responses in the inferior olive to stimulation of the cerebellar and cerebral cortices in the cat. J. Physiol. (Lond.) **187**, 553—574 (1966). [166, 314]
BENKE, B., u. J. HÁMORI: Elektronenmikroskopische Untersuchung der cerebellaren Rindenatropie. Acta neuropath. (Berl.) **5**, 275—287 (1965). [50]
BODIAN, D.: Introductory survey of neurones. Cold Spr. Harb. Symp. quant. Biol. **17**, 1—13 (1952). [196]
BOISTEL, J., and P. FATT: Membrane permeability change during inhibitory transmitter action in crustacean muscle. J. Physiol. (Lond.) **144**, 176—191 (1958). [245]
BRAITENBERG, V., and R. P. ATWOOD: Morphological observations on the cerebellar cortex. J. comp. Neurol. **109**, 1—34 (1958). [2, 9, 13, 223, 224, 312]

BREMER, F.: Contribution a l'étude de la physiologie du cervelet. La fonction inhibitrice du paléocerebellum. Arch. int. Physiol. **19**, 189—226 (1922). [247]

BROCK, L. G., J. S. COOMBS, and J. C. ECCLES: The recording of potentials from motoneurones with an intracellular electrode. J. Physiol. (Lond.) **117**, 431—460 (1952). [192]

BRODAL, A.: Experimentelle Untersuchungen über die olivocerebellare Lokalisation. Z. ges. Neurol. Psychiat. **169**, 1—153 (1940). [38, 255, 256, 312]

— Afferent cerebellar connections. In: Aspects of Cerebellar Anatomy, pp. 82—188. Ed. J. JANSEN and A. BRODAL. Oslo: Johan Grundt Tanum Forlag 1954. [158]

— The Reticular Formation of the Brain Stem: Anatomical Aspects and Functional Correlations. The William Ramsay Henderson Trust Lecture. Edinburgh: Oliver & Boyd 1957. [273, 274, 281, 294, 313]

— In: Das Kleinhirn by J. JANSEN and A. BRODAL. In: Handbuch der mikroskopischen Anatomie des Menschen, vol. 4/8 Nervensystem, pp. 1—323. Ed. W. v. MÖLLENDORF, and W. BARGMANN. Berlin-Göttingen- Heidelberg: Springer 1958. [32]

— O. POMPEIANO, and F. WALBERG: The Vestibular Nuclei and Their Connections, Anatomy and Functional Correlations. Edinburgh-London: Oliver & Boyd 1962. [234, 252, 274, 281, 292, 294]

—, u. A. TORVIK: Über den Ursprung der sekundären vestibulocerebellaren Fasern bei der Katze. Eine experimentell-anatomische Studie. Z. ges. Neurol. Psychiat. **195**, 550—567 (1957). [232]

— F. WALBERG, and T. BLACKSTAD: Termination of spinal afferents to inferior olive in cat. J. Neurophysiol. **13**, 431—454 (1950). [167, 215, 300, 304, 305, 312]

BROOKHART, J. M.: The cerebellum. Handbook of Physiology, Sect. I, Neurophysiology, II, pp. 1245—1280. Washington (D.C.): American Physiological Society 1960. [235, 247]

—, and E. FADIGA: Potential fields initiated during monosynaptic activation of frog motoneurones. J. Physiol. (Lond.) **150**, 633—655 (1960). [286]

— G. MORUZZI, and R. S. SNIDER: Spike discharges of single units in the cerebellar cortex. J. Neurophysiol. **13**, 465—486 (1950). [188]

— — — Origin of cerebellar waves. J. Neurophysiol. **14**, 181—190 (1951). [188]

BUSCH, H. F. M.: Anatomical aspects of the anterior and lateral funiculi at the spinobulbar junction. In: Organization of the Spinal Cord. Ed. J. C. ECCLES and J. P. SCHADÉ: Progress in Brain Research, vol. 11, pp. 223—237. Amsterdam-London-New York: Elsevier 1964. [294]

CAJAL, S.-R.: See S. RAMÓN Y CAJAL.

CANNON, W. B., and A. ROSENBLUETH: The Supersensitivity of Denervated Structures, pp. 245. New York: Macmillan Co. 1949. [190, 281]

CARREA, R. M. E., M. REISSIG, and F. A. METTLER: The climbing fibers of the simian and feline cerebellum. J. comp. Neurol. **87**, 321—365 (1947). [37]

CHAMBERS, W. W., and J. M. SPRAGUE: Functional localization in the cerebellum. I. Organization in longitudinal corticonuclear zones and their contribution to the control of posture, both extrapyramidal and pyramidal. J. comp. Neurol. **103**, 105—129 (1955 a). [227]

— — Functional localization in the cerebellum. II. Somatotopic organization in cortex and nuclei. Arch. Neurol. Psychiat. (Chic.) **74**, 653—680 (1955 b). [227]

COLONNIER, M., and R. W. GUILLERY: Synaptic organization in the lateral geniculate nucleus of the monkey. Z. Zellforsch. **62**, 333—355 (1964). [42]

CONDÉ, H.: Analyse electrophysiologique de la voie dentato-rubrothalamique chez le chat. J. Physiol. (Paris) **58**, 218—219 (1966). [270]

COOMBS, J. S., D. R. CURTIS, and J. C. ECCLES: The interpretation of spike potentials of motoneurones. J. Physiol. (Lond.) **139**, 198—231 (1957). [72, 79]

— J. C. ECCLES, and P. FATT: The specific ionic conductances and the ionic movements across the motoneuronal membrane that produce the inhibitory postsynaptic potential. J. Physiol. (Lond.) **130**, 326—373 (1955 a). [91, 146, 192]

COOMBS, J. S., J. C. ECCLES, and P. FATT: Excitatory synaptic action in motoneurones. J. Physiol. (Lond.) **130**, 374—395 (1955 b). [192]

COURVILLE, J., and A. BRODAL: Rubro-cerebellar connexions in the cat: An experimental study with silver impregnation methods. J. comp. Neurol. **126**, 471—485 (1966). [283]

CREPAX, P., e F. INFANTELLINA: L'attività elettrica del limbo isolato di corteccia cerebellare di gatto. Boll. Soc. ital. Biol. sper. **31**, 1229—1231 (1955). [188, 189]

CROSBY, E. C., T. HUMPHREY, and E. W. LAUER: Correlative Anatomy of the Nervous System, pp. 1—731. New York: Macmillan Company 1962. [226]

CURTIS, D. R., and J. C. ECCLES: Synaptic action during and after repetitive stimulation. J. Physiol. (Lond.) **150**, 374—398 (1960). [111, 171, 270]

— J. W. PHILLIS, and J. C. WATKINS: The depression of spinal neurones by γ-amino-n-butyric acid and β-alanine. J. Physiol. (Lond.) **146**, 185—203 (1959). [245]

—, and J. C. WATKINS: The pharmacology of amino acids related to gamma-aminobutyric acid. Pharmacol. Rev. **17**, 347—391 (1965). [245]

DAVIS, R.: Comparison of physiological and pharmacological properties of neurones in red nucleus and ventrolateral thalamic nucleus following brachium conjunctivum stimulation. XXIII Internat. Congr. Physiol. Sci. Abstr. 998, Tokyo (1965) [276]

DENNY-BROWN, D., J. C. ECCLES, and E. G. T. LIDDELL: Observations on electrical stimulation of the cerebellar cortex. Proc. roy. Soc. B **104**, 518—536 (1929). [247]

DEURA, S., and R. S. SNIDER: Corticocortical connections in the cerebellum. In: Morphological and Biochemical Correlates of Neural Activity. Ed. M. M. COHEN and R. S. SNIDER, pp. 142—177. New York: Harper & Row 1964. [166]

DE VITO, R. V., A. BRUSA, and A. ARDUINI: Cerebellar and vestibular influences on Deitersian units. J. Neurophysiol. **19**, 241—253 (1965). [247]

DOW, R. S.: The electrical activity of the cerebellum and its functional significance. J. Physiol. (Lond.) **94**, 67—86 (1938). [188]

— Cerebellar action potentials in response to stimulation of various afferent connections. J. Neurophysiol. **2**, 543—555 (1939). [176]

— The evolution and anatomy of the cerebellum. Biol. Rev. **17**, 179—220 (1942). [215, 226, 300]

— Action potentials of cerebellar cortex in response to local electrical stimulation. J. Neurophysiol. **12**, 245—256 (1949). [55]

—, and G. MORUZZI: The Physiology and Pathology of the Cerebellum. 675 pp. Minneapolis: University of Minnesota Press 1958. [2, 188, 215, 257, 300]

EAGER, R. P.: Efferent cortico-nuclear pathways in the cerebellum of the cat. J. comp. Neurol. **120**, 81—104 (1963 a). [239, 242, 251]

— Cortical association pathways in the cerebellum of the cat. J. comp. Neurol. **121**, 381—393 (1963 b). [178]

— The mode of termination and temporal course of degeneration of cortical association pathways in the cerebellum of the cat. J. comp. Neurol. **124**, 243—258 (1965). [178, 181, 182]

ECCLES, J. C.: The Physiology of Nerve Cells. 270 pp. Baltimore: John Hopkins Press 1957. [131]

— The Physiology of Synapses. 316 pp. Berlin-Göttingen-Heidelberg: Springer 1964. [70, 72, 109, 111, 136, 171, 174, 235, 243, 245, 289]

— Functional meaning of the patterns of synaptic connections in the cerebellum. Perspect. Biol. Med. **8**, 289—310 (1965). [175, 222, 242]

— J. I. HUBBARD, and O. OSCARSSON: Intracellular recording from cells of the ventral spino-cerebellar tract. J. Physiol. (Lond.) **158**, 486—516 (1961). [111, 297, 303]

— R. LLINÁS, and K. SASAKI: Excitation of cerebellar Purkinje cells by the climbing fibers. Nature (Lond.) **203**, 245—246 (1964). [68, 156, 239]

— — — The inhibitory interneurones within the cerebellar cortex. Exp. Brain Res. **1**, 1—16 (1966 a). [62—64, 66, 67, 69, 82, 86, 111, 136, 187, 188, 190]

ECCLES, J. C., R. LLINÁS, and K. SASAKI: Parallel fiber stimulation and the responses induced thereby in the Purkinje cells of the cerebellum. Exp. Brain Res. **1**, 17—39 (1966 b). [54—58, 63, 64, 81, 83, 86, 91, 93, 100—102, 104, 107, 109, 187]

— — — The mossy fiber-granule cell relay in the cerebellum and its inhibition by Golgi cells. Exp. Brain Res. **1**, 82—101 (1966 c). [80, 116, 130, 135, 145, 146, 153, 187, 188, 190—192, 285]

— — — The excitatory synaptic action of climbing fibers on the Purkinje cells of the cerebellum. J. Physiol. (Lond.) **182**, 268—296 (1966 d). [65, 68, 80, 83, 93, 156, 157, 159, 160, 161, 162, 163, 174, 225, 239, 256, 259, 283, 305, 309]

— — — The action of antidromic impulses on the cerebellar Purkinje cells. J. Physiol. (Lond.) **182**, 316—345 (1966 e). [58, 63, 64, 65, 68, 70, 72, 74, 75, 76, 77, 78, 79, 82, 84, 87, 89, 90, 91, 93, 102, 105, 106, 108, 109, 144, 149, 176, 184, 185, 187, 188]

— — — Intracellularly recorded responses of the cerebellar Purkinje cells. Exp. Brain Res. **1**, 161—183 (1966 f). [63, 81, 83, 85, 91, 146, 148, 187, 188, 192, 193, 217, 225]

— — —, and P. E. VOORHOEVE: Interaction experiments on the responses evoked in Purkinje cells by climbing fibers. J. Physiol. (Lond.) **182**, 297—315 (1966). [70, 92, 168, 169, 170, 172, 173, 175]

— O. OSCARSSON, and W. D. WILLIS: Synaptic action of Group I and II afferent fibers of muscle on the cells of the dorsal spino-cerebellar tract. J. Physiol. (Lond.) **158**, 517—543 (1961). [301]

— K. SASAKI, and P. STRATA: The profiles of physiological events produced by a parallel fiber volley in the cerebellar cortex. Exp. Brain Res. **2**, 18—34 (1966). [58, 63, 64, 72, 82, 86, 93, 100, 102, 103, 104, 106, 112, 113, 115, 153]

— — — The potential fields generated in the cerebellar cortex by a mossy fiber volley. Exp. Brain Res. **3**, 58—80 (1967 a). [69, 74, 80, 116, 130, 131, 132, 137, 138, 141, 143, 145, 153, 154, 155, 187, 191]

— — — A comparison of the inhibitory actions of Golgi cells and of basket cells. Exp. Brain Res. **3**, 81—94 (1967 b). [58, 82, 91, 116, 149, 151, 152, 153, 191, 220]

— R. F. SCHMIDT, and W. D. WILLIS: Inhibition of discharges into the dorsal and ventral spinocerebellar tracts. J. Neurophysiol. **26**, 635—645 (1963). [301]

EMMELIN, N., and F. C. MAC INTOSH: The release of acetylcholine from perfused sympathetic ganglia and skeletal muscles. J. Physiol. (Lond.) **131**, 477—496 (1956). [151]

ESTABLE, C.: Notes sur la structure comparative de l'écorce cérébelleuse, et derivées physiologiques possibles. Trab. Lab. Invest. Biol. Madrid **21**, 169—256 (1923). [94]

FADIGA, E., and J. M. BROOKHART: Monosynaptic activation of different portions of the motor neuron membrane. Amer. J. Physiol. **198**, 693—703 (1960). [286]

FATT, P., and B. KATZ: Spontaneous subthreshold activity at motor nerve endings. J. Physiol. (Lond.) **117**, 109—128 (1952). [270]

FOX, C. A.: The structure of the cerebellar cortex. In: Correlative Anatomy of the Nervous System, pp. 193—198. Ed. E. C. CROSPY, T. H. HUMPHREY and E. W. LAUER. New York: Macmillan Company 1962. [225]

—, and J. W. BARNARD: A quantitative study of the Purkinje cell dendritic brachlets and their relationship to afferent fibers. J. Anat. (Lond.) **91**, 299—313 (1957). [4, 9, 11, 13, 45, 49, 52, 53, 94, 108, 196, 198]

—, and E. G. BERTRAM: Connections of the Golgi cells and the intermediate cells of Lugaro in the cerebellar cortex of the monkey. Anat. Rec. **118**, 423 (1954). [27]

— D. E. HILLMAN, K. A. SIEGESMUND, and C. R. DUTTA: The primate cerebellar cortex: A Golgi and electron microscope study. In: Progress in Brain Research, vol. 25. Ed. C. A. FOX and R. S. SNIDER. Amsterdam-London-New York: Elsevier 1967. [108, 116, 118, 119, 123, 127, 133, 150, 153, 182, 215, 219, 225]

— K. A. SIEGESMUND, and C. R. DUTTA: The Purkinje cell dendritic branchlets and their relation with the parallel fibers: Light and electron microscopic observations. In: Morphological and Biochemical Correlates of Neural Activity, pp. 112—141.

Ed. M. M. Cohen and R. S. Snider. New York Harper & Row 1964. [13, 45, 49, 55, 69, 70, 178, 202]

Freygang, W. H.: An analysis of extracellular potentials from single neurones in the lateral geniculate nucleus of the cat. J. gen. Physiol. **41**, 543—564 (1958). [165]

—, and K. Frank: Extracellular potentials from single spinal motoneurones. J. gen. Physiol. **42**, 749—760 (1959). [165]

Frezik, J.: Associative connections established by Purkinje axon collaterals between different part of the cerebellar cortex. Acta morph. Acad. Sci. hung. **12**, 9—14 (1963). [178, 181, 197]

Friede, R.: Quantitative Verschiebungen der Schichten innerhalb des Windungsverlaufes der Kleinhirnrinde und ihre biologische Bedeutung. Acta anat. (Basel) **25**, 65—72 (1955). [9, 13, 15]

Furukawa, T., and E. J. Furshpan: Two inhibitory mechanisms in the Mauthner neurones of goldfish. J. Neurophysiol. **26**, 140—176 (1963). [150]

Gernandt, E., and S. Gilman: Descending vestibular activity and its modulation by proprioceptive, cerebellar and reticular influences. Exp. Neurol. **1**, 273—304 (1959). [294]

Granit, R.: Receptors and sensory perception. 366 pp. New Haven: Yale University Press 1955. [247]

—, and C. G. Phillips: Excitatory and inhibitory processes acting upon individual Purkinje cells of the cerebellum in cats. J. Physiol. (Lond.) **133**, 520—547 (1956). [65, 71, 147, 158, 165, 166, 169, 171, 188, 190, 191, 306]

— — Effect on Purkinje cells of surface stimulation of the cerebellum. J. Physiol. (Lond.) **135**, 73—92 (1957). [71, 188]

Grant, G.: Spinal course and somatotopically localized termination of the spinocerebellar tracts: An experimental study in the cat. Acta physiol. scand. **56**, Suppl. 193, 5—42 (1962). [33, 134, 256]

—, and O. Oscarsson: Mass discharges evoked in the olivocerebellar tract on stimulation of muscle and skin nerves. Exp. Brain Res. **1**, 329—337 (1966). [304, 305, 306]

— —, and I. Rosén: Functional organization of the spinoreticulo-cerebellar path with identification of its spinal component. Exp. Brain Res. **1**, 306—319 (1966). [304]

Gray, E. G.: Axo-somatic and axo-dendritic synapses of the cerebral cortex: An electron microscope study. J. Anat. (Lond.) **93**, 420—433 (1959). [45]

— The granule cells, mossy synapses and Purkinje spine synapses of the cerebellum: Light and electron microscope observations. J. Anat. (Lond.) **95**, 345—356 (1961). [32, 45, 69, 119, 125, 128, 133]

— A morphological basis for pre-synaptic inhibition? Nature (Lond.) **193**, 82—83 (1962). [42]

Hámori, J.: Identification in the cerebellar isles of Golgi II axon endings by aid of experimental degeneration. Electron Microscopy 1964. Proceedings of Third European Regional Conference, vol. B, pp. 291—292. Ed. M. Titlbach. Prague: Publishing House of Czechoslov. Acad. Sci. 1964. [127]

— and J. Szentágothai: The "Crossing Over" synapse. An electron microscope study of the molecular layer in the cerebellar cortex. Acta biol. Acad. Sci. hung. **15**, 95—117 (1964). [15, 45, 47—50, 52, 53, 55, 69, 204, 314]

— — The Purkinje cell baskets: Ultrastructure of an inhibitory synapse. Acta biol. Acad. Sci. hung. **15**, 465—479 (1965). [11, 17, 95, 97, 118, 150, 151]

— — Identification under the electron microscope of climbing fibers and their synaptic contacts. Exp. Brain Res. **1**, 65—81 (1966 a). [30, 32, 38, 40, 41, 58, 59, 60, 61, 98, 99, 142, 156, 182, 225]

— — Participation of Golgi neurone processes in the cerebellar glomeruli: An electron microscope study. Exp. Brain Res. **2**, 35—48 (1966 b). [24, 61, 68, 123, 125, 127, 136, 142, 153, 220, 221]

— — Modes of termination of current Purkinje axon collaterals: An electron microscope study. Exp. Brain Res. 1967 (in the press). [214]

HARREVELD, A. VAN, J. CROWELL, and S. K. MALHOTRA: A study of extracellular space in central nervous tissue by freeze-substitution. J. Cell Biol. **25**, 117—137 (1965). [202, 204]

HERNDON, R. M.: The fine structure of the Purkinje cell. J. Cell Biol. **18**, 167—180 (1963). [9]

HIROTA, I., M. YOSHIDA, and M. UNO: Antidromic and orthodromic responses in the relay neurones of the thalamic ventrolateral nucleus by cortical stimulation. (In course of publication, 1967.) [290, 291]

HOLMQVIST, B., O. OSCARSSON, and I. ROSÉN: Functional organization of cuneocerebellar tract in cat. Acta physiol. scand. **58**, 216—235 (1963). [134, 302]

HONGO, T., E. JANKOWSKA, and A. LUNDBERG: Effects evoked from the rubrospinal tract in cats. Experientia (Basel) **21**, 525—528 (1965). [288, 289]

HUBBARD, J. I.: Repetitive stimulation at the mammalian neuromuscular junction, and the mobilization of transmitter. J. Physiol. (Lond.) **169**, 641—662 (1963). [111, 171]

HURSH, L. B.: Conduction velocity and diameter of nerve fibers. Amer. J. Physiol. **127**, 131—139 (1939). [242]

ITO, M., T. HONGO, and Y. OKADA: Vestibular-evoked postsynaptic potentials in Deiters neurones. (In course of publication, 1967 a.) [252]

— — M. YOSHIDA, Y. OKADA, and K. OBATA: Intracellularly recorded antidromic responses of Deiters neurones. Experienta (Basel) **20**, 295—296 (1964 a). [235, 252]

— — — — — Antidromic and trans-synaptic activation of Deiters neurones induced from the spinal cord. Jap. J. Physiol. **14**, 638—658 (1964 b). [235, 294]

—, and N. KAWAI: IPSP-receptive field in the cerebellum for Deiters neurones. Proc. Jap. Acad. **40**, 762—764 (1964 c). [237]

— —, and M. UDO: The origin of cerebellar-induced inhibition and facilitation in the neurones of Deiters and intracerebellar nuclei. XXIII Internatl. Cong. Physiol. Sci. Abstr. 997, Tokyo (1965 a). [238]

— — — The origin of cerebellar-induced inhibition of Deiters neurones. III. Distribution of the inhibitory zone. (In course of publication, 1967 b). [237, 238]

— — — , and S. MANO: Axon reflex activation of Deiters neurones through the cerebellar afferent collaterals. (In course of publication, 1967 c.) [249, 250, 252, 253, 254, 275, 280]

— — —, and N. SATO: Cerebellar-evoked disinhibition in Deiters neurones. (In course of publication, 1967 d.) [244, 246, 248, 249, 283]

— K. MATSUNAMI, M. NOZUE, and N. SATO: Properties of the inhibitory postsynaptic potentials which Purkinje cell axons produce in Deiters neurones. (In course of publication, 1967 e.) [243]

— K. OBATA, and R. OCHI: Initiation of IPSP in Deiters and fastigial neurones associated with the activity of cerebellar Purkinje cells. Proc. Jap. Acad. **40**, 765—768 (1964 d). [238]

— — — The origin of cerebellar-evoked inhibition of Deiters neurones. II. Temporal correlation between the trans-synaptic activation of Purkinje cells and the inhibition of Deiters neurones. Exp. Brain Res. **2**, 350—364 (1966 a). [184, 238, 239, 240, 252, 253, 255, 256]

— R. OCHI, and K. OBATA: Antidromic and trans-synaptic excitation of inferior olive neurones. (In course of publication, 1967 f.) [163, 164, 247, 259, 283]

—, and T. OSHIMA: Electrical behaviour of the motoneurone membrane during intracellularly applied current steps. J. Physiol. (Lond.) **180**, 607—635 (1965 b). [270]

— M. UDO, and S. MANO: Long inhibitory and excitatory pathways converging on reticular neurones. (In course of publication, 1967 g.) [272, 273, 274, 281, 282, 294, 295, 296, 297]

—, and M. YOSHIDA: The cerebellar-evoked monosynaptic inhibition of Deiters neurones. Experientia (Basel) **20**, 515—516 (1964 e). [184, 235]

ITO, M., and M. YOSHIDA: The origin of cerebellar-induced inhibition of Deiters neurones. I. Monosynaptic initiation of the inhibitory postsynaptic potentials. Exp. Brain Res. **2**, 330—349 (1966b). [184, 235, 236, 242, 249, 252, 259]

— —, and K. OBATA: Monosynaptic inhibition of the intracerebellar nuclei induced from the cerebellar cortex. Experientia (Basel) **20**, 575—576 (1964f). [184, 186, 235, 239, 242, 268]

— — — N. KAWAI, and M. UDO: Purkinje cell inhibition of cerebellar nuclei. (In course of publication, 1967h). [184, 235, 239, 241, 256]

JAKOB, A.: Das Kleinhirn. In: Handbuch der mikroskopischen Anatomie des Menschen, vol. 4, pp. 674—916. Ed. W. v. MÖLLENDORFF. Berlin: Springer 1928. [27, 60, 99, 229, 242]

JANSEN, J.: Efferent cerebellar connections. In: Aspects of Cerebellar Anatomy, pp. 189—248. Ed. J. JANSEN and A. BRODAL. Oslo: Johan Grundt Tanum Forlag 1954. [226]

—, and A. BRODAL: Experimental studies on the intrinsic fibers of the cerebellum. II. The cortico-nuclear projection. J. comp. Neurol. **73**, 267—321 (1940). [227]

— — Aspects of Cerebellar Anatomy. Oslo: Johan Grundt Tanum Forlag 1954. [33, 34, 227, 262]

— — Das Kleinhirn. In: Handbuch der mikroskopischen Anatomie des Menschen, vol. 4/8 Nervensystem, pp. 1—323. Ed. W. v. MÖLLENDORFF and W. BARGMANN. Berlin-Göttingen-Heidelberg: Springer 1958. [1, 33, 34, 60, 227, 234, 262, 264, 304]

—, and J. K. S. JANSEN: On the efferent fibers of the cerebellar nuclei in the cat. J. comp. Neurol. **102**, 607—623 (1955). [229]

JANSEN, J. K. S.: Afferent impulses to the cerebellar hemispheres from the cerebral cortex and certain subcortical nuclei. Acta physiol. scand. **41**, Suppl. 143, 1—99 (1957). [176]

—, and C. FANGEL: Observations on cerebro-cerebellar evoked potentials in the cat. Exp. Neurol. **3**, 160—173 (1961). [176]

— K. NICOLAYSEN, and T. RUDJORD: Discharge pattern of neurones of the dorsal spino-cerebellar tract activated by static extension of primary endings of muscle spindles. J. Neurophysiol. **29**, 1061—1086 (1966). [305]

—, and T. RUDJORD: Dorsal spinocerebellar tract: Response pattern of nerve fibers to muscle stretch. Science **149**, 1109—1111 (1965). [221, 301, 305, 307]

KATZ, B., and R. MILEDI: Propagation of electric activity in motor nerve terminals. Proc. roy. Soc. B **161**, 443—482 (1965). [242]

KAWAI, N., M. ITO, and M. NOZUE: Postsynaptic influences on the vestibular descending and superior nuclei from the primary vestibular nerve and the cerebellum. (In course of publication, 1967.) [274, 281, 282, 294]

KIRSCHE, W., H. DAVID, E. WINKELMANN u. I. MARX: Elektronenmikroskopische Untersuchungen an synaptischen Formationen im Cortex cerebelli von Rattus rattus norvegicus, Berkenhoot. Z. mikr.-anat. Forsch. **72**, 49—80 (1965). [119]

KOHNO, K.: Neurotubules contained within the dendrite and axon of Purkinje cell of frog. Bull. Tokyo med. dent. Univ. **2**, 411—442 (1964). [11, 19]

KRAVITZ, E. A., S. W. KUFFLER, and D. D. POTTER: Gamma-aminobutyric acid and other blocking compound in Crustacea. III. Their relative concentration in separated motor and inhibitory axons. J. Neurophysiol. **26**, 739—751 (1963). [245]

— P. B. MOLINOFF, and Z. W. HALL: A comparison of the enzymes and substrates of gamma-aminobutyric acid metabolism in lobster excitatory and inhibitory axons. Proc. nat. Acad. Sci. (Wash.) **54**, 778—782 (1965). [245]

KRNJEVIĆ, K., M. RANDIĆ, and D. W. STRAUGHAN: Pharmacology of cortical inhibition. J. Physiol. (Lond.) **184**, 78—105 (1966). [245]

KUBOTA, K., and J. M. BROOKHART: Recurrent facilitation of frog motoneurones. J. Neurophysiol. **26**, 877—893 (1963). [286]

KUFFLER, S. W., and C. EDWARDS: Mechanism of gamma-aminobutyric acid (GABA) action and its relation to synaptic inhibition. J. Neurophysiol. **21**, 589—610 (1958). [245]

KUNO, M.: Quantal components of excitatory synaptic potentials in spinal motoneurones. J. Physiol. (Lond.) **175**, 81—99 (1964). [269]

KURIYAMA, K., B. HABER, B. SISKEN, and E. ROBERTS: The γ-amino-butyric acid system in rabbit cerebellum. Proc. nat. Acad. Sci. (Wash.) **55**, 846—852 (1966). [245]

LANDAU, E.: Zweiter Beitrag zur Kenntnis der Körnerschicht des Kleinhirns. Anat. Anz. **65**, 89—93 (1928). [28]

— La cellule synarmotique. Bull. Histol. appl. **9**, 159—168 (1932). [28]

— La cellule synarmotique dans le cerevelet humain. Arch. Anat. (Strasbourg) **17**, 273—285 (1933). [28]

LAPORTE, Y., and A. LUNDBERG: Functional organization of the dorsal spino-cerebellar tract in the cat. III. Single fiber recording in Fleschig's fasciculus on adequate stimulation of primary afferent neurones. Acta physiol. scand. **36**, 204—218 (1956). [305]

LLINÁS, R.: Mechanisms of supraspinal actions upon spinal cord activities. Differences between reticular and cerebellar inhibitory actions upon alpha extensor motoneurone. J. Neurophysiol. **27**, 1117—1126 (1964). [176, 177, 277, 286, 298]

—, and J. BLOEDEL: Frog cerebellum: Absence of long term inhibition upon the Purkinje cell. Science **155**, 601—603 (1967). [64]

LÖWENTHAL, M., and V. HORSLEY: On the relations between the cerebellar and other centers (namely cerebral and spinal) with special reference to the action of antagonistic muscles. Proc. roy. Soc. B **61**, 20—25 (1897). [235]

LORENTE DE NÓ, R.: Vestibulo-ocular reflex arc. Arch. Neurol. Psychiat. **30**, 245—291 (1933). [252, 298]

— A study of nerve physiology. In: Studies from the Rockefeller Institute for Medical Research, vol. 132, Chapter 16 (1947). [57]

LUGARO, E.: Sulle connessioni tra gli elementi nervosi della corteccia cerebellare. Riv. sper. Freniat. **10**, 297 (1894). [27, 229]

LUND, S., and O. POMPEIANO: Descending pathways with monosynaptic action on motoneurones. Experientia (Basel) **21**, 602—603 (1965). [286, 288, 294]

LUNDBERG, A.: Ascending spinal hindlimb pathway in the cat. In: Progress in Brain Research, vol. 12, pp. 135—163. Ed. J. C. ECCLES and J. P. SCHADÉ. Amsterdam-London-New York: Elsevier 1964. [223, 301, 304]

—, and O. OSCARSSON: Functional organization of the dorsal spino-cerebellar tract in the cat. IV. Synaptic connections of afferents from Golgi tendon organs and muscle spindles. Acta physiol. scand. **38**, 53—75 (1956). [301]

— — Functional organization of the dorsal spino-cerebellar tract in the cat. VII. Identification of units by antidromic activation from the cerebellar cortex with recognition of five functional subdivisions. Acta physiol. scand. **50**, 356—374 (1960). [3, 218, 302]

— — Functional organization of the ventral spino-cerebellar tract in the cat. IV. Identification of units by antidromic activation from the cerebellar cortex. Acta physiol. scand. **54**, 270—286 (1962). [34, 218, 303, 304]

—, and G. WINSBURY: Functional organization of the dorsal spino-cerebellar tract in the cat. VI. Further experiments on excitation from tendon organ and muscle spindle afferents. Acta physiol. scand. **49**, 165—170 (1960). [221, 301]

MABUCHI, M., and T. KUSAMA: The cortico-rubral projection in the cat. Brain Res. **2**, 254—273 (1966). [286]

MAGNI, F., and W. D. WILLIS: Identification of reticular formation neurones by intracellular recording. Arch. ital. Biol. **101**, 681—702 (1963). [272]

— — Cortical control of brain stem reticular neurones. Arch. ital. Biol. **102**, 418—433 (1964 a). [294, 295]

— — Subcortical and peripheral control of brain stem reticular neurones. Arch. ital. Biol. **102**, 434—448 (1964 b). [298]

MAJOROSSY, K., M. RÉTHELYI, and J. SZENTÁGOTHAI: The large glomerular synapse of the Pulvinar. J. Hirnforsch. **7**, 415—432 (1965). [42]

MASSION, J.: Contribution à l'étude de la régulation cérébelleuse du système extra-pyramidal. Contrôle réflexe et tonique de la voie rubrospinale par le cervelet. Bruxelles: Arscia; Paris: Masson & Cie. 1961. [276]

—, et D. ALBE-FESSARD: Dualité des voies sensorielles afférentes contrôlant l'activité du noyau rouge. Electroenceph. clin. Neurophysiol. **15**, 435—454 (1963). [276]

MEAD, C. O., and H. VAN DER LOOS: Experimental synapto-chemistry of the rat cere-bellar glomerulus. Anat. Rec. **148**, 311 (1964). [127]

MISKOLCZY, D.: Über die Endigungsweise der spinocerebellaren Bahnen. Z. Anat. Ent-wickl.-Gesch. **96**, 537—542 (1931). [32, 33, 37]

— Endigungsweise der olivocerebellaren Faserung. Arch. Psychiat. Nervenkr. **102**, 197—201 (1934). [37]

MORIN, F., and E. D. GARDNER: Spinal pathways for cerebellar projections in the monkey *(Macaca Mulatta)*. Amer. J. Physiol. **174**, 155—161 (1953). [167]

—, and B. HADDAD: Afferent projections to the cerebellum and the spinal pathways involved. Amer. J. Physiol. **172**, 497—510 (1953). [167]

— G. LAMARCHE, and A. Z. OSTROWSKI: Responses of the inferior olive to peripheral stimuli and the spinal pathways involved. Amer. J. Physiol. **189**, 401—406 (1957). [305]

MORUZZI, G.: Problems in Cerebellar Physiology. Springfield (Ill.): Ch. C. Thomas, Publ. 1950. [235, 247]

— Esperimenti e considerazioni sull' elettronarcosi cerebellare. Arch. Sci. biol. (Bologna) **41**, 91—104 (1957). [188]

NELSON, P. G., and K. FRANK: Extracellular potential fields of single spinal motoneu-rones. J. Neurophysiol. **27**, 913—927 (1964). [79]

NYBERG-HANSEN, R., and A. BRODAL: Sites and mode of termination of rubrospinal fibers in the cat. An experimental study with silver impregnation methods. J. Anat. (Lond.) **98**, 235—253 (1967). [288]

—, and T. A. MASCITTI: Sites and mode of termination of fibers of the vestibulospinal tract in the cat. An experimental study with silver impregnation methods. J. comp. Neurol. **122**, 369—387 (1964). [288, 294]

OBATA, K.: Pharmacological study on postsynaptic inhibition of Deiters neurones. XXIII Internat. Congr. Physiol. Sci. Abstr. 958, Tokyo (1965). [243]

— M. ITO, R. OCHI, and N. SATO: Pharmacological properties of the postsynaptic inhi-bition by Purkinje cell axons and the action of γ-aminobutyric acid on Deiters neurones. Exp. Brain Res. **4**, 43—57 (1967). [243, 245]

OCHI, R.: Occurrence of postsynaptic potentials in the inferior olive neurones associated with their antidromic excitation. XXIII Internat. Congr. Physiol. Sci. Abstr. 944, Tokyo (1965). [259, 283]

OSCARSSON, O.: Functional organization of the ventral spinocerebellar tract in the cat. II. Connections with muscle, joint and skin nerve afferents and effects on adequate stimulation of various receptors. Acta physiol. scand. **42**, Suppl. 146, 1—107 (1957). [303, 306]

— Three ascending tracts activated from Group I afferents in forelimb nerves of the cat. In: Progress in Brain Research, vol. 12, pp. 179—196. Ed. J. C. ECCLES and J. P. SCHADÉ. Amsterdam-London-New York: Elsevier 1964. [218]

— Functional organization of the spino- and cuneocerebellar tracts. Physiol. Rev. **45**, 495—522 (1965). [34, 256, 303, 304]

— Functional significance of information channels from the spinal cord to the cerebel-lum. Proc. Symposium on Neurophysiological basis of normal and abnormal motor activities. New York: Rockefeller Univ. Press 1967. [303, 304, 305]

—, and I. ROSÉN: Response characteristics of reticulocerebellar neurones activated from spinal afferents. Exp. Brain Res. **1**, 320—328 (1966). [304, 306]

—, and N. UDDENBERG: Identification of a spinocerebellar tract activated from forelimb afferents in the cat. Acta physiol. scand. **62**, 125—136 (1964). [303]

OSCARSSON, O., and N. UDDENBERG: Somatotopic termination of spino-olivo-cerebellar path. Brain Res. **3**, 204—207 (1966). [309, 315]

OTSUKA, M., L. L. IVERSEN, Z. W. HALL, and E. A. KRAVITZ: Release of gamma-amino-butyric acid from inhibitory nerves of lobster. Proc. nat. Acad. Sci. (Wash.) **56**, 1110—1116 (1966). [245]

— E. A. KRAVITZ, and D. D. POTTER: The γ-aminobutyric acid (GABA) content of cell bodies of excitatory and inhibitory neurones of lobster. Fed. Proc. **24**, 399 (1965). [245]

PALAY, S. L.: The structural basis for neural action. In: Brain Function, vol. II, pp. 69—107. Proc. Second Conference, 1962, RNA and Brain Function. Ed. M. A. B. BRAZIER. Los Angeles: University of California Press 1964. [150]

PAPPAS, G. D., E. B. COHEN, and D. P. PURPURA: Electron microscope study of synaptic and other neuronal interrelations in the feline thalamus. 8th Internat. Congr. of Anatomists, Wiesbaden, p. 92. Stuttgart: Georg Thieme 1965. [42]

PENSA, A.: Osservazioni e considerazioni sulla struttura della corteccia cerebellare dei mammiferi. Mem. R. Accad. naz. Lincei, Cl. Sci. Fiz. Mat. e Nat., Ser. VI, **5**, 25—50 (1931). [28]

POLLOCK, L. J., and L. DAVIS: The reflex activities of a decerebrate animal. J. comp. Neurol. **50**, 377—411 (1930). [247]

POMPEIANO, O.: Responses of electrical stimulation of the intermediate part of the cerebellar anterior lobe in the decerebrate cat. Arch. ital. Biol. **96**, 330—360 (1958). [247]

— Cerebellar control of flexor motoneurones. Arch. ital. Biol. **100**, 467—509 (1962). [286]

—, and A. BRODAL: Experimental demonstration of a somatotopical origin of rubro-spinal fibers in the cat. J. comp. Neurol. **108**, 225—251 (1957). [264, 286]

—, and E. COTTI: Analisi microelecttrodica delle proiezioni cerebellodeitersiane. Arch. Sci. biol. (Bologna) **43**, 57—101 (1959). [247, 310]

PURPURA, D. P., T. L. FRIGYESI, J. G. MCMURTRY, and T. SCARFF: Synaptic mechanisms in thalamic regulation of cerebello-cortical projektion activity. In: The Thalamus. pp. 153—170 Ed. D. P. PURPURA and M. D. YAHR. New York and London: Columbia University Press 1966. [292]

RALL, W.: Electrophysiology of a dendritic neurone model. Biophys. J. **2**, 145—167 (1962). [79]

RAMÓN Y CAJAL, S.: Histologie du Système Nerveux de L'Homme et des Vertébrés. Tome II. 993 pp. Paris: Maloine 1911. [1, 11, 13, 22, 26, 27, 28, 32, 36, 37, 43, 45, 60, 61, 69, 107, 113, 118, 119, 123, 165, 178, 182, 196, 198, 215, 225, 229, 232, 262, 263, 267]

— Les preuves objectives de l'unité anatomique des cellules nerveuses. Trab. Lab. Invest. biol. Univ. Madr. **29**, 1—137 (1934). [1]

— Studies on vertebrate neurogenesis, pp. 432. Translated by Lloyd Guth. Springfield (Ill.): Ch. C. Thomas 1959. [113]

RINVIK, E., and F. WALBERG: Demonstration of a somatotopically arranged cortico-rubral projection in the cat. J. comp. Neurol. **120**, 393—407 (1963). [264, 286, 288]

ROSIELLO, L.: Sull' origine delle fibre muschiose del cerveletto. Riv. Neurol. **10**, 437—455 (1937). [37]

SACCOZZI, A.: Sul nucleo dentato del cervelletto. Riv. sper. Freniat. Arch. ital. Mal. nerv. ment. **13**, 93—99 (1887). [229]

SALCANICOFF, L., and E. DE ROBERTIS: Subcellular distribution of the enzymes of the glutamic acid, glutamine and γ-aminobutyric acid cycles in rat brain. J. Neurochem. **12**, 287—309 (1965). [244]

SASAKI, K., and P. STRATA: Responses evoked in the cerebellar cortex by stimulating mossy fiber pathways to the cerebellum. Exp. Brain Res. **3**, 95—110 (1967). [116, 130, 133, 139, 140, 141, 153, 307]

SCHEIBEL, M. E., and A. B. SCHEIBEL: Observations on the intracortical relations of the climbing fibers of the cerebellum. J. comp. Neurol. **101**, 733—760 (1954). [30, 32, 36, 37, 38, 39, 58, 60, 61, 68, 156, 181, 225]

SCHEIBEL, M. E., and A. B. SCHEIBEL: The inferior olive: A Golgi study. J. comp. Neurol. **102**, 77—132 (1955). [165]

— — Structural substrates for integrative patterns in the brainstem reticular core. In: Reticular Formation of the Brain, pp. 31—55. Ed. H. H. JASPER et al. Boston and Toronto: Little, Brown & Co. 1958. [298]

— — Patterns of organization in specific and nonspecific thalamic fields. In: The Thalamus, pp. 13—46. Ed. D. P. PURPURA and M. D. YAHR. New York and London: Columbia University Press 1966. [264]

— — A. MOLLICA, and G. MORUZZI: Convergence and interaction of afferent impulses on single units of reticular formation. J. Neurophysiol. **18**, 309—331 (1955). [294]

SCHIMERT (SZENTÁGOTHAI), J.: Die sekundare Degeneration der Endbäumchen und Kollateralen im Zentralnervensystem. Ergänzungsh. Anat. Anz. **87**, 312—319 (1939). [37]

SEDGEWICK, E. M., and T. D. WILLIAMS: Responses of single units in the inferior olive to stimulation of the limb nerves, peripheral skin receptors, cerebellum, caudate nucleus and motor cortex. J. Physiol. (Lond.) **189**, 261—280 (1967). [305]

SHERRINGTON, C. S.: The mammalian spinal cord as an organ of reflex action. Proc. roy. Soc. **61**, 220—221 (1897). [235]

— Experiments in examination of the peripheral distribution of the fibers of the posterior roots of some spinal nerves. Phil. Trans. B **190**, 45—286 (1898). [235]

— Man on his Nature, pp. 413. Cambridge: Cambridge University Press 1940. [308]

SNIDER, R. S.: Alterations which occur in mossy terminals of the cerebellum following transection of brachium pontis. J. comp. Neurol. **64**, 417—435 (1936). [33, 37]

—, and A. STOWELL: Receiving areas of the tactile, auditory and visual systems in the cerebellum. J. Neurophysiol. **7**, 337—357 (1944). [304, 312]

SPENCER, W. A., and E. R. KANDEL: Electrophysiology of hippocampal neurones. IV. Fast prepotentials. J. Neurophysiol. **24**, 272—285 (1961). [79]

SUDA, I., and T. AMANO: An analysis of evoked cerebellar activity. Arch. ital. Biol. **102**, 156—182 (1964). [166]

SWETT, J. E., S. INOUE, and Y. FUJITA: Cerebellar evoked responses to low threshold muscle afferents. XXIII Internat. Congr. Physiol. Sci. Abstr. 1057, Tokyo (1965). [166]

SZENTÁGOTHAI, J.: Kisérlet az idegrendszer szöveti elemeinek természetes rendszerezésére (An attempt of a "natural systematization" of nervous elements). Magy. Tud. Akad., Biol. orv. Tud. Osztal. Közl. **3**, 365—412 (1952). [196]

— Somatotopic arrangement of synapses of primary sensory neurones in Clarke's column. Acta morph. Acad. Sci. hung. **10**, 307—311 (1961). [34, 302]

— Anatomical aspects of junctional transformation. In: Information Processing in the Nervous System, pp. 119—136. Ed. R. W. GERARD and J. W. DUYFF. Proc. Internat. Union Physiol. Sci., vol. 3, XXIII Internat. Congr., Leiden. Amsterdam: Excerpta Medica Foundation 1962 a. [33, 42, 123, 234]

— Discussion. In: Information Processing in the Nervous System, pp. 443—446. Ed. R. W. GERARD and J. W. DUYFF. Proc. Internat. Union Physiol. Sci., vol. 3, XXIII Internat. Congr., Leiden. Amsterdam: Excerpta Medica Foundation 1962 b. [196]

— Ujabb adatok a synapsis funkcionális anatómiájához (New data on the functional anatomy of synapses). Magy. Tud. Akad., Biol. Orv. Tud. Osztal. Közl. **6**, 217—227 (1963). [93, 108, 113, 115, 207, 209]

— The use of degeneration methods in the investigation of short neuronal connexions. In: Progress in Brain Research, vol. 14: Degeneration Patterns in the Nervous System, pp. 1—32. Ed. M. SINGER and J. P. SCHADE. Amsterdam-London-New York: Elsevier 1965 a. [30, 37, 92, 93, 94, 95, 108, 113, 307]

— Complex synapses. In: Aus der Werkstatt der Anatomen, pp. 147—167. Ed. W. BARGMANN. Stuttgart: Georg Thieme 1965 b. [119]

—, u. K. RAJKOVITS: Über den Ursprung der Kletterfasern des Kleinhirns. Z. Anat. Entwickl.-Gesch. **121**, 130—141 (1959). [37, 38, 39, 61, 68, 156, 165, 181, 305]

SZENTÁGOTHAI-SCHIMERT, J.: Die Bedeutung des Fasenkalibers und der Markscheiden-dicke im Zentralnervensystem. Z. Anat. Entwickl.-Gesch. **111**, 201—223 (1941). [161, 242, 256]

TAKAHASHI, K.: Slow and fast group of pyramidal tract cells and their respective mem-brane properties. J. Neurophysiol. **28**, 908—923 (1965). [270, 289]

TAKAHIRA, H., and A. C. NACIMIENTO: Properties of the burst response of cerebellar Purkinje cells. XXIII Internat. Congr. Physiol. Sci. Abstr. 934, Tokyo (1965). [166]

TAXI, J.: Étude au microscope électronique de synapses ganglionnaires chez quilques Vertébrés. Proceedings IV Inter. Congr. Neuropath., vol. II, pp. 197—203. Ed. H. JACOB. Stuttgart: Georg Thieme 1962. [129]

TERZUOLO, C. A.: Cerebellar inhibitory and excitatory actions upon spinal extensor motoneurones. Arch. ital. Biol. **97**, 316—339 (1959). [176, 277, 286, 298]

—, and T. ARAKI: An analysis of intra- versus extra-cellular potential changes associated with activity of single spinal motoneurones. Ann. N. Y. Acad. Sci. **94**, 547—558 (1961). [72, 79, 165]

TÖMBÖL, T.: Short neurons and their synaptic relations in the specific thalamic nuclei. Brain Res. **3**, 307—326 (1967). [264, 267]

TOYAMA, K.: The 'disfacilitation' of the red nucleus neurones. XXIII Internat. Congr. Physiol. Sci. Abstr. 1044, Tokyo (1965). [176]

— N. TSUKAHARA, K. KOSAKA, and K. MATSUNAMI: Electrophysiology of the excitatory innervation from the nucleus interpositus to the red nucleus. (In course of publica-tion. 1967 a.) [269, 279]

— —, and M. UDO: The nature of the cerebellar influences upon the red nucleus neu-rones (In course of publication, 1967 b.) [256, 267, 268, 277, 287, 288]

TSUKAHARA, N.: Common activation of the red nucleus and the thalmus from the cere-bellar nucleus. XXIII Internat. Congr. Physiol. Sci. Abstr. 993, Tokyo (1965). [267]

—, and K. KOSAKA: The mode of cerebral activation of red nucleus neurones. Experienta (Basel) **22**, 193—194 (1966). [267, 286, 287]

— — The cerebral corticofugal control of red nucleus neurones. (In course of publica-tion, 1967 a.) [267, 289]

— K. TOYAMA, and K. KOSAKA: Intracellularly recorded responses of red nucleus neurones during antidromic and orthodromic activation. Experientia (Basel) **20**, 632—633 (1964 a). [267, 268, 287]

— — — Electrical activity of the red nucleus neurones investigated with intracellular microelectrodes. Exp. Brain Res. (In press 1967 b.) [267, 268, 269, 289]

— — —, and M. UDO: Disfacilitation of red nucleus neurones. Experientia (Basel) **21**, 544 (1964 b). [176]

ULE, E.: Über die zentrale Kleinhirnrinde als möglichen Ursprungsort der Kletterfasern. Z. Zellforsch. **46**, 286—316 (1957). [37]

UNO, M., M. YOSHIDA, and I. HIROTA: The mode of cerebello-thalamic relay trans-mission investigated with intracellular recording from cells of the ventrolateral nucleus of the thalmus. (In course of publication, 1967.) [270, 271]

WALBERG, F.: Descending connections to the inferior olive: An experimental study in the cat. J. comp. Neur. **104**, 77—174 (1956). [289, 312]

—, and J. JANSEN: Cerebellar cortico-vestibular fibers in the cat. Exp. Neurol. **3**, 32—52 (1961). [233, 234, 238, 242, 249, 250]

WILSON, V. J., and P. R. BURGESS: Disinhibition in the cat spinal cord. J. Neurophysiol. **25**, 392—404 (1962). [187, 247]

— M. KATO, R. C. THOMAS, and B. W. PETERSON: Excitation of lateral vestibular neu-rones by peripheral afferent fibers. J. Neurophysiol. **29**, 508—529 (1966). [298, 310]

YOSHIDA, M., K. YAJIMA, and M. UNO: Different activation of the two types of the pyramidal tract neurones through the cerebello-thalamocortical pathway. Experi-entia (Basel) **22**, 331—332 (1966). [272, 289, 290]

YOUNG, J. Z.: A Model of the Brain. Oxford: Clarendon Press 1964. [196]

Subject Index

Subject Index